Purnell's A-Z of Family Health

A guide to coping with illness and accident in the home

Dr A.S. Playfair

A Charles Herridge Book

First published in Great Britain
in 1982 by Purnell Books, Paulton,
Bristol, BS18 5LQ

Produced by Charles Herridge Ltd.,
Tower House, Abbotsham, Devon

Illustrations by Dee McLean
and Clive Spong
by courtesy of Linden Artists Ltd.,
London

Typeset by Toptown Printers Ltd.
Barnstaple, N. Devon

Printed in Great Britain

ISBN 361 05086 0 (cased edition)
ISBN 361 05087 9 (limp edition)

Emergency Entries

Pages containing emergency entries carry this symbol ◥

Abdominal Injuries

A heavy blow to the abdomen can disrupt an organ inside, causing some internal bleeding. Surprisingly, once the immediate pain has passed there may be only minor symptoms for a short while (minutes or hours). Later progressive discomfort, pain and weakness with signs of shock (p. 183) may develop. Beware also of the so-called 'pattern bruise' on the skin where the blow was received. This is the bruise imprint left by an item of clothing through which the blow was received: it could be from a belt buckle or even the lattice design of a string vest. Any blow strong enough to raise such a mark is strong enough to have damaged an underlying organ. If in doubt make the patient lie down and either call a doctor or an ambulance to take him to hospital. It is better not to give him anything by mouth until doubt has been resolved.

A cut into the abdominal wall is a much more definite emergency. While awaiting the ambulance, have the victim lying down in what might be described as a half folded position. The muscles of the abdominal wall go in several directions, but the major fibres run from the lower end of the rib cage down to the bones of the pelvis. The elastic pull of the muscle tends to gape such an incision wide open. This will be worsened if the patient is stretched out flat, but lessened if you have set him so that pelvis and rib cage are made to approach each other. If anything projects through the wound do not try to push it back; merely make your dressing (p.93) very ample and take care that the bandage is not so tight as to cause pressure.

Abortion

Abortion means the ending of a pregnancy when the foetus is expelled before it is likely to be viable, that is before the twenty-eighth week of the pregnancy. In fact many occur at about the twelfth week.

Some of the placenta (the organ which allows nourishment and oxygen to pass from the mother's blood to that of the foetus) gets detached from its site on the inside wall of the uterus, and the first signs of this are vaginal bleeding and perhaps, but not always, a little pain. At this stage the condition is a *threatened abortion.* With treatment, which is mainly rest in bed with sedatives, it may settle down and the

HALF-FOLDED POSITION

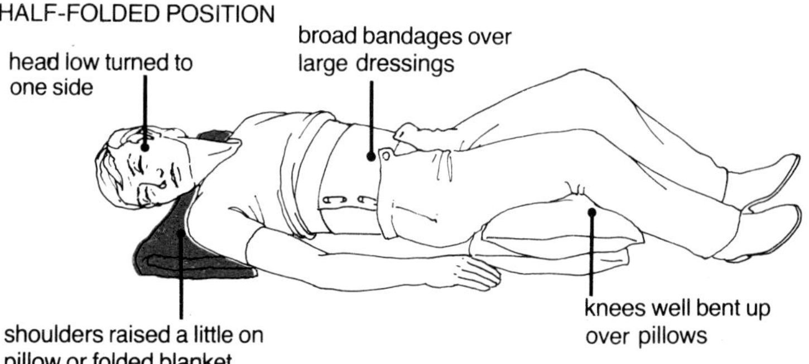

pregnancy continues. In that case one can reassure the mother that there is no reason to suspect damage to the baby. However, if a great part or all of the placenta gets detached, with more bleeding, this becomes an *inevitable abortion.* The baby and the placenta and the associated membranes are expelled and the abortion is *complete,* resembling a miniature labour. Sometimes however it is *incomplete,* some of the material remaining inside the uterus with a continuation of bleeding. Then the mother needs the obstetrician's help to evacuate the uterus completely.

Generally no cause is found for the abortion. Inevitably (and inaccurately) the unfortunate mother asks herself what she has done to provoke it. There is no evidence that 'strain' is a factor: that time she was frightened, or she lifted a heavy weight had nothing at all to do with it. There are some medical factors, such as a very severe fever or kidney trouble, which might play a part. Rare mechanical causes are a developmental abnormality of the uterus, its gross malposition, or the presence inside it of a large fibroid (p.112). The cervix (the neck of the uterus) occasionally is lax: sometimes this can be treated by the gynaecologist inserting stitches, which will be removed later when the pregnancy is at its end. Another possibility is that there is a low amount of the chemical which, during pregnancy, circulates in the blood to safeguard the firm attachment of the placenta.

What is certain is that any pregnant women who experiences bleeding at any point of her pregnancy should report this at once to her doctor.

'Abortion' and 'miscarriage' mean the same thing. However popular use, or misuse, has often let the word 'abortion' stand for the deliberate termination of a pregnancy. The law of Britain is quite definite here. Therapeutic termination can be performed legally if two doctors agree that a continuation of the pregnancy would threaten (a) the physical health of the woman, (b) her mental health, or (c) the security of her family, or that there is a strong likelihood that the baby would be born with severely handicapping abnormalities.

Abrasion *see* Wounds

Abscess

An abscess is a collection of pus localised somewhere in the body. It is an unpleasant mess of microbes (some alive, some killed by white blood cells), of white blood cells (some alive, some killed by microbes), of chemical protectors produced by the body and of the microscopic debris of tissues damaged and broken up in the battlefield where infection and body defences have been fighting.

The amount of pus can be quite small, as at a finger tip or in a boil (p.54), or it can develop deeply, in some internal organ and become very big before it is diagnosed. Antibiotics are often insufficient as treatment as they cannot reach the microbes adequately. The pus must escape. Often it does this by bursting spontaneously through to the nearest surface (not necessarily the skin in the really deep ones). The doctor, however, may wish to spare the patient much suffering by incising the abscess and letting the pus out.

There are two lessons for the patient with an abscess near the skin. The first is not to try to squeeze the stuff out: this is painfully inefficient and may spread the damage deeper. The second is that many doctors disapprove of hot poultices, not only as being useless but also because they make the skin soggy and vulnerable.

Accidents

Most accidents in the home are due to inaction, to lack of planning or correction. With hindsight and analysis the huge majority of accidents are found to be foreseeable possibilities and, therefore, avoidable possibilities.

The elderly are particularly vulnerable, for their liability to falls is extremely high. Seventy per cent of home falls, and as much as ninety per cent of deaths from these falls are in those aged above sixty-five. As for accidents to children, statistics show that ninety-nine per cent of them resulted in cuts and falls and that in ninety-five per cent of these cases the children were actually in the charge of one or both parents at the time.

Prevention is the keynote and here is a brief summary of some of the important points to consider.

Floors: No slippery, highly polished or uneven surfaces; no loose mats; carpet edges secured; no trailing flexes.

Stairs: Well lit; banisters and handrails.

Kitchen: Whenever possible working surfaces on either side of and at same height as cooker and sink; door opening and transit areas to be clear of working spaces; cupboards and shelves of easily reachable height and depths; cooker/flames clear of draught from window; do not let saucepan handles project beyond the cooker; good lighting onto work areas; good view onto children's play area.

Bathrooms and 'wet areas': Flat bottomed bath; grab rail for the elderly; electric switches and apparatus remote from wet contacts.

Electricity and lighting: Easily reached switches and plugs, but covered to protect small children; apparatus earthed; no overloading of sockets; correct fuses in plugs; no exposed wires or frayed leads; repairs only by qualified experts; switch off apparatus not in use and pull out plug; lights that switch on and off from either end of stairway or of the paths between bedroom and lavatory; for old people especially, a light switch near the bed.

Fires: Sparkguard over open fires; no mirror over the mantelpiece; chimneys swept regularly; good air circulation around heaters; no clothing or materials draped on heaters; non-flammable clothes for children and the elderly; plenty of ashtrays; no smoking in bed; matches kept away from children; seek advice on fire extinguishers and fire blankets — and follow it.

Storage: Household and garden chemicals in cupboards inaccessible to children; keep medicines in special place equally inaccessible (p. 155); all substances correctly labelled; clear up any spilt material in garages or work sheds; no clutter in store rooms; paraffin and petrol in correct metal containers.

Correct tools: Do not 'save time' by using the wrong tool for a job; do not hop on a chair instead of getting a ladder or steps.

Acne

Acne is one of Nature's unkindest tricks. These disfiguring spots appear around puberty, just at the age when the sufferer is beginning to be aware of his appearance (and that of the opposite sex).

A protective oil called sebum is produced by small glands in the skin and passes through fine ducts to act as lubricant and softener. It happens that in adolescence quite different glands in the body secrete certain hormones (chemical messengers carried through the blood stream) in large amounts to stimulate sexual development. One undesirable side effect of these hormones is to speed up cell and sebum formation within the skin duct linings, to such an extent that the ducts can become narrowed and blocked. The excess sebum cannot escape; it is caught within the duct, distending it and causing local inflammation and infection. This forms the red spots, the 'blackheads' and sometimes the little pus abscesses which characterise acne. They appear on the face, the neck, the back or the shoulders.

Self conscious, the poor victims become shy of showing themselves. It is extremely small comfort to be reassured that they will 'grow out of it in time'. They seek an immediate cure. The first thing they must learn is to keep their hands off the spots. Squeezing out sebum or pus with finger nails is very likely to worsen the condition and to leave unpleasant scars. But the good normal friction of frequent washing with soap and water is an excellent start to treatment.

As for medication, it is wise not to try to seek it for oneself at the chemist or through friends' advice but to get the help of the doctor and then to follow the prescription exactly. Sometimes attention to diet and to vitamins is suggested. The results are disappointing except that avoidance of chocolate or cocoa and of excessive amounts of fats may help.

Local applications to the skin aim to clear the blockage at the exit of the gland ducts and so mobilise the flow of sebum. They include various lotions and also an abrasive preparation to be rubbed on the skin. One of them can reduce sebum production. Ultra violet light (which, of course, includes sunlight) can also open up the ducts by making the skin peel. All these must be used only with medical guidance.

The doctor may prescribe a certain type of antibiotic. It is still not entirely clear how this works, for the problem is not simply one of controlling infection, yet very often it proves effective. A relatively large amount may begin the treatment, and then, as the skin improves, this is decreased to a smaller maintenance dose. Treatment has to be continued for quite a time and both doctor and patient face the problem that it is not always good for the body in general to be on a long sustained intake of antibiotics. A happy compromise is generally achieved.

Acute and Chronic

Medical men are still not resigned to hearing their patients use the term 'chronic' as if it were a superlative. When a patient settles in the consulting room chair to complain that the pain, or the cough, or the indigestion is 'chronic' he is trying to say that it is awful, severe, intense, in other words that it is acute, and at once a difficulty arises.

For the doctor a condition is 'acute' when its onset is sudden and its duration is short. It may be severe or it may be mild. Appendicitis is an acute illness. So is the common cold. The word is derived from the latin *acutus*, meaning 'sharp pointed'.

'Chronic' on the other hand comes from the Greek *Khronos*, meaning 'time'. It is used for long lasting illnesses, which generally are slow in developing. This could be said of most rheumatic and arthritic states. The man who for years has a wheezy chest with coughing probably has chronic bronchitis. Someone suddenly stricken with fever, cough, pain on breathing and breathlessness may have acute pleurisy.

Sitting on the fence between these two is the expression 'subacute'. This very useful word lets the doctor describe something which has appeared rather fast and then lingered on longer than expected, or vice versa. It is rather indefinite but at least it sounds nicely scientific.

Adder Bite *see* Snakebite

Addiction to Drugs

There are two meanings of the word 'drug'. Originally it covered any medicinal substance. Now it is frequently used to describe preparations taken, without medical need, to heighten spirits or to change mood. This second meaning also implies dangerous substances to which the user becomes addicted. He develops a craving for them, requires increasing doses, and suffers unpleasant symptoms if they are suddenly withdrawn. These drugs can be put in three groups, 'soft', 'psychedelic' and 'hard', though their dividing lines are by no means rigid.

Addiction can involve anybody, yet often the patient (and it is an illness, not a sin) is someone who is unsuccessful at work, with problems in personal relationships, who finds it hard to make friends. Facing emotional or social crisis he might be persuaded to try drugs, and then perhaps moving gradually from the milder to the more potent ones, be unable to give them up.

Soft drugs include stimulant 'pep pills' like *amphetamines* or sedatives like *barbiturates*. Amphetamines give a false feeling of confident well being, with energetic wakefulness. When this wears off the victim may feel a reactionary depression which invites him to take another dose. Alternate moods of elation and sadness, irritable or erratic behaviour, thirst but poor appetite might be the mark of this addict. The pep pill victim in a crisis often behaves with the loquacious irrationality of a drunken man. Cope with this by talking to him with friendliness, but be wary lest he become violent.

Sedatives on the other hand are generally depressing, and in large repeated dosage will give a slow slurred speech and drowsiness. If the addict collapses suddenly, put him in the recovery position for unconsciousness (p.210) and rapidly get medical help.

Psychedelic drugs primarily affect the mind. The common type is *cannabis* which comes from the flowers or the resin of hemp, a plant similar to hops. Resin (much the stronger form) is dark brown; the flowers are cut up, mixed with vegetable matter and look like a mixture of tobacco and dried grass.

Smoked as cigarettes or in a pipe cannabis generally creates a happy sense of power and relaxation, while the smoker has a fatuous, dreamily contented look, his speech may be slurred and, like a drunk, he may be unsteady and uninterested in his surroundings. Sometimes he may experience hallucinations. The addict is sometimes detectable by his mood, by reddened eyes and by the characteristic acrid smell of cannabis about his person.

Apart from its immediate action cannabis could in the long term harm other functions of the body. For instance, scientific studies have demonstrated its bad effects on brain tissue, on sexual potency and on the production of spermatozoa by the testicles.

Those who argue that the law against smoking 'pot' interferes with civil liberties often point to the permitted sales of alcohol and cigarettes. An answer to this could come in parable form. If a garden is already beset with potentially harmful weeds, difficult to control, this is no excuse for the introduction of yet another type.

Lysergic acid or *LSD*, another psychedelic drug, comes in various tasteless forms as capsules, tablets, powders or liquids. Very small doses can give two or three hours of strong effect followed by slowly waning effect with intermittent bouts of normality for twenty-four hours or more. Sights, colours, sounds and smells are perceived intensely and this can be accompanied by a variety of twisted emotions of delight, ecstasy, disgust or terror. Judgment can be so impaired that, for instance, the taker can have the notion of being able to float down from a height.

An addict found in such a crisis must be kept under close watch with attempts at reassurance, but the minimal physical interference. He should be restrained only if it is necessary to prevent him harming himself. This could be difficult and dangerous if delusions of being attacked make him counter attack violently.

Of the 'hard' drugs, *heroin*, derived from an oriental poppy, is a grisly example. It is usually injected by the user into his veins, with crude and contaminated apparatus. Apart from the effect of the drug itself the consequence may be abscesses, blood poisoning or clotting in the vessels.

The typical addict is concerned to maintain his supplies, by frequent telephoning or absences from home. His appetite, his speech and his personal appearance deteriorate; he gives up his previous friends, interests and activities. Under the effect of heroin the taker is dreamy and detached, often lying down and relaxed, unable to concentrate and resenting disturbance. As the effect wears off, an addict who cannot get another dose becomes fidgety and restless, he sneezes, and has running eyes and nose. Later his condition worsens — sweating with a raised temperature and pulse rate, he is exhausted but unable to sleep. Attacked by stomach cramps, diarrhoea and vomiting, he suffers from severe prostration. He urgently needs medical help: the doctor may be able to give him a heroin substitute to ease the immediate position. The very difficult and long problem of trying to wean the addict from his drug and to cope with his psychological state now follows.

Another danger of hard drugs is the way they can depress respiration. The unconscious victim on a large dose may cease breathing and need artificial respiration (p.26).

This brief, necessarily incomplete survey may suggest that addiction is only to one or other type of drugs. The user of 'soft' drugs however is a potential user of the more serious 'hard' ones. A 'pusher', the criminal pedlar of drugs, may try to use cannabis as the thin edge of the wedge which will get his victim eventually on to more serious, more addictive and more lucrative wares like heroin. He then has a dependent customer with ever increasing needs for many months before disaster or death, or even cure, removes him.

Any discussion on addiction would lack reality if it did not also mention alcoholism (p. 13) and smoking (p. 188).

Adenoids *see* Tonsils and Adenoids

The Aged *see* The Elderly

Alcohol

If you want to minimise the effect of drinks at a party remember this:

1. Alcohol is absorbed from the stomach fairly fast.

2. Alcohol also passes to the bowel beyond the stomach from whence it is absorbed considerably faster.

3. The faster alcohol is absorbed, the more potent its effects. Sobriety is easier with slow absorption.

4. Stodgy food in the stomach slows alcohol absorption through the stomach wall. It also slows the passage of alcohol into the bowel.

5. So before your party you should eat stodgy food such as milk and bread and butter.

Alcoholism

We should not regard alcoholism as if it were a crime with moral stigma. It is an illness and must be handled as such if any help is to be effective.

The illness has insidious beginnings, for one cannot mark just at what point he or she who was a 'social drinker' slips into becoming an alcoholic. Those who have lost, or are losing, control over alcohol begin to be untruthful (to themselves as well as to others) about how much they take. They 'jump the gun' by having drinks before others at reunions or parties; they start drinking earlier and earlier in the day. They turn to alcohol to celebrate success, to bolster themselves for effort or difficulties, and to comfort themselves for disappointments. Anyone can become an alcoholic; there are no definite personality types marked out as likely victims.

The alcoholic is one who depends on drinking to an extent which disturbs his mental, personal, social and economic well-being. Dependence can be psychological and physical. The psychological factors involve problems with personal relationships or business affairs. But alcohol is no stimulant. In fact it depresses. One of its first effects is to damp down the controlling centres of the mind. The drinker feels less inhibited and more relaxed. He becomes falsely confident. (It is this which makes even small amounts of drink so dangerous in a car driver.)

It is later that physical dependence could take over; the body (and not just the mind) demands the effect of drink. The alcoholic now no longer partakes for pleasure or for mental relief, but to avoid the distress of not drinking. Sustained drinking harms stomach, brain, liver and heart muscle. In the late stages the victim's memory has blanks; he is shaky and feels sick; he is unreliable and vague. Often he hopes to relieve these symptoms by further drinking.

In earlier stages alcoholics do not recognise that they have a problem: they are confident of being able to stop drinking any time they wish. It is hard for close relatives and friends, even with tact and sympathy, to make them realise how they are moving into a threatening situation. Those alcoholics who seek treatment will do so late.

The response of the doctor will show no moral judgment, only a desire to help someone in difficulties. He will not expect the use of will power, for in this respect the patient has no will power. To a great extent the alcoholic has borne psychological loneliness: often he has introspectively come to dislike himself. Once treatment begins with the right medical approach and with help from his family he finds he no longer is fending for himself. In the fight against his troubles he has found allies; some self respect returns.

Living with an alcoholic can be a hideous, almost unbearable, strain to the family, yet the importance of its sympathy cannot be overstated. The Al-Anon organisation offers support and advice to families.

For some patients group therapy in a clinic or hospital specialising in alcoholism will reassure by showing how many others have a similar illness.

The Alcoholics Anonymous group makes a great contribution on these lines. Its members (in all parts of the country) are redeemed alcoholics who 'speak the language' of the patient. With no demand for entrance fee or subscription they pilot him through his difficulties and give constant support.

One of the key beliefs of A.A. is that it is impossible to succeed unless the patient *wants* to be cured. They ask him to follow the principles of 'Never take the first drink' and the daily renewed resolution: 'I shall not have a drink today'.

Cure is slow and long and, unfortunately, one recognises that relapses could be expected even after very long abstinences. However, if they happen this set back is no sign of irretrievable failure.

The ex-alcoholic always remains a potential alcoholic. Abstinence must be total and for ever. He cannot aim to become a mild 'social drinker' again. The life long risk of relapse remains with even the smallest glass of sherry. In this sense there is no 'cure' for alcoholism. But the possibility of achieving fully controlled and contented abstinence is a real one.

Allergy

Allergy is an excessive sensitivity of the body to one or more substances which, to most people, are quite harmless. These substances are so varied that they include dust, pollen, bee venom, fungus spores, antibiotics, feathers, plants, cloth fibres, furs, cosmetics, detergents, foods and even metals. Inhaled, eaten or in contact with the skin they provoke the cells of some tissues to liberate histamine or similar chemicals. This histamine has a number of unpleasant effects. It widens blood vessels; furthermore it makes them permeable so that some of the plasma, the liquid component of the blood, oozes out. The tissues concerned become swollen and boggy. Another of its actions is to cause spasm of some of the 'smooth' muscles. These are the ones which act automatically, independent of the will, in such organs as the stomach, the bowels or the breathing tubes.

These are the features involved in producing symptoms of hay fever, asthma, nettlerash or eczema in babies (each of which has its section in this book). Very rarely allergy hits all the body with a severe explosive reaction, called anaphylaxis. The victim develops a severe rash, his blood pressure falls, he gets breathless, waterlogged lungs and severe palpitations; sometimes he will vomit.

Why anyone acquires allergy is not known. Heredity does play a part. Sensitivity is not all. So called 'non-specific' contributory factors play their parts: smoke (and smoking), cold winds or dampness can all help to precipitate an attack. So can mental strains, and emotions like fear or excitement.

To cope with the allergic state obviously the first thing is to try to avoid the harmful substance — if one knows what it is. This is not as easy as it sounds, as so many factors can be operating. The doctor may begin by skin tests, applying or injecting weak extracts of the suspected substances: if anyone produces a wheal surrounded by reddening, that substance can be pronounced guilty. Sometimes a desensitising course helps: injections of weak extracts of the relevant substance are given at intervals, with gradually increasing doses. The body in this way may build up a resistance. As far as foods are concerned it may be possible to trace the offending components by what is known as 'elimination diets'. The patient begins with a regimen excluding everything which is likely to give allergic trouble. It does not make very interesting menus, but little by little, one at a time, other items are added and the appearance of untoward symptoms is noted. This ought to be done under medical guidance and with the cautionary knowledge that in many of today's foods there lurk possible sensitisers such as colouring, flavouring or preservatives.

For the treatment of an allergic attack antihistamines (p.19) and corticosteroids (p.79) are useful, but they do need a doctor's decision and supervision.

Alopecia *see* Baldness

Anaemia

Anaemia is one of the most misused words. It does not mean 'thin blood'. It is not the most probable cause of feeling tired. It does not always need iron medicines. But it always means that there are inadequate red blood cells.

The task of the red blood cells is to carry oxygen. As blood passes through the circulation in the lungs it picks up oxygen and holds it in loose chemical combination. Red cells in their millions are swept through the arteries and their branches until they reach every tissue in microscopically minute vessels (the capillaries) so thin that they can barely pass through them. As they jostle and squeeze along inside the capillaries the oxygen they carry moves to the adjoining tissues.

Red blood cells are made in bone marrow. They have a finite life of about four months only, and every second we produce about two million of them. The red cells contain, and derive their colour from a pigment called haemoglobin. It is to this that the oxygen is attached chemically when it passes in from the lungs.

At least three things in food are needed for the production of normal red cells: iron, vitamin B12 and folic acid. Vitamin C also plays some part. The average mixed diet of western man contains enough of these under ordinary circumstances.

Anaemia is a reduction of the number of red cells in the circulation or of the haemoglobin they contain, and consequently of the oxygen-carrying capacity of the blood. Sudden severe bleeding is an obvious example. The body responds by throwing in its reserves and the marrow becomes busier than before. Far more common is a quiet insidious loss of haemoglobin, from hidden, unnoticed, or slightly regarded bleeding. Piles or a stomach ulcer, for instance, can bleed very mildly and slowly but continuously so that the cumulative loss becomes large. Many women in their child-bearing years have heavy menstrual periods with therefore an iron loss which is beyond replenishment from a normal diet. These conditions need treatment not only for themselves but also for the iron deficit they create.

Some other illnesses of stomach and bowel could interfere with the absorption of iron from food, and occasionally there are people who live on such a restricted diet that they deny themselves the necessary iron. The red blood cells then have a low haemoglobin content.

A quite different problem arises when something interferes with the bowels' absorption of vitamin B12 from the diet: normally the stomach secretes what is known as 'the intrinsic factor', which is needed for this absorption. In pernicious anaemia the intrinsic factor is deficient. The development of red cells is upset and their number is reduced. A similar state of affairs happens when folic acid is inadequate in the diet.

Some illnesses and infections (like malaria) and some toxic chemicals (like lead) destroy the red cells in the circulation. Others reach further back and damage them as they are being formed in the marrow. Sometimes the marrow fails.

These forms of anaemia can be diagnosed by straightforward laboratory tests and most of them are very amenable to treatment. This treatment, of course, must be specific to the original cause.

If you 'feel anaemic' or appear pale, you may not lack iron; you may just need a holiday. On the other hand you may need vitamin B12 injections or treatment to piles. You will need investigating. Do not drop into your chemist or your travel agent. Go to see your doctor.

Angina *see* Heart Troubles

Animal Bites *see* Bites

Anorexia Nervosa

Anorexia Nervosa affects particularly females in the teenage group; only rarely do adults and males suffer from it. The patients are afraid of fattening foods especially of carbohydrates (starches and sweets). They reduce their diet to a dangerous minimum and seek a loss of weight far beyond any concept of fashionable slimming.

It is not because they dislike eating that they avoid food, but because they are really frightened and distressed by any weight gain. Commonly they have a completely false notion of their body size, picturing themselves much bigger than they are. They may wear thick and loose clothes which are in keeping with their misconceptions and which, perhaps, they use unconsciously to hide their true figures from the world.

Doctors believe that this attitude stems from stresses of home relationships, from demands which the patient feels are made upon her by family or husband. She unconsciously rejects responsibilities arising from moving into adolescence and sexuality. In a way she equates the size of the human body with the facing of life's problems.

She becomes alarmingly wasted. She will probably cease having menstrual periods after the weight loss, though sometimes this happens right at the onset of the illness. The intense fear of overeating often makes her go to extremes like taking regular and excessively large doses of laxatives or trying to subsist on grapefruit only. She may make herself vomit after eating. With this come intermittent bouts of compulsive overeating, to be followed by a deep sense of guilt and stringent attempts to atone. She may be rather withdrawn or sullen.

The illness clearly is a dangerous one. Wasting of the alimentary tract may eventually give a real loss of appetite. Fatal starvation has occasionally happened. More common is the lowering of resistance to infections or toxic changes of body chemistry.

It is very difficult to make these patients realise that they are ill. Once weight loss has become great many need hospital treatment. Here proper feeding (and close supervision), with suitable medicines to help the emotional side, will bring weight back towards normal. But this could prove inadequate unless at the same time they are given a deep and sympathetic exploration of psychological problems. This may have to be followed up closely with careful help for several years. One society, Anorexic Aid, offers support to supplement medical treatment.

Antibiotics

A century back a few bacteriologists described the way certain microbes could disturb the growth of others by using the word 'antibiosis' and from this was derived the word 'antibiotic'. It is a substance produced by the growth of some fungi or bacteria, capable of killing others or interfering with their growth.

The antibiotic era began in 1928 when Alexander Fleming noticed that the accidental presence of mould *(penicillium notatum)* in a laboratory culture interfered with the growth of the bacteria. It took another thirteen years before the chemical concerned, christened penicillin, was isolated and suitably prepared for use on patients with infections. This was the first of the very large armoury of antibiotics now available.

The word is now extended to include many other chemicals from micro-organisms and also those which research has produced synthetically. Different antibiotics work in different ways, damaging the cell walls of the inner structure of the bacteria. Some kill the bacteria and others slow down their growth. Some are useful against a big range of bacteria (broad spectrum antibiotics) and others against only a limited number (narrow spectrum). The doctor selects the one appropriate to the patient's illness.

The antibiotic path has not been consistently smooth. Many forms of bacteria which used to succumb to certain antibiotics now show a firm resistance to them. The nature of this resistance is quite often misunderstood: one may hear someone saying: 'I have become resistant to penicillin.' This does not really make sense. Any resistance lies not in the patient but in the particular bacteria which infect him. If later he has a quite different infection, then penicillin might well be just right to cure him.

There are several causes for this bacterial resistance. Perhaps some strain of microbes, originally resistant to an antibiotic, have increased in prevalence and taken over from another strain which was not resistant. Sometimes profound, sudden changes, called mutations, occur spontaneously in microbes, altering their response to antibiotics. Or the microbes may have developed a resistance because the illness was treated by antibiotics taken in doses too small and over too short a time to eradicate them from the patient.

Can antibiotics be harmful? Occasionally the body develops a sensitivity to a certain antibiotic and the patient will come out in a rash the next time he takes it. Some antibiotics attack not only the harmful invaders, but also some of the harmless or even useful bacteria which lie in the bowels. The absence of the latter now gives yet other micro-organisms lurking there the chance to flourish and multiply and cause troubles like diarrhoea. A few antibiotics may sometimes do unpleasant things like causing staining and poor growth of children's teeth or, more seriously, depressing the bone marrow's production of blood cells.

Doctors are well aware of these problems and guard against them. In extreme cases they may have to call upon an antibiotic with a possible bad side effect when this is the only one likely to control a really dangerous infection. In no way should we overlook how any bad points of antibiotics are enormously over-shadowed by all the good they do and all the lives they save.

Patients must play their part, take the full amount prescibed, for all the time instructed. They must never cut a course short just because they feel better. And they should never treat themselves to any odd antibiotic which happens to lie as a residue in the medicine cupboard; they would be very likely to take a preparation unsuited to their illness. Such haphazard behaviour is just the way to make ensuing laboratory tests invalid and also to create yet another antibiotic resistance.

Anticoagulants

Sometimes a patient refers to anticoagulants prescribed to him as designed to 'thin the blood'. This is a careless way of describing drugs which reduce the clotting power of the blood. They are used when there has been abnormal clotting which is likely to worsen or where there is a foreseeable risk of clotting. Examples of these are *some* types of vein inflammation (phlebitis), or the blockage by a clot of an artery of the heart muscle (coronary thrombosis). For rapid action in emergencies the patient receives anticoagulants by injection. The usual maintenance treatment is by tablets.

They must be taken exactly as instructed. This is one of the cases where precision of dose is very important. Too much anticoagulant carries the risk of provoking untoward bleeding, for instance from stomach, bowel or bladder, or showing as bruise-like spots under the skin. The clinician, in cooperation with his laboratory colleagues, monitors the effect of the prescribed anti-coagulant by regular tests of the patient's blood and adjusts doses accordingly.

The patient may be asked to carry with him details of his anticoagulant, of its current dose and of blood tests, marked on a card, available to any medical man called to attend him. If he were to need an emergency operation the surgeon must be forewarned that the normal clotting processes are in abeyance and counter this. Also some other drugs, of which aspirin is one, increase the effect of anticoagulants and should be avoided by the patient.

On the other hand a patient may inadvertently decrease the power of his anticoagulant by taking a multivitamin preparation which includes vitamin K.

Taken with meticulous attention to these rules anticoagulants are immensely useful and sometimes lifesaving drugs.

Antihistamines

The symptoms of allergy (p.14) are caused by liberation in the body of a substance called histamine. Antihistamines are drugs which block this effect and therefore stop or, at least, reduce the symptoms. This may seem an ideal treatment for allergies but it is not a complete solution. Asthma, for instance, does not respond to antihistamines. The drug is at its most effective in conditions like nettlerash (p.162) or hay fever (p.127). It had a brief and undeserved vogue as treatment for the common cold. To be sure it may decrease the watery discharge from the nose, but it can overdo this and leave the nose's lining membrane very dry and vulnerable to further infection. Some antihistamine preparations have proved useful in combating sea and car sickness, and certain forms of dizziness.

The many antihistamine preparations available are generally prescribed as tablets or capsules. They all have the disadvantage of making the patient somewhat drowsy, a side effect which would be intensified if he took sedatives or alcohol at the same time. He should be wary of working on machines or driving a car while on antihistamines. Some pharmaceutical firms claim that their brand of antihistamine is less likely to cause drowsiness. However, each patient's response to this type of drug can be so individual that a little trial and error testing between brands may prove necessary.

Antihistamine is also presented in creams and ointments to be used on allergically affected skin. It works quite well this way, but so often can bring about a skin sensitivity that many dermatologists advise against their use.

Antiseptics

An antiseptic is a substance which destroys bacteria or arrests their growth. The name intimates that it is used on the human body. Its sister word 'disinfectant' is best reserved for chemicals used about the home on *things* rather than on *people* (to whom they might be harmful).

The perfect antiseptic has the following virtues: it is very active against many types of bacteria and it works fast; it is long acting and it remains effective in the presence of body fluids like pus, blood or serum; it is not only painless on open wounds, but also quite harmless to the tissues and it does not inactivate the defensive, protective, white blood cells; it is not strongly absorbed into the body; it does not stain and either it is odourless or it has a pleasant smell.

No such marvellous preparation exists. We are limited to those which come as near as possible to this ideal. We must not be misled by advertisements relating how laboratory tests prove that Brand X kills millions of germs rapidly. It might well do this in a test tube, but can it keep up that standard in human tissues?

It was about a century ago that Lord Lister made the first extensive use of antiseptics by having phenol (carbolic acid) sprayed over operation sites during surgery. This was dramatically successful, but by now we have far superior antiseptics and realise how damaging phenol can be in strong or repeated applications. Other substances we should forget as antiseptics are alcohol (too weak), boric acid (too weak, liable to cause a rash, dangerous to babies if absorbed), tincture of iodine (too harmful to tissues, too painful, staining) and peroxide of hydrogen (too weak, too brief in effect).

Here, in alphabetical order, is a selection from today's antiseptics (some of the trade or proprietary names are given in brackets): Benzalkonium chloride (Roccal); Cetrimide (Cetavlon); Chlorhexidine (Hibitane); Chloroxylenol (Dettol, Supersan). There are also preparations with two antiseptics, such as the one which combines cetrimide and chlorhexidine (Savlon). All these are excellent products and there are several more. Many of them come not only as liquid but also in ointment or cream form. Cetrimide ½% cream (Cetavlex) is very useful on dressings to avoid their sticking to the wound.

Whatever antiseptic you chose, *you must read the instructions* about how much to dilute and how to apply it. The cheerful notion of 'the more the better', leading to a hefty dollop from the bottle into a splash of water may create a solution more fit to deal with the kitchen sink than a human being.

Skins can become sensitive to any antiseptic after repeated use. Also many rashes have nothing at all to do with infections, and the blind use of antiseptics on an undiagnosed rash is asking for trouble.

You do not use antiseptics in ordinary first aid measures. You reserve them for 'second aid', that is anything beyond an immediate emergency, or for simple home treatment. If a doctor or nurse is going to see the injury very soon, leave out the antiseptic which might interfere with his management. But soap and water, for cleaning the skin round a wound is an extremely good substitute. Antiseptics are at their most useful when medically prescribed for an infected condition after the doctor has assessed the situation.

So when does one use antiseptics in everyday life? The truth is: rarely.

Anxiety State

All of us get anxious or fearful at times, and feel no shame at this. The condition is different with those patients who are diagnosed as having a form of neurosis (p.163) called 'anxiety state'. In this illness the anxiety is not a reasonable one. The sufferer may recognise what causes his fears and be able to talk about it. But the degree of fear is quite out of proportion and quite inappropriate to its source. Very often, though the patient does not know why he is anxious, deep down something is nagging at him. It may be related to past experiences or to present features. His conscious mind, unwilling to face them, has relegated them to the unconscious mind. But they are still at work with nefarious effects. Sometimes they are connected with phobias of special things like heights, rail travel, crowds or even the harmless cat.

Sudden fear in real danger produces well recognised changes: the heart beats faster and stronger, blood pressure rises, the skin is pale and sweating, pupils widen, the mouth goes dry, the muscles tense. All these are very useful to the body in an emergency, gearing it for what has been well described as 'flight or fight'. In anxiety state the same things can happen in much diluted form. The effects are similar but far less intense. On the other hand they are long sustained, over weeks or months, creating unremitting physical and mental distress. It is worse when the patient does not recognise the cause.

Many are the symptoms, and they all reduce efficiency in daily life. Work and concentration suffer. So may rest, the patient having great difficulty in relaxing and going to sleep. He may become depressed and feel weak. Palpitations and attacks of dizziness or fast breathing may alarm him. In severe cases he may be assailed by sudden bouts of tremor or of blind panic. Inevitably these can lead to new anxieties concerning his general health, his heart or his sanity. A vicious circle has set in.

The doctor finds it difficult to break this circle. He knows that, even after a careful physical examination, it is useless to tell the patient that 'nothing is wrong'. Attempts to reassure by following up with special manoeuvres like X-ray examinations, electrocardiographs or blood tests are unlikely to help when they all prove to be normal; the unfortunate patient reckons that his case must be serious to need all these checks.

Treatment, besides sympathy allied to reassurance, consists of trying to explain and trying to find out why. It is not easy to get a patient to understand the anxiety process, and psychotherapy, often long drawn out, may be a primary need to disclose hidden causes. In the meantime sedatives and modern tranquillizers can give very valuable support.

Apoplexy *see* Strokes

Appendicitis

The appendix is a vestigial organ of no use at all. Its appearance has been compared to that of a small worm; about 7cm long and the thickness of a pencil, it is a tube pouching from the caecum (which is the beginning of the large intestine, low on the right side of the abdomen).

Infection and inflammation of the appendix is generally related to its being blocked by becoming kinked

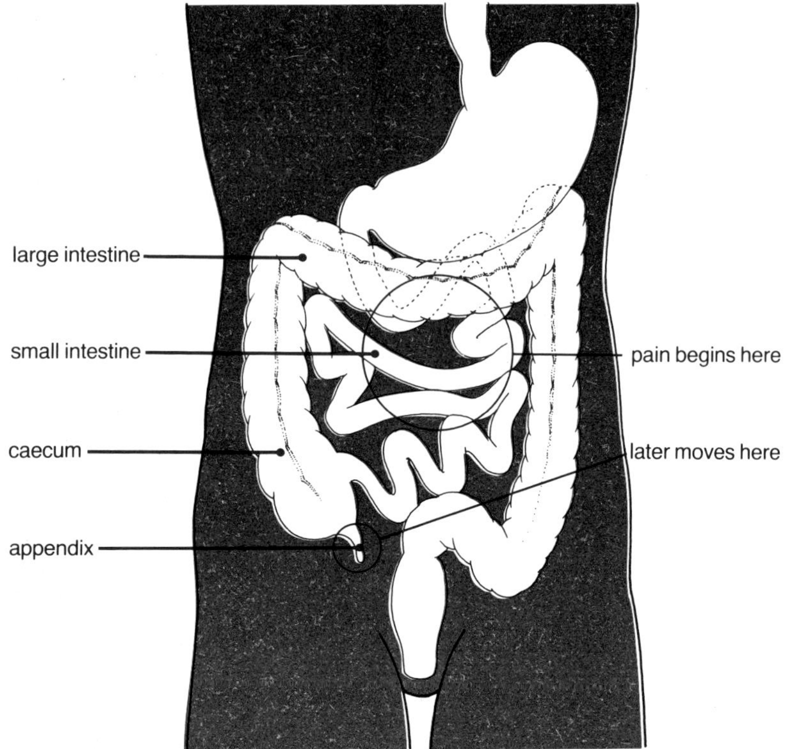

or by some of the waste matter in the bowel getting within its narrow tube and hardening there. This is the first stage of the trouble. Within a few hours it gives symptoms typical of colic (p.75). The pain begins suddenly, is intermittent and in the middle of the abdomen. This is the typical site for colic pain of many causes. The patient may feel and may be sick and his appetite is poor, but otherwise he will not at this point appear very ill.

Some hours later the appendix becomes inflamed: its weakened muscle can no longer contract and squeeze against the obstruction, and the colic ceases. But now a new pain takes over, that caused by the inflammation itself irritating the tissues around the appendix. It changes site and is no longer colicky but constant. Temperature and pulse rate begin to rise, the tongue becomes coated, the breath may be tainted and the patient seems ill.

This classical history, however, can vary a lot, especially as the appendix does not always lie straight down from the caecum as illustrated but may be folded back around or behind it. Then the site of the second pain can be different. Also such features as fever, nausea or the second type of pain can be quite mild or absent. As for bowel action this can range from constipation to slight diarrhoea.

Children have a tendency to develop appendicitis fast with marked pain and vomiting. Old people on the other hand may misleadingly have the mildest of symptoms while the condition develops slowly but inexorably. Even the doctor's examination can sometimes givc puzzling features and diagnosis may not be straightforward.

If diagnosis is not yet clear, the doctor may decide to have the patient in hospital either for close supervision or for definite operation. Removing a healthy appendix is by far the lesser evil than leaving in one which is getting worse. It may become gangrenous as its blood supply becomes impaired. It may form an abscess. It may rupture and cause peritonitis, infection of the membranes lining the abdominal cavity. The risk of rupture is high if the unwary give a so called 'opening medicine' to the sufferer.

The double lesson is obvious. If there is a possibility of appendicitis do not wait but get medical advice. And never ever give a purgative to someone suffering from a undiagnosed abdominal pain.

Arthritis

The suffix '-itis' means inflammation and the 'arthr-' part of this word means joint, both being derived from the Greek. Arthritis then means little more than inflammation of joints, and of these there are many forms, many causes.

To begin with we consider in an elementary way the make up of a typical healthy joint like the knee. The

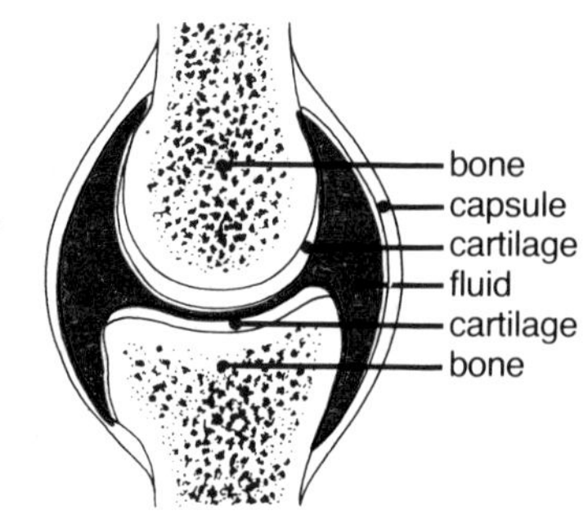

two bones move upon each other with minimal friction thanks to a layer of very smooth, shiny cartilage at the end of each. This is enhanced by the lubricating effect of 'synovial fluid' held within a thin, surrounding 'synovial membrane'. The whole is bounded by a thicker, firmer capsule. Finally the joint is made strong and stable, yet mobile, by its associated muscles and ligaments.

Rarely arthritis may arise from various types of bacterial infection sometimes with pus forming in the joint. Such attacks develop relatively fast with fever and prostration. Tuberculosis can also attack a joint; happily this infection has decreased greatly over the last years.

Another form of arthritis is the well known enemy gout (p. 125). However the two more common scourges are the quite distinct entities of rheumatoid arthritis and osteoarthritis.

Rheumatoid Arthritis

This wretched illness, which tends to involve many joints, can appear at any age, but generally between twenty five and fifty. (There is a form called Still's Disease which attacks children. Though its features are severe, often needing hospitalisation, it generally clears up completely.) Women are affected three or four times as frequently as men. Researchers suspect quite a number of factors, such a virus infection, as the cause but definite proof is lacking. Its onset may be due to what is known as 'auto-immunity', which can be described as a special allergy or sensitivity of the patient to some of his own tissues. Anxiety and mental stresses may play a part, if not in causing rheumatoid arthritis, at least in worsening it.

As a rule several joints are inflamed at the same time. Any can suffer, but chiefly those of the fingers and toes, the wrists, ankles and elbows. Onset is gradual with joints becoming painful, swollen and warm. They are stiff, especially after rest.

The synovial membrane becomes thickened. Later the cartilage softens and becomes eroded. Even later the ends of the bones suffer some damage. The condition is generally long lasting until eventually the inflammation subsides. However, in severe cases the joints by then have undergone so much scarring that they have become fixed in great deformity.

The hands in such serious and sustained attacks are crippled with fingers abnormally bent and knobbly and the wrists extremely restricted in their range of movement. The muscles serving these joints have weakened and are wasted from lack of use. These are extreme cases. In many others, especially where treatment has begun early, the condition settles with little or no handicap.

An important part of any treatment is attending to the patient's general health, clearing any untoward features like dental caries or anaemia.

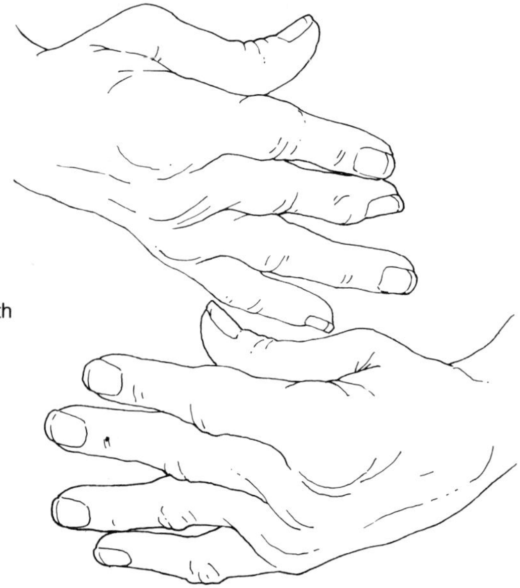

In severer forms of rheumatoid arthritis the hands and fingers can suffer great deformities with swellings at the stiffened joints.

Any inflamed structure needs rest as the first part of its treatment, and so it is with joints. They need to be quiet, to minimise the risk of deformity. For bad cases doctors may prescribe splints shaped to hold the joints in their most useful positions. Splinting will not cause stiffening, but by reducing inflammation will reduce damage. At the same time, even if this sounds a contradiction, the associated muscles are kept in trim by physiotherapy and exercises given as soon as inflammation and pain have been reduced. Sometimes the joints can be helped by physiotherapy using infra-red rays, short wave diathermy or hot wax baths, in short, methods of giving a penetrating but soothing heat.

Aspirin (p.28) still holds a very high place for it is not just a pain reliever; it can reduce inflammation considerably. In the last decade a whole new set of useful drugs with similar anti-inflammatory action have become available. Corticosteroids (p.79) also can be dramatically effective. Unfortunately there is always a price to pay. Many of these preparations can irritate the digestive tract or have other unpleasant side effects, so they are used carefully and strictly according to medical instructions.

Orthopaedic specialists can use two surgical methods on joints which have become severely deformed. Arthroplasty is remodelling to restore most, if not all, movement. The term includes setting in an artificial joint of metal to return smoothness and freedom of action. On the other hand arthrodesis consists of fixing the joint permanently in its best position; it no longer moves, but it is no longer painful.

Osteoarthritis

This is not really an inflammatory condition like rheumatoid arthritis, but the result of damage and of wear and tear. Therefore many doctors prefer to call it osteoarthrosis, the '-osis' suffix meaning merely a diseased condition. As joints get older they undergo some degree of degeneration; in the osteoarthritic joint this process has been intensified through stresses and strains. Constant heavy use of one joint from a certain occupation (e.g. heavy gripping and twisting) may be a factor, as well as some past injury. Carrying a heavy human body can be quite a task for hip and knee joints which are more likely to be affected in the obese.

Inside the joint the cartilage degenerates, thins and slowly wears away down to the bone. The bone ends harden, roughen and develop knobbly projections which can cause pain and restrict joint action. The onset is very gradual; little by little moving the joint becomes less and less easy. Any pain tends to be worse in cold and damp weather, yet these factors are only aggravating ones and do not cause the changes.

Osteoarthritis is potentially not as disabling as rheumatoid arthritis. Indeed it may exist without causing trouble. Many of us as we grow older have these joint changes without realising it until a chance X-ray examination discloses them.

If the diagnosis is established, what is the treatment? As long as we are symptom free we need take no special measures except to respect the joints and not subject them to further avoidable stresses. This may involve a reducing diet for the overweight, but in no other way would a special diet help.

Where pain and stiffness are present preparations like aspirin can be useful, but the corticosteroids are not likely to help since their action is essentially to reduce inflammation. Courses of physiotherapy can sometimes relieve symptoms. The patient should remain as active as he can within the bounds of avoiding discomfort or pain. Where a joint has become badly disorganised surgeons may try arthroplasty and arthrodesis just as they do for rheumatoid arthritis. Quite often the unfortunate patient has both rheumatoid arthritis and osteoarthritis co-existing. The former causes the damage which eventually creates the changes of the latter.

Finally, those who end up in either condition with grossly handicapped joints can regain a great deal of activity or independence by using some of the many gadgets designed to help the handicapped (p. 126).

Artificial Respiration

It is unsatisfactory to learn artificial respiration from a book. The methods ought to be learnt from organisations which give classes in first aid (see p. 112). What follows here is better than not learning at all, but please let every reader aim to attend a suitable course. *Particularly important is the fact no one should ever practice on a real person:* practice is made on one of the lifelike manikins available at classes.

Give artificial respiration only when natural breathing has stopped. Do not try it when someone has collapsed but is still breathing.

Breathing may stop in drowning, after choking (p. 70), electric shock (p. 100) or some types of poisoning

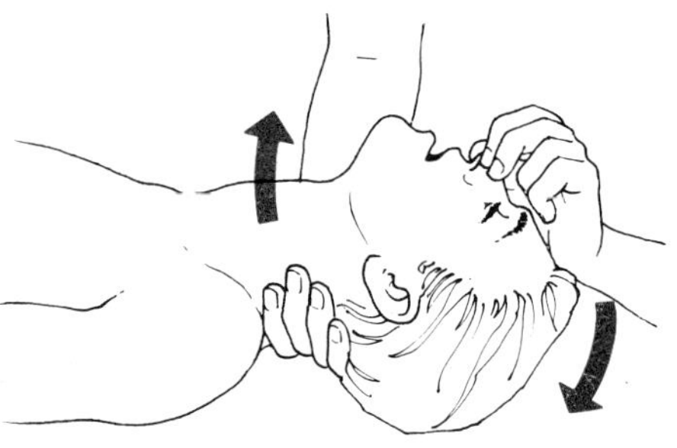

hand under neck lifts it slightly; head falls back, mouth falls open

finger and thumb pinch nose; wrist on forehead tilts head

Two different ways of getting the head positioned: use that which proves more effective or convenient.

OR

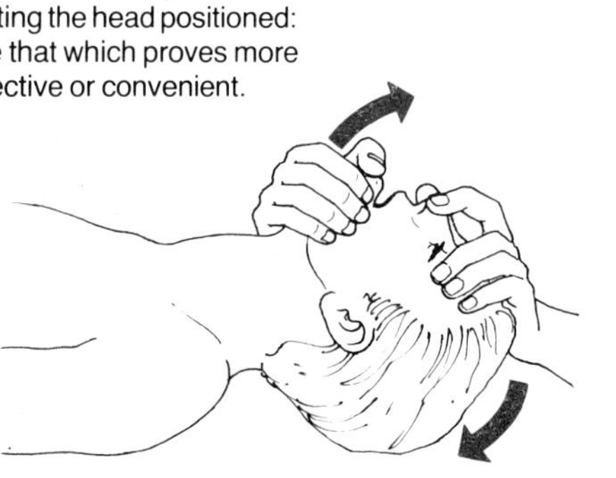

palm on forehead bends head back; finger and thumb close nose

jaw pushed forward and mouth kept open (avoid resting hand on neck)

(p. 171). In cases of drowning do *not* attempt to drain water from the lungs. This will waste time, for air will bubble past any water in the air tubes.

The Method

1. Very rapidly: clear the mouth and throat of any obstruction (false teeth, vomit, mud, blood) by scooping your finger round the back of the mouth.
2. Very rapidly: (a) get the victim on his back; (b) tilt the head fully back at the neck so that the nostrils look upwards, push the jaw forwards, and get the mouth open (this position ensures a clear airway and must be maintained throughout); (c) pinch the nose shut.
3. Take a deep breath in; seal your lips fully over the victim's open mouth; blow into the mouth firmly but gently, and your air entering his lungs should make his chest rise.
4. Lift your mouth off and take in a new breath. As you do this turn your head sideways to confirm that the victim's chest has risen; it should now be falling again letting the air out.

The first three or four breaths should be given fast to 'top up' the victim's oxygen. After that let the breathing rhythm become natural, allowing the victim's chest to descend fully before immediately inflating again. This rhythm will be about twelve times a minute.

You must continue thus until either the victim shows signs of breathing for himself or an expert takes over. In all cases of recovery keep a very close watch lest the victim's breathing ceases again.

If possible, summon help to loosen his clothing and to cover the lower part of his body.

Other important points are:

- It is easy to forget to maintain the backwards tilt of the head as you proceed: keep this always in mind.

- In the case of a small child your lips may seal over both mouth and nose, and the nose is not pinched shut.

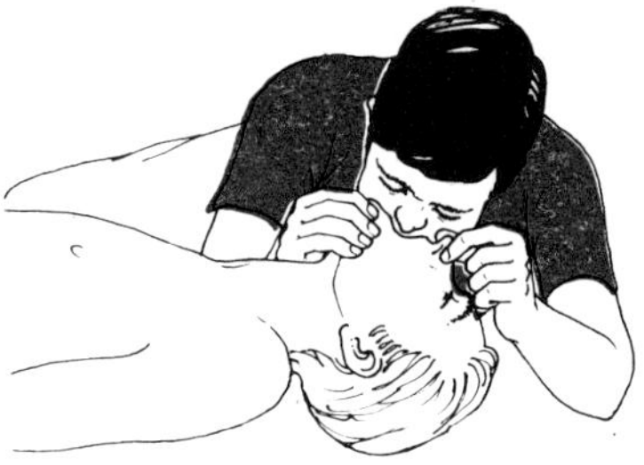

Above: take a deep breath in; seal your lips fully over the victim's open mouth; blow into the mouth firmly but gently.

Below: lift your mouth off and take in a new breath; turn your head sideways to check that the victim's chest has risen (it should now be falling again, letting the air out).

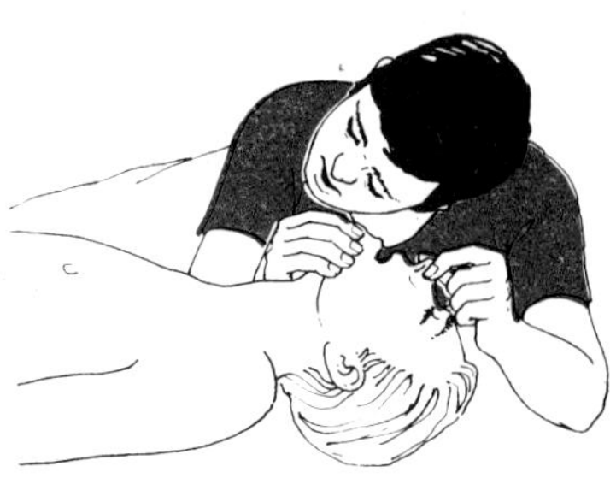

● Forceful breathing is an error: aim to get the chest moving smoothly. With young victims, breathe only with the energy needed to make the chest rise. To a small baby give only small puffs: you will find a baby's natural rate is faster, in the order of thirty a minute.

● If the victim vomits, quickly turn his head to one side and scoop the mouth clear. Then resume artificial respiration, with the first three or four breaths quick ones.

Successful artificial respiration should restore the victim's colour and pulse. If it fails then perhaps not only his breathing but also his heart beat has stopped. In that case he will need heart compression (by pressure on the breastbone) as well. However, this must not be tried by anyone who has not attended a class and demonstration on the subject. This is a further reason for enrolling for a course on first aid.

Asphyxia *see* Choking

Aspirin

Aspirin was first presented to the world in 1898 by the German firm Bayer who derived its name from the shrub Spiraea, a plant rich in salicylates which is the chemical background of this drug. They announced it to doctors as a preparation '...which will certainly take a predominant place in the medical treasury'.

They were right. For over eighty years aspirin has been successfully relieving pain, reducing inflammation, lowering fevers and decreasing rheumatic troubles.

To some extent its excellence has been marred by the fact that a few people are ultra-sensitive to it and develop rashes or stomach upsets after taking it. And a great number of others still do not take the tablets in the manner advised, broken up or dissolved in water or milk. Swallowing the tablets whole and dry is asking for trouble. It is for this reason that in the last decade the drug paracetamol has tended to supersede it as pain killer. Yet that too has its unfortunate side effects and many doctors still believe aspirin to be superior and more versatile.

The pain relieving effect of aspirin is attained in thirty to forty minutes and maintained for about five hours. For rapid relief of occasional pain and headache it is excellent (unless one happens to be sensitive to it). But it should not be taken regularly and in large doses (i.e. more than two or three tablets at a time) without medical advice for then it may give untoward effects like head noises, bleeding from the stomach or reduced clotting power of the blood.

The pharmaceutical name is Acetylsalicylic Acid and these words may be found in the small print on the containers of some pain killers marketed under trade names by firms who may wish to disguise the fact the aspirin is a component (perhaps the only one) of their product. The term may be further obscured into the form Acidum Acetylsalicylicum or even o-Acetoxybenzoic Acid. There is little point buying dearer aspirin under special brand names when, under its own name, from a good chemist, it is as good and cheaper.

It is available in 'junior' form, pleasantly flavoured and in small doses, for children. It can be obtained in capsules or mixtures which reduce any risk of stomach upsets. Some tablets with delayed action protective coating (this time to be swallowed whole) when taken at bedtime will act only some hours later — a help to those who have conditions likely to wake them painfully in the middle of the night.

Asthma

The asthmatic attack can be triggered off by different factors, which may act separately or in combination. Allergy (p.14) is the major one but irritation (e.g. smoky atmosphere or fog), infection (e.g. a cold) and also emotion can play their parts. An attack may begin from the patient's exposure to some substance to which he is sensitive, but if it is severe and he is in distress the superadded emotion of fear could well worsen the situation.

Two components of the lungs airways are involved. They are the fine muscle fibres ringing the air tubes and the lining membrane. During an attack three things happen to block the tube and make breathing difficult: (1) the muscles tense and narrow the tube; (2) the lining membrane thickens considerably; (3) the membrane secretes thick mucus, filling what little space is left. The patient has great trouble getting air in and out of his lungs — especially out, since the muscular work for expiration has to be greater than for inspiration. His breathing is laboured, distressed and wheezy. On this point let us realise that children with colds and chest infections often wheeze. Not every wheezing child is necessarily an asthmatic.

An asthmatic attack can last but a few minutes or it may extend to hours. If the prescribed remedies do not

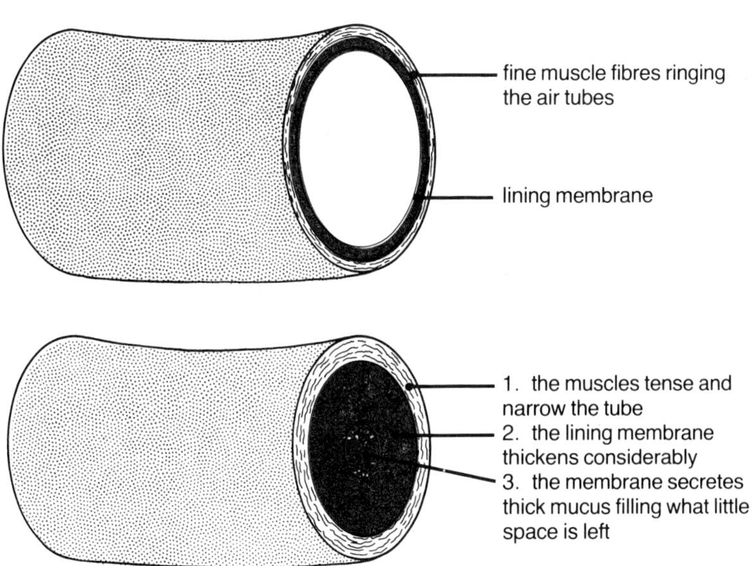

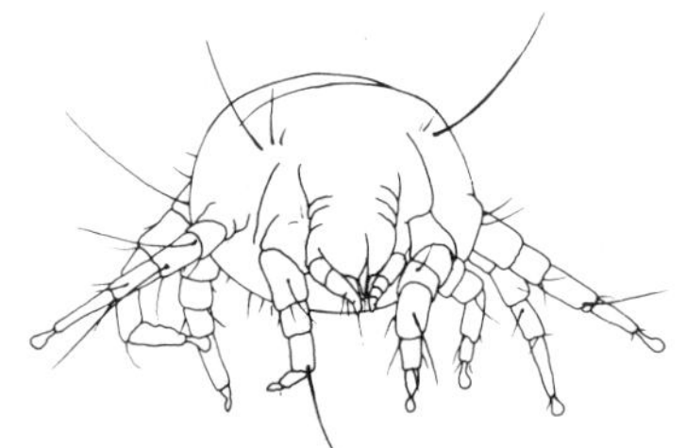

The house dust mite, culprit of much asthma, very greatly enlarged.

work, a doctor ought to be called. Sometimes the attack may extend to many hours or even into days, the so-called *status asthmaticus,* and the patient becomes worse and worse with oxygen deprivation; medical help is certainly needed urgently.

Prevention takes the first line in treatment. The sufferer avoids any substances to which he has been shown to be allergic. Foods, spices, animals, feathers, plants, pollens, moulds and house dust feature in the great list of possibilities. Concerning house dust it has been shown that a minute invisible mite in dust, and not the dust itself, is often responsible.

If the asthmatic is sensitive to feathers he must not use these in pillow or duvet fillings. It is not enough to give him a pillow of sponge rubber and leave feathers in the one alongside him. In an emergency pillows can (under the pillow case) be put within plastic bags which are then sealed with Scotch tape.

Any infection (including those of teeth) ought to be treated vigorously.

Sometimes exercises are taught to improve chest movements for more effective breathing; one major point is that in any attack the patient should not struggle against the tightness he feels in the upper part of the chest, but direct his breathing movements to waist level.

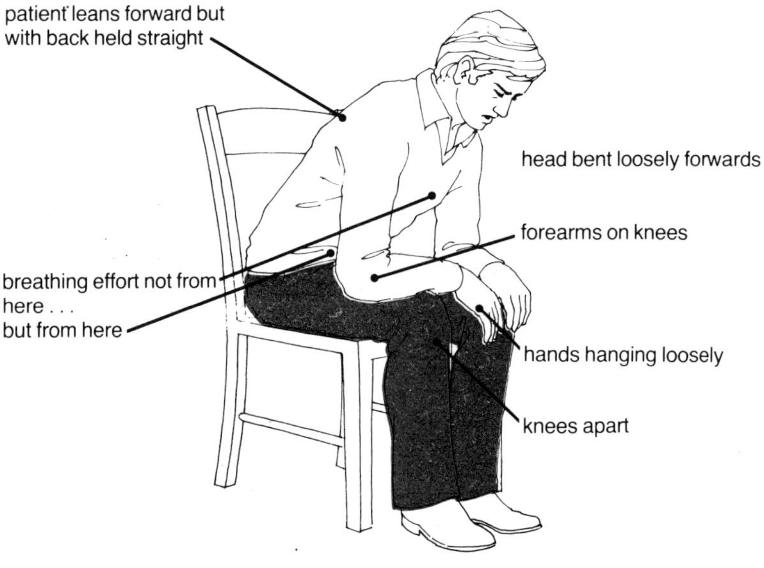

patient leans forward but with back held straight

head bent loosely forwards

forearms on knees

breathing effort not from here . . .

but from here

hands hanging loosely

knees apart

Attempts to desensitise against allergy (see p. 14) are sometimes tried but all too often prove disappointing.

First aid for an asthmatic attack.
Get the patient to relax physically and mentally. A calm attitude of confidence with advice clearly given helps greatly. Let him sit as in the illustration, leaning forward and totally relaxed except for (a) his back which he keeps straight to help the mechanics of breathing and (b) concentrating breathing movements at the lower chest and waist.

Let in fresh (but not cold) air. If he has tablets or inhalers prescribed for such attacks make sure he uses them, but be certain this be according to the doctor's instructions and do not let him take an overdose.

Cardiac asthma is a bad name for a certain type of sudden heart failure. It has nothing to do with ordinary asthma.

Athlete's Foot *see* Tinea

Baby Sitting

It just is not good enough to be satisfied that 'someone is there' while you, the parents, are out. How well known to you is that someone? Have there been meetings before? Does she come through a reliable recommendation? Above all, how known is she to the child? If at all possible let the child, even the smallest baby, see her, communicate with her, play with her at least once before the baby sitting occasion. Let her arrive early and help to feed the child or put him to bed. Let him learn that she is familiar with him, his parents and the home.

Should she be allowed a friend with her? The same rules apply to the friend as to the sitter. One might argue that a companion is a help and reassurance for her: equally one might say that the friend could be a distracting presence, taking her mind, eyes and ears away from the child. Use your judgment. Let the baby sitter know at what time you will return; then be fair and do not be late.

The counsels which follow may seem drastic. They cover the very rare emergencies, those for which planned action is essential.

Does she know first aid? A book on the subject could be provided.

Are the fires protected with guards?

She keeps the door locked and the lights on at the front of the house. If someone calls she does not open but enquires through the door or from a window. She does not explain that she is baby sitting.

Kept by the telephone are written details of where the parents are and how they can be contacted. Any special instructions, such as giving medicines, are also written out, not just explained verbally. Numbers for emergency (e.g. the doctor) are clearly marked.

If the telephone rings she should answer. This ensures that you could, if necessary, telephone to her. If someone else rings she should do no more than say that you are out and take, *in writing,* the name of the caller, the time, and any message. She should not get into conversation.

If you have no telephone let her have a written note about the neighbour who has agreed to let his be used or about the nearest call box.

In case of fire she must know of two routes of escape if possible (e.g. by the front door and by the back door or window). Her immediate task is to get the child out of the house without spending time to dress him in more than a blanket, or to bring out pets and toys. She closes the door behind her and alerts the fire brigade.

In case of gas escape she also takes the child out, but she leaves the door open and notifies the police for emergency call to the gas company.

One last point: remember that if she is younger than sixteen the law does not hold her responsible for the child's care and safety. You, the parents, are the responsible ones.

Backache

Back Injuries

Pain in the back following a blow or fall is generally due to minor injury, but the consequences of neglecting and badly handling the occasional fractured spine can be so permanently horrible that no victim of such an accident should be moved until full and expert assessment has been made (see Fractures, p.117).

General Back Pain

Any thoughts on general backache should begin by considering all the structures whose malfunction could be responsible. Stomach ulcers can, rarely, give a left back pain. Pleurisy is a common cause, and so are kidney and gall bladder disease. Troubles of the ovaries and the uterus may give low back pain. Far less common is the pain caused by aneurysm (a bulging, with weakening of its wall) of the aorta (the major blood vessel) in the abdomen. Even shingles (p.182) can give a pain in the back, mystifying in the few days which precede the characteristic rash.

By far the most common reason is to be found in the muscle, skeletal, and nerve systems which dominate structure and function of the back.

The backbone consists of a series of bones set one upon the other to form a semi-rigid structure which spans from neck (linking with the skull) to buttocks (linking with the bony pelvis). Each vertebra interlocks with its neighbours by means of many apposition surfaces, vulnerable to the ills which can befall all joints. Irregular excrescences of bone from every vertebra are points of attachments for ligaments and muscles which help to bind, support and move the torso. These too are subject to strain and damage. Furthermore each vertebra is designed as a stout bony ring through which the spinal cord of nerves passes down from the brain. At every vertebral level the spinal cord sends out and receives nerves serving the body. This nervous system benefits from the protection of hard bone, but spaces are small and any positional abnormality risks hurting the delicate nerve tissues. The triad of muscle, bone and nerve forms a splendid compromise of stability and mobility when all is in order, but the tight design of its components leaves little or no room for any one of them to vary without causing pressure and therefore pain.

A full dissertation on back pain merits a book on its own, and that would show how uncertain and con-

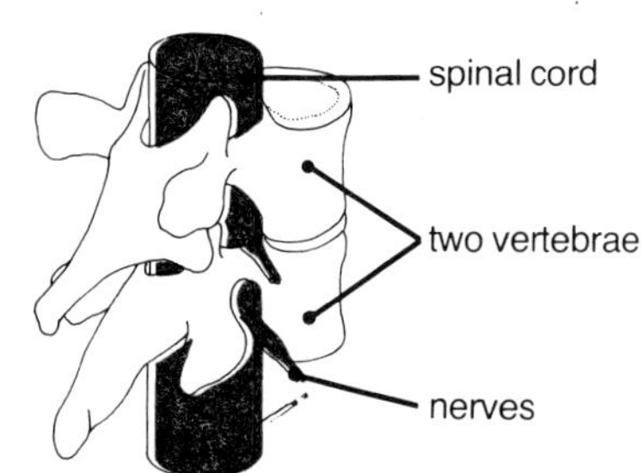

jectural we remain on many points. *Fibrositis* (p. 112) of the back muscles might explain some symptoms, but any muscle integrated with inflamed nerve or bone tends to go into painful spasm. As for the term *lumbago,* all it means is a lower backache so as a path to understanding it is useless. *Strained ligaments* about the back and pelvis may arise from general flabbiness after a serious illness, or may be related to overweight. It can bother women in pregnancy or after childbirth, since ligaments tend to relax during pregnancy.

Sciatica means pain extending along the back of the thigh and down to the back of the leg, along the course of the sciatic nerve, which is the biggest nerve in the body. A great deal in relation to backache can irritate the sciatic nerve, or its roots as they arise from the lowest two vertebrae and the region of the pelvic bone just below them. Tumours and inflammation of these bones can do it. Arthritic changes at the vertebral joints can exert severe pressure, as could even mild displacement of the vertebrae.

By far the most common cause of irritation of the sciatic nerve is the *displaced intervertebral disc.* The disc is a small buffering cushion of elastic cartilage which lies between each vertebra. A sudden strain can make part of the disc slip a little out of place, and press up against a nerve. The typical strain is some action like lifting or pulling a heavy weight while the back is bent forward. Even a heavy cough has been known to do it.

The pain can be very disabling and long lasting. It has a mechanical cause and the treatment is correspondingly mechanical, aided by taking pain-relieving tablets. Rest, stretched on a very firm mattress for days (or weeks)

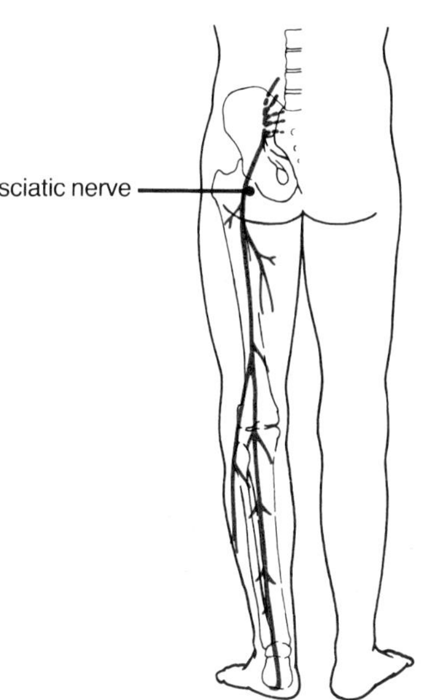

is generally recompensed by the disc correcting its position; all bending must be avoided. If the patient is able to move about, he must guard his back by constantly keeping it straight, watching this carefully as he walks, gets in and out of bed, or sits. His chairs should have straight back and a relatively high and narrow seat. A small cushion at the lower back can help. He must avoid the popular 'squashy' low armchair, with its deep seat, which compels him to sit in a half folded position.

The more severe attacks may need support from a surgical belt, or physiotherapy, including stretching of the spine.

Sometimes, fortunately rarely, a really difficult, long standing case can come to surgical treatment to have an obstinately static piece of disc removed from its protrusion against the nerve root.

Prevention of Backache

Sleep on a firm mattress.

Lose any surplus weight.

Hold yourself straight at all times. (Imagine you are suspended by a cord at the top of your head, with your feet just off the ground).

Study the diagrams. In lifting try to keep your trunk as nearly vertical as you can, and stand close to the object you are tackling.

Baldness

Baldness is bad luck. This at least is true in most of the cases we see. Recession of hair from the forehead line, at the temples and at the crown is common in men after middle age. It is not a sign of poor health, but it may be related to natural hormonal changes. There is some inherited factor here; the tendency to balding, which some-

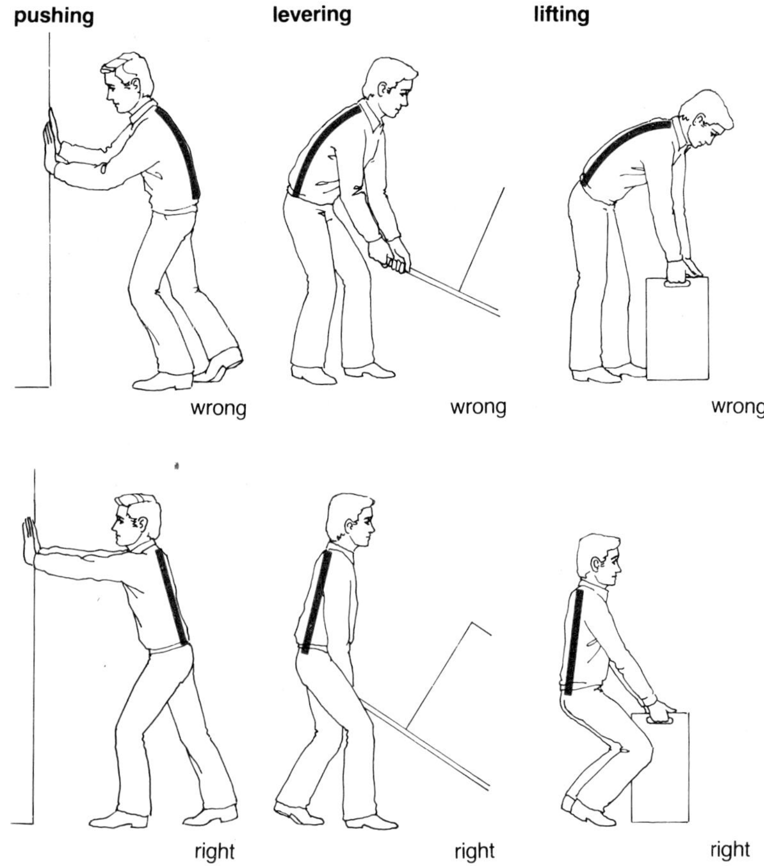

times happens to younger men, can be familial. Women normally do not go bald in this way; when they are older they may have a general thinning of hair.

This normal type of hair decrease is quite unaffected by treatment. No amount of lotions, shampooing or scalp massage will bring the hair back. Nor can the blame be put on wearing hats, worry, poor diet or dandruff.

Alopecia is the general medical name for hair loss. There is one unusual type called *alopecia areata,* in other words patchy baldness. This can happen at any age and shows one or more round or oval areas of hair loss giving a rather 'moth eaten' appearance. Why it happens is not at all clear, but sometimes it is associated with mental stresses. In the huge majority of cases the hair returns spontaneously in some months and the patient may give the credit to any 'hair tonic' or patent 'cure' he happens to be using at the time.

Of course there are some definite illnesses which can bring about hair loss. Ringworm of the scalp is a form of tinea (p.206) which breaks off hairs. Thinning of hair, as opposed to actual baldness, may be related to general constitutional conditions like anaemia or thyroid deficiency. Some severe fevers can lead to baldness; so can certain drugs which have the side effect of stopping hair growth. All these will recover when the illness is over or when the drug is discontinued.

Do not get worried when hair comes out as you comb and brush; this is not abnormal. The deep follicles in the scalp, which are the points from which hairs grow; wax and wane in activity and in their resting phases they can quite naturally lose their products.

If general health is suspect then a doctor's advice should be sought, but in most cases the line to take is to be philosophical or expectant and not to spend money on alleged cures.

Bandages *see* Dressings

Baths to the Sick or Disabled

When a patient is fit enough to get up for his bath you should make it as easy as possible for him. Get the bathroom warm, with window closed, and have the bath filled at a suitable temperature. Prepare all the necessary soap, brush, towels, bath mat and clean clothes. Have a chair handy. Where appropriate let the patient clean his teeth and visit the lavatory before he has his bath.

Even if he does not need help with undressing, drying, dressing or getting in and out of the bath and wishes to be alone, keep within hearing and do not let the door be locked. A child should not be left. Once the bath is over, help the patient back to bed.

A patient who finds movement difficult can get into a bath by means of boards set as seats across the top (see illustrations overleaf), suitably protected from slipping by side flanges (a). In some cases this can be made with a broad seat at the top and two steps below on which the patient moves down in stages (b). This is removed during the bathing and replaced when the patient wants to get out, so that he can come up sitting on each step in turn. Another simple form is within the bath, with the angle of its side pieces adjustable to the size of the bath tub (c). If plastic covered and with rubber tips to the feet it will not scratch the enamel.

On the base of the bath a rubber mat with both surfaces patterned in indentations prevents slipping. A thick, rough towel can act as an emergency substitute.

Do not let the water away before helping your patient out; its buoyancy makes it easier to lift him. A rail set firmly on the walls by the bath helps him to get in and out. This should be at a higher level than the top of the bath tub, and at an angle rather than parallel to wall or floor. The frame which fits on the taps to lie across the top of the bath tub may look impressive but is difficult for those with weakened arms and legs to manage.

More sophisticated and considerably more expensive are the many patterns of hoists in which the patient sits to be lifted up, swung round and lowered. None of this apparatus should be obtained without first consulting the doctor and those experienced in their design. In some cases where the need is essential it may be possible to obtain aids through the social services.

Bedmaking

Now that fitted sheets and loose duvets are available bedmaking can be beautifully easy. But for the many of us who retain the common forms of linen making up the bed has its finesses.

The Empty Bed

Working from below upwards:

The mattress should be firm.

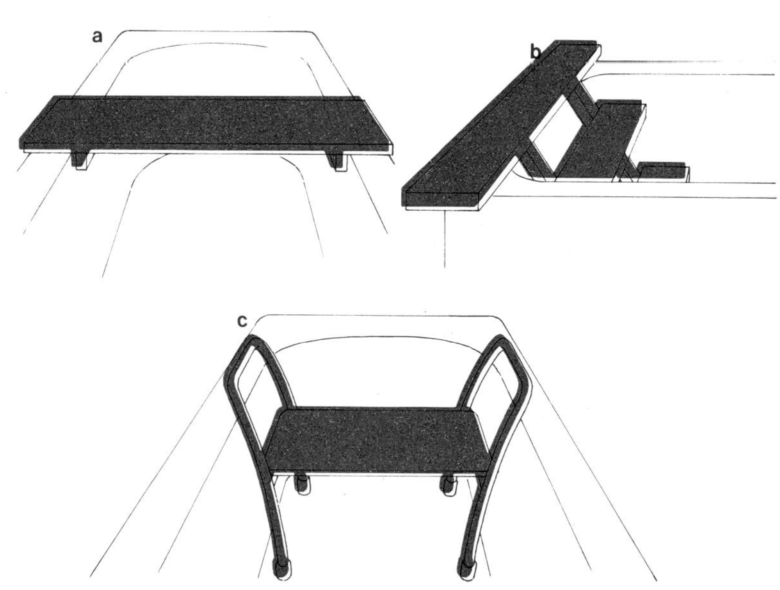

Softness and sagging give a preliminary impression of comfort which soon disappears. A water mattress needs a very strong bed with extra support to its base and can give problems of 'flopping' as the patient moves. The underblanket should be small enough to lie flat and is not tucked in.

Place the bottom sheet centrally, being guided by its ironed crease. Tucking the ends in 'hospital corner' fashion is not essential but gives a neat professional finish. The diagram is self-explanatory. If you start this at the top it is then easy to draw the sheet down, even and taut, towards the bottom. Finish by tucking the sides in under the mattress.

Where there are troubles with incontinence a plastic sheet is placed in the appropriate position. This is covered by the draw sheet which is about six feet long — this length to go across the bed. Width, to fit under the trunks and buttocks of the patient need be only about three feet. If you get its upper end where the lower part of the pillows will cover it this reduces the likelihood of slipping and creasing. One end of the width is tucked under one side of the mattress and the free long end is folded in neat pleats under the other side. This allows reserves of fresh sheeting to be pulled through when required.

Now put in the pillows according to your patient's need. The top sheet comes next, again with care to place it centrally. Over this go one or more blankets, which reach to the top of the patient's chest. As you tuck in the top sheets and the blankets make sure you leave them loose enough for the patient's comfort. Making a small pleat across them at the bottom allows room for the feet. Only the lower ends have 'hospital corners'. Put on the

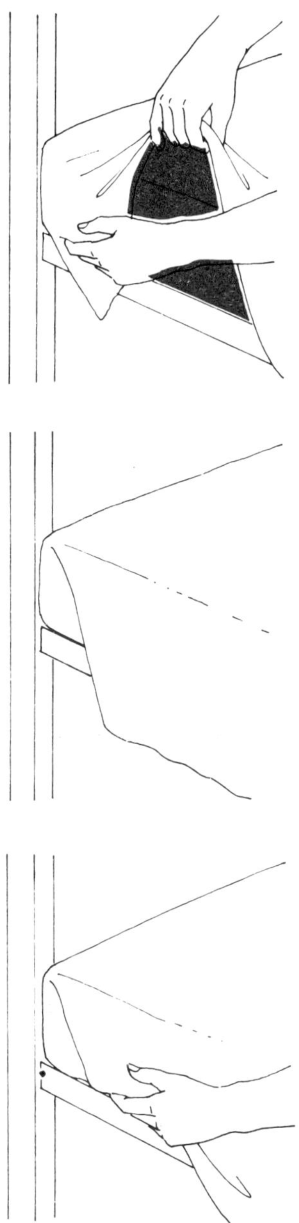

counterpane and fold back the upper ends of the top sheet and blankets over it.

With the Patient in Bed

Let the patient know what you are going to do and, since you are about to uncover him partly, see that the room is warm and close the window. Have a receptacle ready for the soiled linen. Get all the fresh linen on a chair or table near the bed. Have a free chair standing nearby.

Untuck the bedclothes all round from under the mattress. Fold down the counterpane from its top to its bottom. Remove it and put it on the chair. Do the same with the top blanket. Leaving the other blanket to cover the patient remove the top sheet from beneath it. Remove all pillows but one (unless the patient's illness demands that they remain).

Roll the patient to one side and support him there, making sure he keeps covered by the blanket. Where you have a draw sheet you roll him away from the end which will be pulled out. Pull out a fresh area of drawsheet and fold it up towards the patient's back. Now turn the patient to his other side. Pull the new drawsheet surface across the bed and tuck the used part under the mattress. As you handle the drawsheet you clear away any crumbs or other debris and smooth all surfaces. Roll the patient onto his back again.

Put the top sheet back over him and remove the blanket from under it. Tuck in the sheet. Put both blankets over the patient and tuck them in and finish with the counterpane. Finally replace and adjust the pillows.

You can do all this single handed but it is much easier with someone to help you. Do not forget to open the window again.

Bedpan, Urinal and Commode

To those confined to bed the need for bedpans or urinals is a nuisance, but this can be mitigated by a good routine in their use. Do not keep these articles in the bedroom: bring them in from the bathroom when they are wanted. And when the patient asks for one try not to keep him waiting.

It should be brought in dry, slightly warmed and covered with a paper towel or a cloth. Let a man use a urinal in privacy if he can, but if he is too ill for this help by putting it in position. After he has used it take it away at once, again covered, to be emptied in

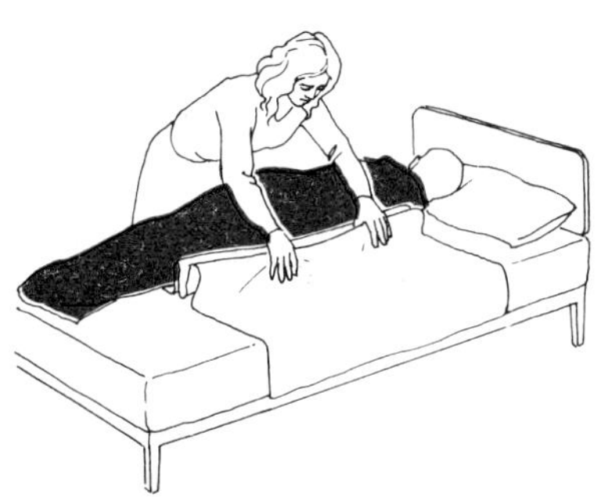

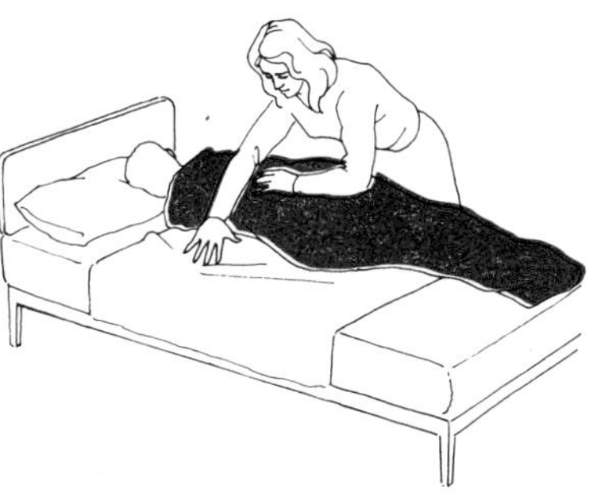

the lavatory. Wash it and leave it inverted to drain and dry out.

The bedpan is rather more troublesome. Begin by making sure the room is warm and, if necessary, the windows closed. Bring sufficient lavatory paper, already torn from the roll. Loosen the top bedclothes and adjust the pyjamas or nightgown. Now stand alongside the bed; help the patient onto the bedpan by putting one arm under the buttocks to lift them slightly, sliding the pan in position with the other hand. Here you may need someone to assist if the patient is heavy or helpless. Unless the patient's condition forbids this leave the room and close the door but remain within calling distance.

After the patient has finished you return to lift him gently off the bedpan, which you carefully place on the floor, covering it again. If the patient can, let him clean himself; otherwise you do this for him, turning him gently to one side. Settle the patient down comfortably; and take the bedpan to the lavatory to empty and wash it.

Now wash your hands and bring the patient soap, water and towel to wash his own hands. Then open the windows.

Urinals and bedpans are on sale at chemists, but they can also be obtained through the social services and from the medical loan depots of the Red Cross. An emergency urinal can be improvised from a large and wide mouthed jar.

For a patient who has to remain long in bed but is able to move or be moved just out of it a commode at the side is the better solution. Most of them have a hinged lid and are shaped like chairs: one can find a design which makes an acceptable and (almost) disguised piece of bedroom furniture.

Bedsores

Any pressure on skin will compress the small local blood vessels; if this is prolonged it severely restricts blood supply and nutrition to that area of the skin, which then becomes devitalised and finally ulcerated.

This abnormal pressure is likely to affect the bedfast who lie or sit on any prominent body area, especially where skin is thinly stretched over bony knobs, as at the base of the back, the hips, the outer edges of ankles, the heels or the elbows. In spite of their name these sores may also appear on people relatively or absolutely immobile in wheel chairs or within plaster casts.

The most vulnerable are the elderly, the frail, the undernourished, the anaemic and those with defective sensation due to nerve injury or disease. Pressure is not the only factor; friction from wrinkled bedsheets or even crumbs will worsen things, and so will moisture from undue perspiration or from incontinence.

The ulcer starts as a red patch, which soon turns blueish; then the skin becomes inelastic and begins to ulcerate. In very bad cases the ulcer deepens to expose underlying fat, muscle and even bone. Once it is established the ulcer is difficult to manage; treatment lies in constant watching and preventative care.

Begin with the patient's diet, which should have adequate protein from meat, cheese or vegetables. Though applying skin lotions and powders has its advocates scrupulous attention to cleanliness and dryness is more important.

Encourage the patient to be as active in bed as is in his power. When he has little or no movement change his position every couple of hours.

From his back turn him regularly onto one or other side, banking soft pillows behind him to keep him comfortable there. If necessary put soft pads under the elbows, or small and soft towels, rolled up, as supports to the lower legs to hold heels or ankles off contact with the bed.

Have the bedsheets smooth and taut. Sheepskin directly under the patient is valuable, for it absorbs moisture and reduces friction. Mattresses or cushions made up of different segments containing air or water are often used for the immobile invalid; some are made to be worked by pumps, so that pressure in (and therefore on) each segment is always altering.

Bedwetting

Incontinence (p.141) is inability to control bowel or bladder action. *Enuresis* is the medical word for the involuntary passing of urine. It can be diurnal ('by day') or nocturnal ('at night'). Bladder control is normally established by the age of two or three, at least by day. Most children are dry by night as well when they are four — or younger.

Parents of bedwetters can be comforted by the fact that between five and ten out of every hundred older children have been bedwetters at some time or other. It troubles boys more often than girls.

Enuresis can be present as persisting 'wetness' since infancy or it may appear suddenly some time after the child has learnt to be 'dry'. There are many possible causes: mental retardation, inadequate training, chronic illness, troubles affecting the nerve supply to the bladder, illnesses (including infections) of the kidney, bladder or genitals. However, all these put together form a quite small minority compared to the most common cause, the child's reaction to some psychological stress.

Yet bedwetting is not a mark of serious mental disturbance: the stress can be a simple affair of childish anxiety about something at school or at home. A quite natural jealousy of the newly born younger brother or sister can lead a child to seek attention by reverting, unconsciously, to babyhood behaviour.

If the doctor is asked to help he may routinely examine the child and the urine for abnormalities; generally he will find none. The doctor's task, and indeed the parents' too, is to approach the child with sympathy and confidence, intimating cooperation towards solving a nuisance problem. The child will be encouraged to hear that as he grows and develops, so will his bladder control. Parents will never punish or blame the child; on the other hand they will always praise him for successes. Some advocate putting coloured stars on a calendar for every dry night; others wonder whether this might not in itself cause a little stress to the child, apprehensive of failure and an unmarked calendar space. They make no palaver of any 'accident' at night but quickly put an impermeable cover over the sheet and give the child dry clothes.

It can be an error to restrict evening drinks severely. A concentrated urine may be as irritating as a large quantity in the bladder.

At night how is the bedroom? Can the child manage on his own? Has he a light switch or electric torch to hand? If he is afraid of the semi-dark, is he allowed to call? Is a pot available or is the route to the toilet easy?

It is a good plan once the child has

been put to bed to let him be awake, reading quietly, for about half an hour. During that time the change in position to the horizontal stimulates the kidney to excrete a great deal of fluid down to the bladder. Then the child gets up, passes urine, and goes back to bed, this time to sleep. Later when the parents retire they may wake him to let him empty his bladder again. It is a mistake for parents to 'lift' and hold him, like a relaxed dormouse, on the toilet or pot; this only deepens the habit of passing urine in a sleepy condition. He must waken thoroughly and not be held.

Parents present all the manoeuvres to the child as ways to help him, rather than as methods of saving them trouble and extra laundry.

By day the child can deliberately 'exercise', not only achieving a sense of control but also naturally increasing the volume of the bladder. He learns to go the toilet not at first feel of bladder pressure, but only when it has become absolutely necessary, when he can wait no longer. Or he can do it by timing. He goes to the toilet every hour in the day and then gradually extends the interval day by day by 15 minutes until it is three hours or more. Another exercise is to stop the stream after he has begun to pass the water, then count ten slowly, before resuming.

Can the doctor prescribe medicines? He may decide that preparations which decrease tension of the bladder wall and increase that of the muscles controlling the bladder exit could help. Also available is the alarm bell, a gadget which rings out loud as soon as the bedclothes become wet, so rousing the child, who then goes to the toilet. This reminds one of closing the stable door after the horse has bolted, yet by association of mind and body sensation it may train the child to wake before the tense bladder has begun to empty.

Bee Stings *see* Insect Stings

Birthmarks

For our purposes the birthmark is either a *mole* or an *angioma*. An angioma is an overexuberant development of skin blood vessels. Generally it is found about the neck and face, though it can appear anywhere on the body. It may be present at birth or develop shortly after. The simplest is the flat, pinkish red or purple 'port wine stain', which does not enlarge, except in proportion to the growth of the child. Since it will not clear spontaneously some doctors advise treatment by measures like diathermy (controlled use of high frequency electricity), but many consider that only a masking cosmetic preparation is appropriate.

The bright red 'strawberry mark' on the other hand is raised from the skin, and may increase in spread. For the majority of cases treatment consists of masterly inactivity under medical observation since it usually regresses to disappear before the child is five years old, leaving only faint scarring of slightly wrinkled skin. Sometimes more definite action for its removal by a specialist is needed when it develops near a structure which matters, such as the eye; scarring then might be a little more marked. Surgical or other treatment could also be necessary for the bigger angioma known as the 'cavernous' type, made up of larger blood vessels. This one is unlikely to clear on its own, and also can cause a problem by bleeding heavily after injury.

Moles are brownish and raised, made up of cells carrying skin pigments. Almost everyone has a few quite small moles on the body. The ones which are large and ugly, especially those which bear hairs, merit removal by a specialist, who probably will advise waiting for this until the child is of school going age.

Ordinary moles are quite harmless. However — and this concerns adults more than children — they have been known to become malignant, that is to develop into a cancer-like tumour. This is rare but any mole which changes its character by becoming darker, or bigger, by changing colour or texture, by bleeding or ulcerating, by becoming inflamed or painful, should be reported at once to a doctor.

Bites *see also* Snakebite

In the domestic scene bites from animals are generally unexpected, from hitherto amenable and loved pets. The victims very often are small children, and the cheek area is usually the attacking animal's target.

Do not let a child get in the habit of embracing or bending down to play with the pet. This can be done without necessarily inculcating unreasonable fear of animals. The child will accept your suitably worded explanation that a dog can be frightened by sudden close movement, that it can misinterpret a quick approach as a threat to its territory. In any case pets do not interpret embraces as do humans.

If a dog threatens you, showing its teeth and barking with menace, stay still and keep looking at it fixedly. Throwing stones may make it move off. If it runs to leap at you try to hit it very hard on the nose. If it makes for your throat protect this with the forearm across it, so that it rams into the back of his open jaws. Bring the edge of your other hand across the back of its neck, to act as a lever against which you now force back the dog's head very hard and sharply.

However trivial the bite (or deep scratch) of an animal it carries the risk of severe infection including tetanus (p.203). It must be seen by a doctor.

Black Eye

see Bruises *and* Eye Troubles

Bladder Troubles *see also* Bedwetting *and* Incontinence

The bladder is subject to many troubles as are all tissues. Only some of its more common misadventures can be considered here. It can become infected ('cystitis'), or contain stones. It can suddenly be unable to empty itself (retention of urine). It may develop tumours.

Cystitis

This is an inflammation of the bladder lining, almost always associated with bacterial infection. It is not merely the bladder which is involved, but also the urethra, that is the tube which takes the urine from the bladder to the outside of the body.

The bacteria could spread from inside the body, perhaps from the bowels which normally and healthily carry those bacteria which are the most common bladder infectors. They could reach the bladder in the urine secreted by an infected kidney. But in a very large proportion of cases

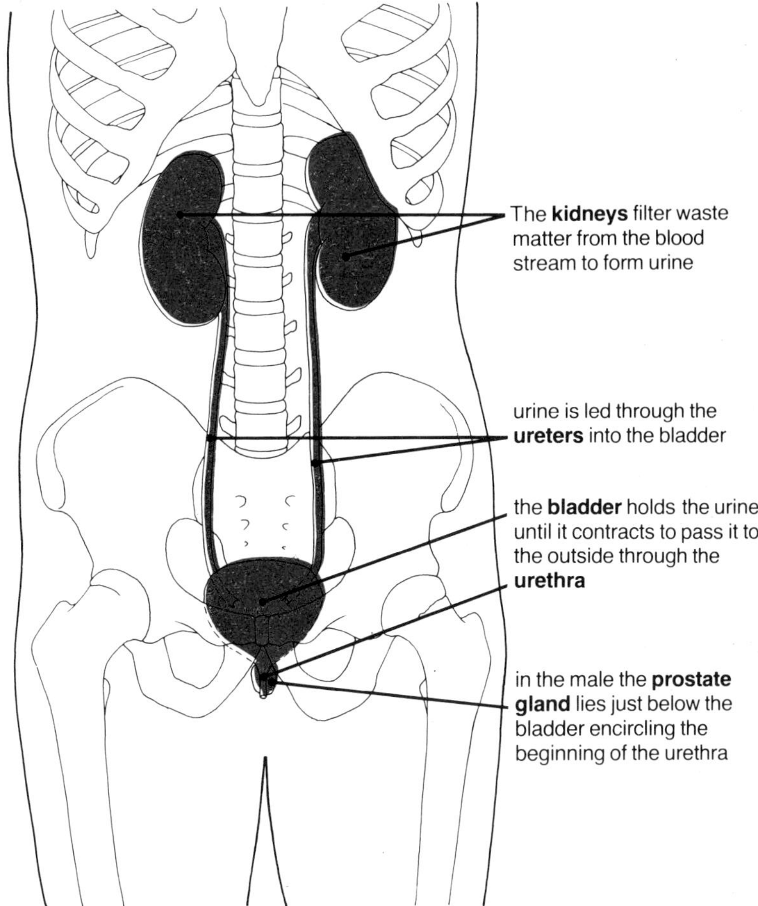

they ascend along the urethra from the germs lying on the skin alongside its opening to the outside.

It is this fact which makes women so much more susceptible to cystitis than men. Not only is the female urethra a very short tube, but also its opening lies close to those of the back passage (the anus) and of the vagina. Any small abnormality, or infection in these parts could be the starting point of germs entering the urethra. Travelling up its moist lining they penetrate the urethral and bladder tissues.

Sexual intercourse may be a cause, especially when it is frequent and, for want of a better word, energetic. A normal feature of intercourse is very mild bruising near the urethral opening. The tissues can cope and repair without trouble, except when subjected to this very often at short intervals. 'Honeymoon' cystitis' is a well recognised condition.

Another possible cause could be an abnormal vaginal discharge such as arises from thrush. The sugar in the urine of a diabetic may play a part. Perhaps a distortion of the urethra from prolapse at the vaginal area could weaken the tissues defences. For some women alcoholic drinks cause congestion around the urethra which might encourage bacterial infection. And one must not overlook carelessness in hygiene as another factor.

The sufferer has to pass urine very frequently. Each time this is extremely painful, and even after it has been completed the bladder still feels raw and full. The urine may appear cloudy and may have a foul odour. Often it is bloodstained.

A woman prone to cystitis can help herself in two ways: by a programme at the onset of an attack and by a routine to try to prevent further attacks.

At the first signs of an attack she begins to drink bland fluids copiously: weak tea, milk, barley water or plain water (coffee, alcohol and strong tea will not do). She manages to get down some four or five pints within three hours. This will include a dose of one teaspoonful of sodium bicarbonate in water, to be repeated three more times at intervals of one hour. (Any patients being treated for kidney or heart conditions should get their doctor's approval before taking the sodium bicarbonate.) If necessary to relieve pain she can also take two tablets of soluble aspirin or of paracetamol at intervals of four to six hours.

In between attacks there are a number of commonsense things to do to keep recurrences at bay. Underwear should be light and nylon avoided as it tends to keep the skin a little too moist and vulnerable. Underwear should be changed once or twice daily, and washed with ordinary soap products, rather than with detergents, and rinsed very thoroughly.

Urine is a good culture medium for any bacteria which reach it, especially if it is stagnant. If she drinks at least six pints a day the bladder will be emptying itself frequently, ridding itself to some extent of bacteria.

After a bowel action she will clean the skin from front to back (never the other way round) using soft toilet paper. She then washes these parts gently with soapy water and dries them with soft dabbing (never rubbing) using discardable tissues. She avoids all vaginal douches or deodorants and locally applied powders; they can irritate the tissues and make them vulnerable.

After intercourse she has a wash, a bath or a shower (this should apply to the male partner as well). And she passes urine as soon as possible.

The doctor may treat cystitis by testing the urine. This test will show the type of bacteria involved and whether it is sensitive to any special antibiotic. Unfortunately it takes a day or two for the test to be completed, so he may use his judgment whether to prescribe the most likely antibiotic while waiting. Other medical precautions could include an examination to make sure there is no abnormality at the vagina or anus.

Though cystitis is a very painful thing, for most people it is generally no more than a wretched nuisance at the time of the attack. However, sometimes the infection can spread up from the bladder to the kidneys, and cause serious trouble there. Any single attack of cystitis merits a medical consultation; a series of recurrent attacks demands it.

Bladder Stones

The stones form in the kidneys and find their way down into the bladder. They have to be very small to do this without being noticed. Any stone which gets jammed at the kidney or in a ureter causes intense colicky pain. It may then free itself and move on. Once in the bladder it can be irritating, causing pain and frequent urination, sometimes with blood. It can predispose to infection and can create yet worse pain if it reaches and gets caught in the urethra.

Some large stones, of course, never do this journey: they remain in the kidney to give trouble there. The kidney is a filtering apparatus, with sophisticated selectivity, so it is understandable that abnormal chemical twists in body chemistry might give the urine excess of some substance, which then comes out of solution as a minute solid particle. The stone then builds up gradually around the particle and grows in size.

Another factor which can lead to stone formation is infection in the kidney. Rarely the urine becomes so concentrated that its chemicals can come out of solution: this is likely to happen in a very hot climate to the unwary resident who sweats heavily and drinks little. Very long immobilisation in bed is known to make the bones less dense, releasing calcium into the blood circulation, to pass into the urine and give stones of calcium salts.

In a large number of cases the services of a specialist are needed to remove the stone, which is too big to go through the urethra. He uses a cystoscope to examine it as it lies in the bladder; this is a tube-like optical instrument with a light, able to be passed through the urethra. It can combine gadgets for catching and also crushing the stone. When this methods does not work an operation is needed to reach into the bladder.

Contrary to optimistic beliefs by patients there is no satisfactory way of dissolving stones. To be sure, those made of a material called cystine will dissolve if medicines are taken to make the urine persistently alkaline, but this type is quite rare.

Retention of Urine

This is the inability to pass urine properly. The stream is slow, hesitant and may even stop entirely in spite of all the patient's efforts. Perhaps the nerve control of relaxation and contraction may be deficient. Perhaps a stone or even a large blood clot has blocked the urethra. Perhaps the inside of the urethra has become scarred and narrowed. Perhaps a large cyst or tumour in that region is pressing on the urethra. The most likely cause by far is enlargement of the prostate which is described on p.174. Any difficulty in passing urine should be reported to the doctor.

Tumours of the Bladder

Warts can grow from the lining of the bladder. Generally they are thin outgrowths, but they can occur in clusters. Trouble arises when they bleed and in treatment the surgeon 'burns' them away (painlessly) using a cystoscope. Even then they need close watching and checking at regular intervals for sometimes they change their benign nature to become cancerous and need immediate further treatment.

Blood in the Urine

If you notice this let your doctor know at once. *See Blood in Wrong Places.*

The Blanket Bath
alias The Bed Bath

You will need a couple of large towels or thin blankets, two smaller towels, nailbrush and soap, talcum powder, warm water (at about 40°C) in a basin and a jug of hotter water to replenish it as you work. Also needed are two face flannels of individual colour or design, for one of them will be used not for the face but for the body. Finally you will have ready a change of clean, warm nightwear. If there is no washbasin in the room have a pail into which to pour used water. Also make sure that the room is warm and the windows are closed.

Begin by taking away the top bedclothes and replacing them with one of the blankets (or larger towels). The second one you roll under the patient.

First wash the face, the ears and the neck with the face flannel, and dry them. Use firm movements rather than small dabbing ones. Each arm in turn is brought over the blanket and washed and dried, with good sweeping movements from the armpit down to the fingers. The hand can be made to lie in the basin of water placed on the bed or placed on a chair alongside it.

Now fold the cover of the patient down to his groin level and wash and dry his chest and abdomen. Pay special attention to the navel. Then cover him again and wash the legs. Take care to dry well between the toes. The genital area and groins come next, and often the patient can do this for himself, and prefers to.

Then roll him over to one side (towards you if there is any risk of his falling out of bed). Wash and dry all of the back and buttocks.

Throughout this as the water in the basin gets dirty, renew it. Whenever the patient's state allows let him wash the different parts for himself. Finish off with talcum powder if he wishes.

Put the clean nightwear on him, remove the blankets or large towels and make up the bed. Tidy away all the materials and open the windows.

Bleeding

The everyday mild bleeding of minor accidents generally stops if the injury is treated as a wound (p.220), but the severe case, with blood pouring out dangerously, is another matter. Here we apply pressure not only to hold back the flow, but also in the hope that this will allow a clot to form.

In an emergency do not delay by looking for a cloth pad; the most immediate equipment is your own hand. Where seconds count do not stop to wash; the patient's body has a limited amount of blood. (See illustration above right.)

1. Immediately either pinch the edges of the wound tightly together with fingers and thumb or press hard down with the palm of the hand. *You must maintain this pressure all the time until you have been able to replace it by the padding and bandage described below.* If you have no one to help this means that for the time being you are left with but one hand to work with. Generally it is not safe to ask the patient to apply the pressure himself; he is not feeling very forceful. Sit the patient or lie him down. If a limb is involved keep it raised, as this helps to reduce the blood flow in it.

2. Find a firm thick pad of gauze or cloth (handkerchief, small towel, scarf, sock) and slip it under your pressing hand.

3. Apply a bandage to take over the pressure of your hand. You must apply this really firmly, and finish by

1

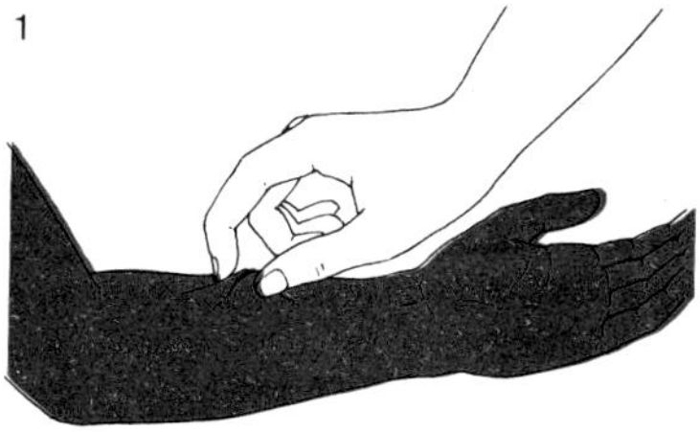

2

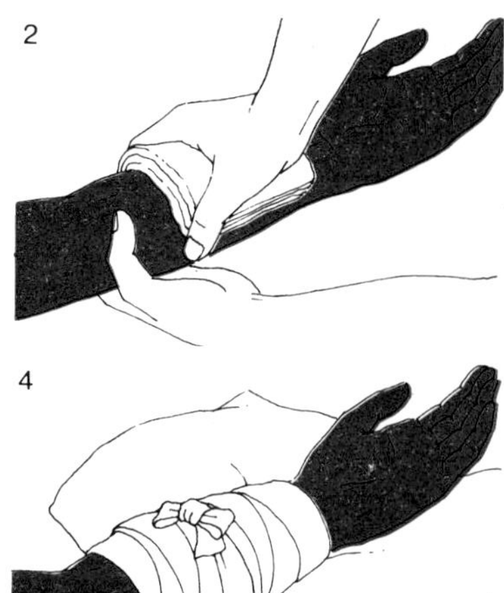

3

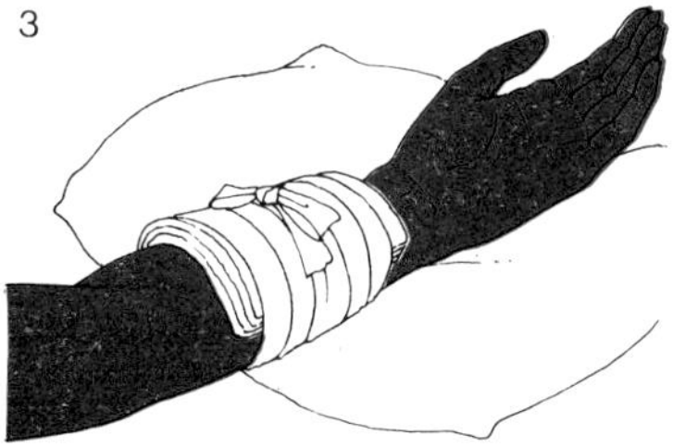

4

BLEEDING FROM A CUT PALM

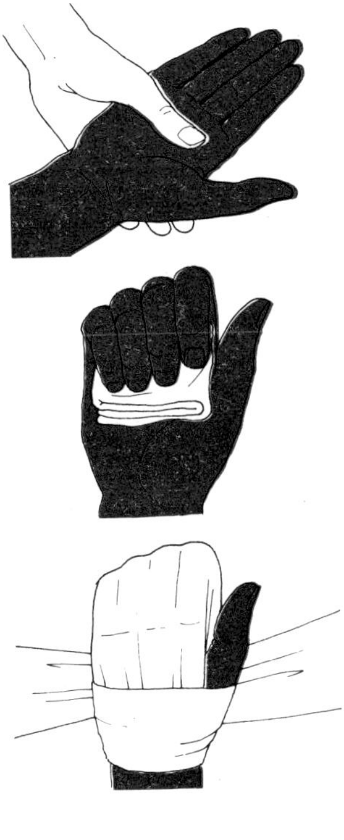

tying the knot onto the pad, where it overlies the bleeding point. (If necessary improvise from a necktie, belt, stocking or scarf.)
Send for medical help or an ambulance and in the meantime use measures against shock (p. 183).

4. Keep watch on the pad and bandage. If blood oozes through do not take them off, but apply another pad and firm bandage over the original ones.

You will note that tourniquets on limbs are not used: they are not only often inefficient, but also can damage underlying tissues. Furthermore they cut off the blood supply not just to the bleeding point but also to the whole limb beyond it.

Bleeding from a Cut Palm

At once seize the hand with your thumb pressing on the cut. Raise the arm. Put on a thick pad and get the patient to clench his fist over it. The whole hand is now bandaged in that position, keeping the thumb free. In this case the knot is tied at the wrist.

Nosebleeding

This nuisance can start after a 'cold' with inflammation of the lining of the nose. Often it may happen to people with slightly hardened blood vessels and raised blood pressure.

Forget anything you may have heard about ice applications, biting corks, pressure on the bridge of the nose, cold objects down the neck, gauze packs to the nostril, or sniffing up fluids. Fortunately the little blood vessel which may burst lies inside the lower and softer part of the nose. Get the patient to pinch the whole of this part firmly between finger and thumb: he must not let go for at least ten minutes. If that is not effective another ten minutes generally succeeds. Urge the patient not to sniff or blow his nose, which might dislodge the clot that has formed.

Make him comfortable for this, sitting up with the elbow on a table. The affair may be messy and a towel as bib is worth while. As some blood tends to trickle into the back of the throat it is sensible to give him a basin to spit into. A very hot room increases congestion of vessels in the nose, so opening a window may help.

Anyone who has repeated nose bleeds should consult his doctor, who may wish to check his blood pressure. In some cases he may even advise cauterising the affected blood vessel; this extremely simple, painless, manoeuvre seals it off and prevents recurrences.

Bleeding from the nose or from the ear which follows a hard blow to the head (not necessarily to the nose) may be a warning of a severe head injury (p. 129).

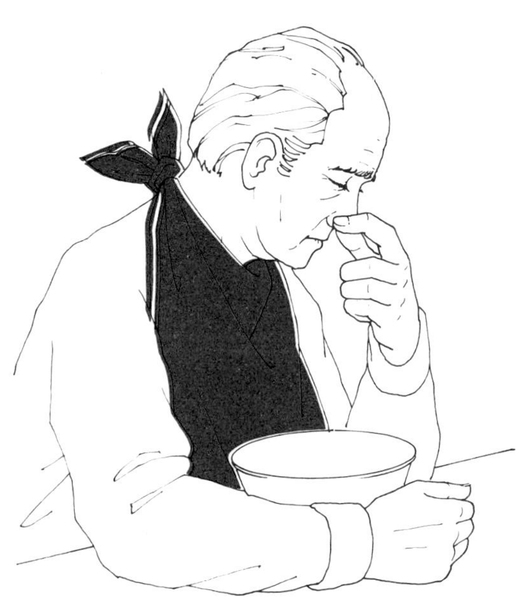

Bleeding Tooth Socket

A tooth socket may bleed severely a few hours after a tooth has been extracted. Sit the patient at a table, with bib and basin (as for nose-bleeding) and let him bite hard onto a thick pad made from gauze or cloth (e.g. handkerchief). This pad should bridge over the socket and not be plugged into it. As he bites he can help by pressing upwards with a hand cupped under the chin, the elbow on the table. This pressing is kept up for at least ten minutes. He must avoid mouth rinsing, which could dislodge the clot.

Watch the pad: let it be big enough to stick out of the patient's mouth; he might unwarily aspirate a small one into the back of his throat.

Blisters

Whenever possible leave a blister alone. It contains plasma, the clear liquid of the blood, which has exuded under the skin from the blood vessels in the area. Tucked within its cover the fluid will generally be safe enough and will in time be absorbed. Cover it with a gentle protective dressing and let time look after it.

Often, however, this is grossly unpractical advice to follow. Blisters form on burns (p.61) or where there has been strong or repeated friction, as on palms after sliding down a long rope or on feet after much walking in unwisely chosen shoes. Then the sheer mechanical presence of the blister interferes with daily living. It becomes necessary to empty it.

Ideally this should be done by a doctor or nurse, but you can get away with it if you are careful. The point is to avoid getting the area infected once its skin cover has been disturbed. Boil a long needle in a small saucepan of water for ten minutes. Meanwhile wash your hands. Then gently but thoroughly clean the blister and surrounding skin with antiseptic (p.19) or soap and water, using clean material. Pour away the water from the saucepan, leaving the needle inside; let it cool. Hold the needle by its blunt end only and do not let the sharp end touch anything but the cleaned blister. Puncture this blister at its base at two diametrically opposite points. Press the material over it to squeeze the fluid out and mop it away. Put a clean dry dressing over the blister.

This will not work well if the blister is several days old, for by then the contents will have become jelly-like.

Blood in Wrong Places

Apart from the phenomenon of normal menstruation the only right place for blood is in the heart and blood vessels. Any blood coming at an unexpected time or from an unexpected place raises a question mark which demands an answer. The cause may be trivial or it may be serious. Let the doctor find out.

Menstruation is a nuisance women have to accept but otherwise it generally gives no trouble. However, heavy periods can cause anaemia. Losses which arise out of normal rhythm or beyond the change of life, when the periods have stopped, could be due to a quirk of hormone activity. They also could be due to tumours. Any bleeding during pregnancy might be fortuitous; it could also indicate a threat of miscarriage. If from a nipple there is a bloodstained discharge this is likely to be due to a small warty formation in one of the milk ducts. But one must make certain the rarer cause of an early breast cancer is not the factor.

Blood in the urine has many possible causes and is always abnormal. Anywhere in the urinary system from kidney to the urethra (see illustration on p.43) infection, tumours or stones can cause bleeding. Blood from the back passage or mixed with the stools is commonly from haemorrhoids (p.127); it may also be due to inflammation or to a tumour of the lowest part of the bowels.

Subjected to the action of digestive juices blood alters its colour to black. Therefore the vomiting of black material or the passing of black stools is a danger signal. Iron medicines can also blacken the stools, but even if the patient is in fact taking iron he should still have a medical check to make sure this is the explanation in his case.

Blood coughed up, even as a few small spots, is another matter for checking. Perhaps the strain of coughing broke a few blood vessels in the upper part of the breathing passages. Perhaps an ulcer or a tumour is present. One must find out.

Anxiety felt from these appearances of blood may keep patients from the consulting room just at the time when they should be getting medical advice. Let them realise that in the majority of cases the causes are not severe and that when they are the sooner they are discovered and treated the brighter the outlook.

Nose bleeding often raises a question. In the elderly especially it could possibly be related to raised blood pressure. One should find out.

Areas of dark bruising under the skin for no obvious reason may be mischance. Sometimes however they indicate an abnormality of blood vessels or of blood cells, and simple tests will give the answer.

Blood Poisoning

Blood is sterile in health and free of bacteria, but constantly it is open to attack from the germs which surround us and which lie on our skin. What happens if bacteria do try to invade, say from an infected wound or from an abscess? Sometimes such an invasion can follow a simple manoeuvre like the extraction of a tooth. Bacteria which gain entry into the blood stream meet a strongly opposing set of defences. They are in hostile territory. The liquid part of the blood (plasma) holds a number of chemicals which make life and multiplication of the bacteria difficult. Also certain forms of the white blood cells counter attack. Some will surround, engulf and kill the bacteria. Others produce chemicals which destroy them. The presence of microbes in the blood is called bacteraemia, and in this battle the defenders are generally victorious. The invasion has failed.

However if the attack is severe, if the microbes are too numerous or too powerful, or if the white cells are deficient in number, then the bacteria overcome the blood's resistance. They multiply rapidly and spread all through the blood stream. Now the condition is that of blood poisoning, medically called septicaemia. If in addition pus or infected clots are formed within the vessels this is known as pyaemia, carrying the risk of abscesses in different parts of the body.

Such a situation is grave, but the advent of antibiotics has very greatly improved the outlook in treatment.

Blood Pressure

We all of us have blood pressure. The

question is how much of it we have.

Consider the hosepipe with which we water the garden. To get a correct and steady flow at the rate we want it we have to adjust the force from the tap according to the width of our hose, to its thickness, to any kinks and to the nozzle at the other end.

The beating heart forces blood through a system of vessels and organs far more complicated than the simple hosepipe. The effect of this forcing is called blood pressure and is dependant not only on muscle strength but also on ease of flow through arteries of varying widths. The steadiness of this force is managed by many inter-connecting controls in the body.

Blood pressure, in terms of the height with which the force would raise a column of mercury, is measured through the simple arm-band gadget used by doctors with its complicated name of sphygmomanometer. It has two values: the 'systolic' represents the force as the heart contracts and the 'diastolic' that as the heart relaxes, dilating before the next contraction. So many factors like age, build, activity and emotion affect these in health that no doctor could be dogmatic as to what is a normal blood pressure. He might quote a systolic of 120 and diastolic of 80 (millimetres of mercury), recordable as 120/80, but he would immediately explain that from individual to individual great variations from these figures are quite within the normal.

A test and reading of blood pressure on a single occasion is of little significance. What the patient had been doing (or thinking) at the time could quite easily alter it temporarily. Checks on different occasions by a qualified person are necessary to reach a meaningful conclusion.

What Causes High Blood Pressure?

The answer is anything but definite. Doctors refer to an abnormally raised blood pressure as 'hypertension' and divide it into two types. 'Primary' (or 'essential') hypertension occurs with no obvious cause. It is the more common type and sometimes is a family matter. In 'secondary' hypertension causes are identifiable: they may be narrowing of arteries, overactivity of part of the adrenal gland or disorders of the kidneys. The kidneys' role in this presents a difficult vicious circle: kidney disease can cause hypertension and hypertension can cause kidney disease.

Other factors can be excess fat in the diet, which affects the thickness of arterial linings, or nicotine from smoking which constricts blood vessels. A sedentary life with little exercise and obesity could add to the trouble. Very rarely a condition producing an increase in blood viscosity will raise the pressure. The oral contraceptive pill may also do this but generally in only a mild way.

Consequences of Hypertension

Hypertension causes the heart to work harder, for example to get blood through narrower vessels. Its muscles enlarge but later, through effort, may degenerate and weaken. Troubles such as angina and heart failure may follow. Kidney disease, as mentioned, could be another consequence. Blood vessels in the retina of the eye may bleed and affect vision. Strokes (p.193) are serious possibilities.

But until these complications or catastrophes happen hypertension gives no specific symptoms. This is why so many examinations by doctors on people who feel quite well include the use of the sphygmomanometer to measure their blood pressure.

Treatment

There are so many links in the causative chain of hypertension that it is not surprising that many types of drugs are used, directed at one or more of these links. The doctor chooses from his tests, his experience and the nature of the patient the most appropriate drug. Treatment is a lifetime affair, with the patient's careful obedience to medical instructions. In addition to medication he will, if he is at all sensible, increase his exercise within the limits medically advised, reduce any overweight, and reject thoughts of smoking.

Blue Baby

The heart can be considered as consisting of two pumps lying side by side, joined to each other. The diagram (a) shows this in an extremely simplified form.

The left hand pump sends blood by arteries to all parts of the body. This blood is bright red, carrying oxygen which is used by tissues for life. Then, darker in colour, the oxygen-depleted blood travels by veins to the right hand pump. This sends it, by other arteries to the lungs to pick up a fresh supply of oxygen. It becomes bright red again and, by other veins moves back to the left hand pump. The cycle is complete and repeats itself with the beats of the pumps.

Rarely there is a developmental defect so that the baby is born with an opening between the two sides of the heart, diagram (b); the contents of the pump mix. This means that not all the oxygen-poor blood manages to reach the lungs. As a consequence what the left pump circulates to the tissues is not fully renewed with an adequate supply of oxygen for the tissues. This is the case of what is often referred to as 'the hole in the heart', but called by doctors 'patent interventricular septum.'

There is another and more complicated possible set of errors in the formation of the heart. It is called Fallot's Tetralogy. Not only is there an

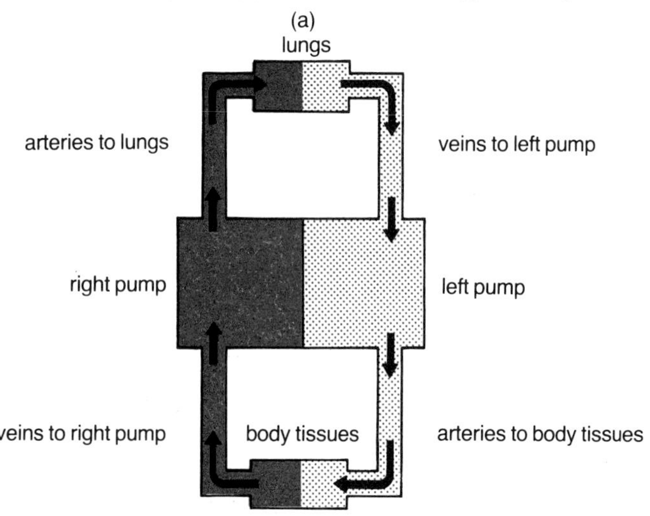

(b)

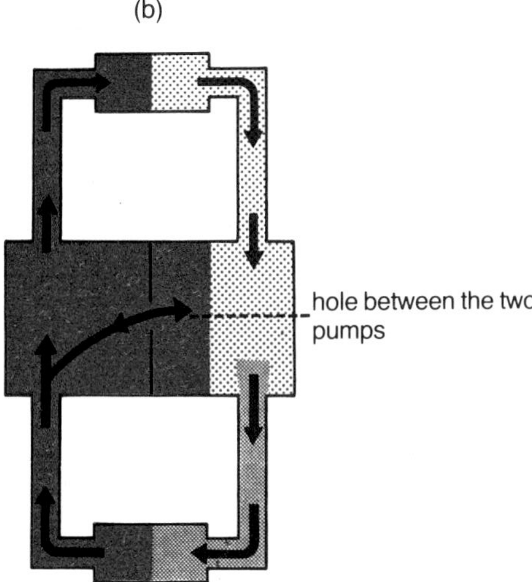

aperture between the two sides of the heart but also the aorta, the first main artery, leaves the heart not from the left but from the right side, diagram (c).

In addition there is a narrowing at the exit of the blood from the right side. It is obviously impossible for the blood to receive a proper supply of oxygen from the lungs and to carry this to the tissues. Another consequence is the thickening of the muscle walls of the right side, a reaction to the stress of

(c)

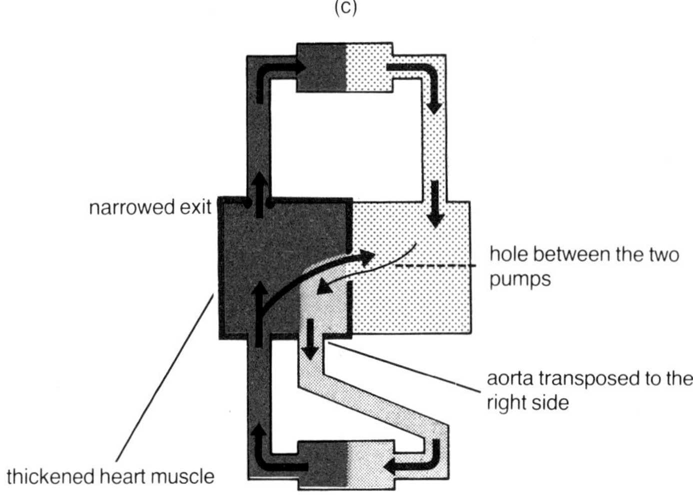

pumping out through a narrow opening.

Babies with such defects may show this at birth or soon after by a blue tinge to the skin and lips, and by breathlessness. These signs may be constantly present or appear during simple efforts like feeding. The child does not thrive well and needs very close care. Feeds should be small and frequent and the very real work of sucking may sometimes have to be relieved by spoon feeding and by early weaning. Any hint of a chest infection or 'cold' merits immediate medical attention lest an antibiotic be needed.

Another possible developmental defect is the persistence of what is known as the ductus arteriosus, diagram (d). Before birth the baby receives its oxygen supply via the placenta from the mother's blood into his blood. At this stage he does not depend on the lungs. Therefore there is a blood vessel which short circuits the lungs, taking blood from the arteries leaving the right pump direct over to the veins about to enter the left pump. At birth this, the ductus arteriosus, closes up and the blood circulates fully through the lungs.

When, rarely, this vessel persists, much of the oxygen-poor blood fails to get through to the lungs and therefore what passes back to the body tissues is oxygen deficient. Some (not all) of these babies also can be 'blue'.

In a system as complex as the heart there can be several other types of congenital deformities. Not all show up by the blue tinge. Not all give serious difficulties. What is encouraging is that in very many cases careful attention with specialist supervision will allow the child to grow old enough to face any necessary corrective heart surgery.

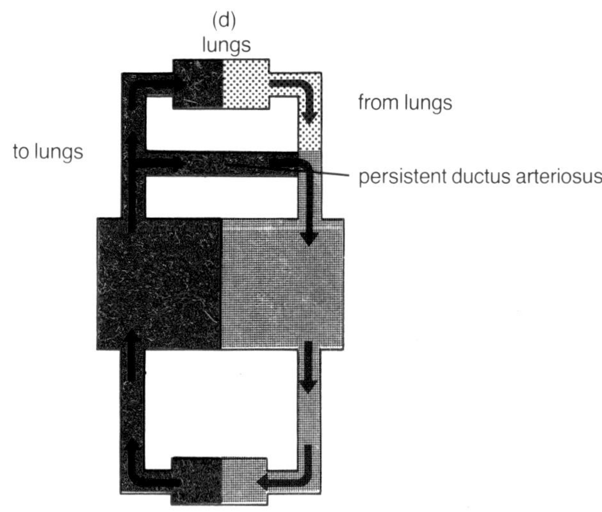

Boils and Carbuncles

Several types of bacteria are normally present on the skin without doing harm, but penetrating deeper through a small crack or abrasion they easily cause a local infection. Sometimes they settle within the depths of the minute ducts which lead to the outside from the skin's hair follicles (recesses from which hairs grow) or sebaceous glands (which produce the natural skin oils). These ducts become blocked, pus forms within and a red spot appears on the skin soon to develop into a little abscess. This is the boil, medically called a furuncle. A carbuncle is larger, caused by spreading infection or from the joining together of several close boils into one big abscess.

These troubles can happen anywhere on the skin: often they appear on the back of the neck, in the lower back or buttocks or by the armpits.

Never, please never, try to pierce or squeeze the abscess yourself. To do so might even create blood poisoning. He who squeezes a boil pushes pus out without realising that at the same time he may be pushing some deeper under the skin to cause worsening damage.

Kept clean and covered many boils will resolve on their own. Otherwise a doctor should be asked to treat. Anybody who gets repeated attacks might question his general skin hygiene or even his general health. Certain conditions, diabetes for instance, can predispose to boils.

Brain Injury *see* Head Injury

Breast Troubles

The size of their breasts is a concern to many women for reasons of appearance and attractiveness, and also as indication of ability to feed their babies. However size is related to the amount of fat in the organ and not to the breast's efficiency as a milk producer. Apparatus and medicaments sold to increase breast size achieve little except the expenditure of money and time. No woman should try them without first consulting her doctor. Medicines or ointments containing hormones could prove harmful. Well fitting brassieres, a good posture and exercise like swimming are certainly the best measures.

Some breasts have a retracted nipple, depressed into the breast surface. This slight maldevelopment is harmless but may make breast feeding difficult. Wearing a special plastic plate within the brassiere during pregnancy is not uncomfortable and may overcome retraction. On the other hand new retraction of a nipple which hitherto had been quite normal could be due to an underlying disease and must be seen by a doctor.

A sore or cracked nipple can be caused by a very vigorous baby at the breast. Here a shaped shield can protect the nipple during feeding. Certain simple applications like zinc and castor oil cream or Friar's Balsam help healing but must be removed before each feed and it is essential to get the doctor's or the midwife's advice.

Infection spreading deep from a nipple, especially if it is cracked, can give mastitis. Part of the breast becomes swollen, flushed, firm and painful and the woman may develop a fever. Fortunately antibiotics are very effective and sometimes their use allows breast feeding to continue if they are begun early enough.

A worse consequence is the breast abscess where the infection forms a pocket of pus deeply. Treatment has to be surgical, with incision to let the pus out, but healing is satisfactory.

A different matter is engorgement of the breasts of a mother who is feeding her baby; here milk production is excessive, the fine tubes to the nipple become blocked and the breasts swell painfully. They are relieved by firm support and by preparations to reduce milk flow.

A breast cyst is a localised lump containing fluid. Until the diagnosis is firmly made it can cause concern lest it be a tumour, therefore it must be seen to at once. Sometimes aspiration of its fluid through a syringe needle is enough to establish its simple nature; sometimes an operation to remove it is needed. A condition known as fibrocystic disease is one which may trouble some women; many cysts form in the breasts which become lumpy and perhaps uncomfortable especially in the days just before a period. Apart from a careful check that no tumour is present no special treatment is needed.

A discharge from the nipple, whether bloodstained or not, demands immediate investigation for it may be caused by a cancer. However, most discharges are due to simple conditions like the one called duct papilloma, consisting of minute warty projections within the milk tubes.

Some tumours like the relatively soft fibro-adenoma are not cancerous but here again careful diagnosis must be made as soon as they are detected.

Cancer of the breast may be suspected by an experienced clinician by the character of the lump but investigations may include X-rays or thermography which shows small temperature variants in different types of normal or abnormal tissues. In very many cases only excision of the lump with immediate microscopic examination will make the diagnosis definite. If the lump proves to be cancer the operation is extended to mastectomy which is removal of the breast. X-ray, hormone and other drug treatment may follow.

The emotional shock to a woman is greatly alleviated by the modern way of full discussion and medical explanation to her and to her husband. Immediately after the operation she will be given exercises to help arm and shoulder movement and she is likely to return home in a few days. A substitute false breast is carefully made to match and feel like the remaining breast. With the support of hospital staff, of her general practitioner and of her family the mastectomy patient is encouraged to return to normal activities including sport.

A rare form of cancer is Paget's Disease of the nipple, where an eczema like rash appears near the nipple and gradually extends over the skin.

In all cases the importance of early treatment for good results must be stressed. This means early diagnosis. And that means sense and speed on the part of the patient.

Self Examination of the Breasts

This is an extremely wise thing for every woman. Though no expert on breast pathology she could detect an abnormality in its early stage, when treatment would have the highest chance of success. If she thinks she finds anything unusual let her report immediately to her doctor. Either he can reassure her (and he will *not* accuse her of hypochondria) or he can initiate investigation at once.

Monthly examination is enough. If you have periods choose the time just after each has ended for the breast is then at its softest and easiest to assess. Otherwise fix a regular date, say the first of each month.

1. Take off all clothing down to the waist. In front of a mirror and in a good light falling evenly from the front examine and compare both breasts, first with the arms down and then with both arms raised. Look for an unusual difference, and unusual shadowing, any puckering or dimpling of the skin or any pulling in of the nipple.

2. Lie on the bed. Place a small pillow under one shoulder and upper back, to tilt your body very slightly; this evens out the tissues of the breast on that side. Using the opposite hand feel with fingers flattened and gently held together (not with the finger tips). Mentally divide the circle of the breast into four quarters. Feel each quarter in turn, moving from the outer edge towards the nipple at the centre. Do this methodically as follows:

With the arm on the side of the breast raised above your head: (a) the inner and upper quarter; (b) the inner and lower quarter.

With the arm on the side of the breast alongside your body: (c) the outer and lower quarter; (d) the outer and upper quarter; (e) this last palpation you continue towards and into the armpit since the breast tissue extends there; (f) then feel the area around the nipple. Now, changing the position of the pillow, repeat the procedure with the other breast.

Breast tissue is nodular, that is mildly irregular in feel. Small lumps you may discover could be no more than this nodularity.

But if you feel anything which raises a doubt, however slight, see your doctor.

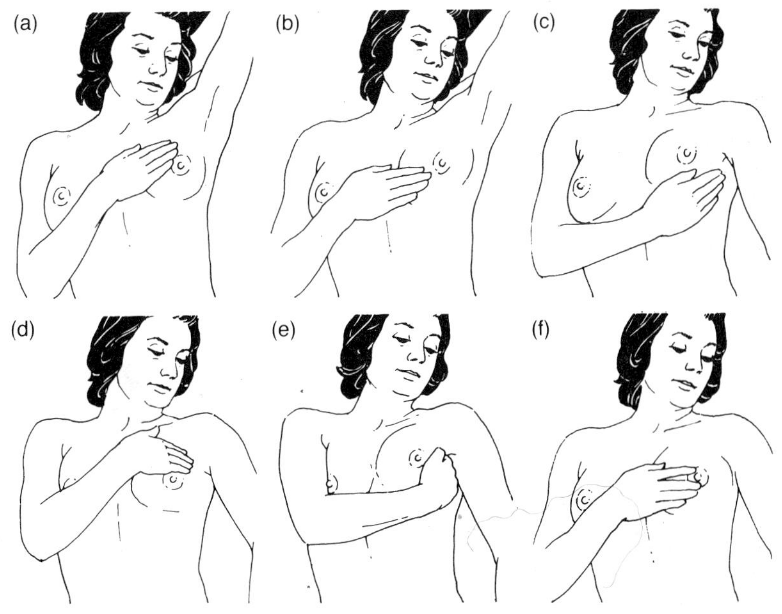

Breath-Holding Attacks

Some parents are victims of a brilliant manoeuvre undertaken by the angry frustrated small child who cannot get his own way. He interrupts his crying to hold his breath. It is almost as if he has worked out that though he is too small, too powerless, to win victory, he can at least either draw concern or provoke anger.

Suddenly he stops breathing. His complexion darkens and goes blue and he gets near to becoming unconscious and falling. To the alarmed adult this appears a dangerous crisis.

The child in fact is quite safe. Automatically his reflexes will take over and he will resume breathing. But by then he may have achieved his purpose of becoming the centre of attentive anxiety. He has created a situation under his control and may use the techinque again and again in the near future.

The parent's countermove is either to ignore the attack completely or to cut it short by subterfuge. Handling the child, scolding him or comforting him will not work. Let the parent act in a way which is quite unrelated to the situation, but surprising or interesting to the child. Let the adult make a sudden move, clap his hands, jump in the air, give a shove to furniture or do anything else that may seem out of place or out of character. Constantly intrigued by the apparently inexplicable world of grown ups the child will stop his trick to assess what is going on and may regain equanimity.

In a short time he will learn that breath holding attacks get him nowhere. Do not think badly of him. We were all rather egocentric at his age.

Bronchitis

In inspiration the chest space increases through the pull of muscles between the ribs and through the windpipe and then through its right and left divisions, the bronchi. These in turn divide into many branching little tubes leading to the final air sacs of the lungs.

Inflammation of the bronchi (bronchitis) can be acute or chronic (see p.10). Infection may reach them as an extension of inflammation of the windpipe.

Acute Bronchitis

The infection is caused mostly by viruses, though bacteria and even some forms of fungus could be responsible. It is an illness in its own right. Sometimes however it forms part of another illness, as with measles or asthma. If the infection spreads deeper down through the smaller air tubes this could lead to pneumonia (p.170).

Simple acute bronchitis presents with a raw feeling behind the breastbone, a cough which starts dry and then in a few days becomes moist with sticky sputum. Temperature may be slightly raised. If there is no complication this all clears in a week or two, though coughing could continue a little longer. Treatment generally aims at easing discomfort, giving rest, warmth, much to drink and something like aspirin. Cough medicines (p.80) may help symptoms but will not in themselves be curative.

Chronic Bronchitis

This is a very sad condition. So often it begins insidiously and slowly worsens to alter the patient's life radically and permanently. So often it could have been avoided if circumstances had been different.

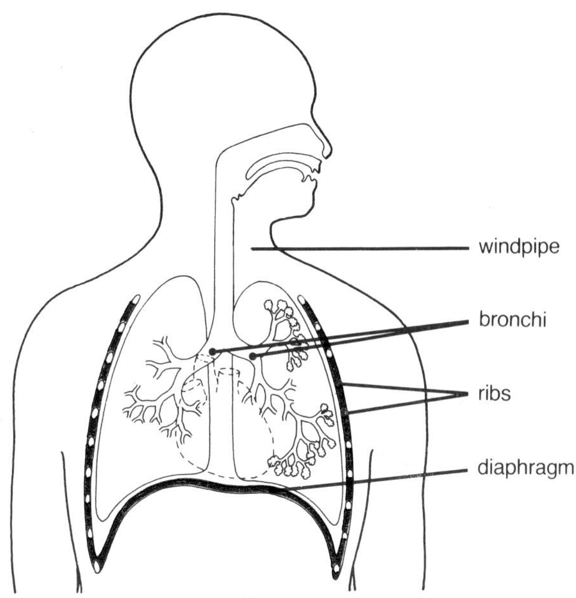

Repeated exposure to damp and dust (certain occupations), to chest infections, to fog and other irritants (smoking!) are major factors. Little by little irreversible changes occur in the lungs. The victim finds himself suffering more and more from attacks of cough with thick sputum, from wheeziness and from breathlessness. It is not easy to pin-point just when someone becomes a chronic bronchitic, but if, looking back over the preceding two or three years, he recognises that for several months each year he has been 'chesty', then he is in danger. The lining membranes of his bronchi could have been greatly damaged.

Very often a state known as *emphysema* is associated with chronic bronchitis. This word means an abnormal accumulation of air in tissues. Emphysema of the lungs is a very special case in which they lose their elasticity and their minute air spaces become greatly distended, reducing their efficiency as breathing apparatus. Comparing the emphysematous lung to a healthy one is rather like comparing a coarse sea sponge to the modern synthetic sponge with its very fine structure of tiny holes. This may be worsened by obstruction of the air tubes with thick secretions.

The patient develops difficulties in breathing in and out, but especially out. His chest may become distended and move poorly. His best ally is the general practitioner who always becomes quite a specialist in chronic bronchitis which is so common in Britain that many have labelled it 'the English disease'. The doctor knows whether to prescribe antibiotics at strategic moments. Drugs to dilate the bronchi may help. In some cases it is worth giving the patient simple exercises to improve the breathing power of his chest; this should be done under medical supervision.

Simple but effective measures can assist. The patient avoids cold or polluted air. His room is warm but ventilated and its air should not be too dry: let him keep a bowl of water in front of the heater. He will get his doctor's advice about correcting overweight. He will report to him any sudden worsening of his state. He avoids infections and seeks his G.P.'s opinion on preventative measures like immunisation against influenza.

Very important advice to the Chronic Bronchitic

If you smoke give it up immediately . . . for ever.

Do not just cut down. Stop it entirely.

ADVICE TO THE CHRONIC BRONCHITIC

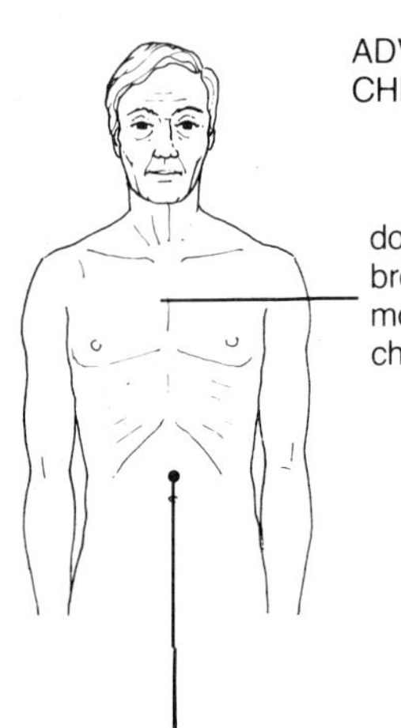

do not consider breathing as moving your chest up here

concentrate on moving the lower part where the bones of the rib cage end as an inverted V

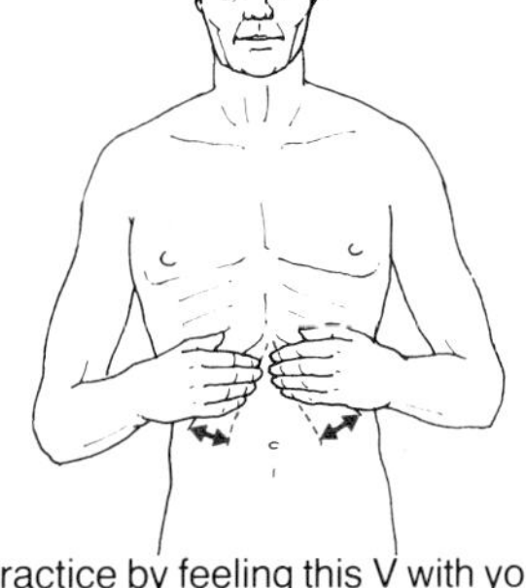

practice by feeling this V with your fingers

breathe deeply to widen it and then for breathing out let all the chest muscles relax to narrow the V

In this way you get the most efficient aeriation of your lungs and the best help from the diaphragm.

Bruises

The bruise is blood which has escaped from ruptured blood vessels and collected just under the skin. The black eye is a good example. Here the blood pigments, through various stages of breakdown, go from blue to green and then to yellow before finally being mopped up by the body's defences and disappearing after some days or weeks.

Sometimes the blood released from the vessels does not stay in their region but, following the law of gravity, tracks down under loose skin, eventually to appear as discolouration at some neighbouring part of the body.

Rarely bruises appear spontaneously without any blow having been noted. Some people, especially women, have unduly fragile small blood vessels which may rupture from a barely noticed pressure. Some illnesses and some drugs can damage certain blood cells. Finally gross and long standing deficiency of vitamin C (very rare in this country) gives the condition of scurvy, accompanied by patches of bleeding and bruising.

First Aid

Most bruises need no treatment, but if an extensive one is likely to form you should put the affected part at rest and apply a cold compress (p.72) which will reduce the amount of blood collecting under the skin. Do this very soon after the injury; it is no use trying it once the bruise has settled.

A really large bruise may accompany a severe injury. As with icebergs, what shows at the surface may be small compared to what is hidden beneath. In bad cases consider the possible risk of shock (p.183).

Another warning concerns the *pattern bruise*. This is the mark left by anything lying against the skin where it received a blow, e.g. belt, strap, buckle or coarse meshed underclothing. If the blow was strong enough to do this it could have been strong enough to tear an internal organ, like lung, kidney or liver. Even though the patient seems well, put him at rest under observation and get medical advice.

Bunions *see* Foot Troubles

Burns

Do not think of the damage done by burns as only to skin surface. It is the heat which penetrates deep into the tissues and stays there which matters. It is this which disrupts the circulation and contributes to severe scarring. Putting out flames and dressing the burns are important, but rapid cooling is essential.

Clothes on Fire

Put the fire out with water if this is immediately available. Otherwise smother the flames with the first thick material handy (rug, towel or even your coat). Cast this, if you can, from head towards feet, to direct the last flames away from the face. Flatten the material down to exclude air. (Do *not* roll the victim round on the floor; this is hard work and dangerous, exposing different zones of his body to the flames before they are extinguished).

Now quickly check the result. Pull away any bits of burnt cloth which still smoulder. (Careful: do not burn yourself; do not start another fire.) Leave in position whatever is stuck to the body: pulling it off may well take skin with it.

For a severe burn get your patient lying down as soon as you can, on the floor if necessary.

Cooling the Burn

Do this at once with ordinary cold water. Tests have shown that ice water is not needed, and in fact may be less helpful.

A small part like a burnt finger tip is held under a running tap. A hand or arm is immersed in a sink or a basin of water. For parts of the body which cannot be immersed (face, chest,

Where burns occur to parts of the body that cannot be immersed, apply thick material soaked in cold water.

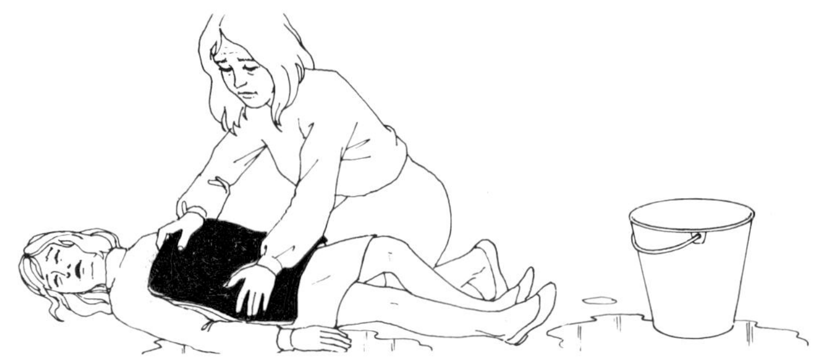

buttocks or abdomen) fold thick material like a towel, soak it in cold water, and apply it so that it generously covers the burnt area. Merely pouring water on the skin is not very effective. What you should *not* do is to immerse a burnt child in a cold bath. Deal only with the part of the body involved.

Keep the cooling going for at least ten minutes. You may find your wet pack so efficient at extracting heat that it gets dry and even warm. If so renew it as necessary. It relieves pain markedly: if pain remains severe continue for second ten minutes.

Even if you come late on the scene, up to half and hour after the accident, you should use the cooling method for the heat is retained under the skin for a long time.

Protecting the Area

A burnt part is likely to swell. Get bangles off a wrist or rings off fingers at once before swelling has them painfully embedded. To some extent the swelling can be reduced by elevating the part, for instance, by resting an arm high on cushions.

Cover the burn with a clean dry dressing (see p.93) and bándage this on lightly. Do *not* try any ointments, sprays or antiseptics.

Shock

This can develop after severe burns, so apply anti-shock measures (p.183). In this case you are allowed to break the 'nothing by mouth' rule by giving a small cupful of sweetened water every ten or fifteen minutes. In severe cases do not delay the patient's receiving hospital treatment by sending for a doctor; call the ambulance.

Chemical Burns

Any harsh chemical is at once washed out, with water. Swamped out might be the better expression. Use tepid and copious streams of water. However do not let the jet be forceful. Wash until no trace of the chemical is likely to remain. As you do this quickly remove contaminated clothes. Then apply a dry dressing.

Chemicals in the eye may be difficult to deal with as the patient in pain will be screwing the lids shut. Tilt his head down towards the injured side,

If chemicals enter the eye, tilt the head down towards the injured side to prevent chemicals spreading to the other eye; gently pour water over the injured eye.

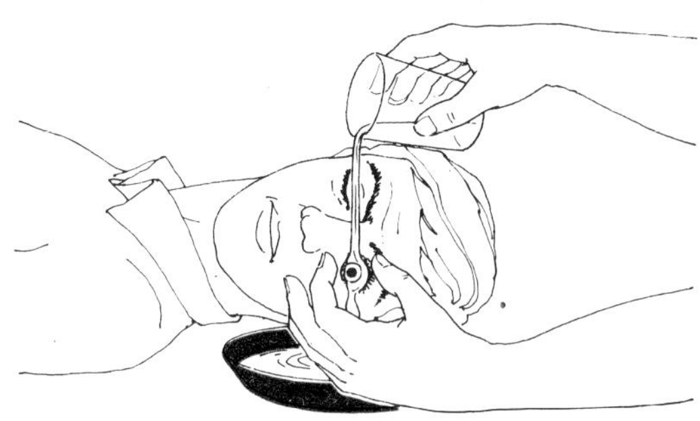

carefully separate the lids and let a stream of water gently over the eye. The position of his head will prevent the water carrying any of the chemical towards the other eye and the rest of his face. Cover the eye largely with a dry pad of gauze or clean linen and get medical advice or send the patient to hospital.

Carbuncles

see Boils and Carbuncles

Cataract

see Eye Troubles

Catarrh

The word catarrh is commonly used to describe a streaming nose, but in medical terminology it defines the inflammation of *any* mucous membrane in the body and the consequent increased discharge of its mucus (note the difference in spelling). A mucous membrane is the delicate lining of any body cavity, including the bowels, the bladder and the air tubes. Mucus is the viscous fluid it normally secretes. Therefore catarrh can apply to all sorts of organs and we are etymologically wrong to restrict it to the nose.

For the nose the right word would be 'rhinitis', and this can be due to allergy (p. 14) or to a viral infection. In allergic cases the discharge is generally copious and watery. With infections very often the viral trouble is secondarily complicated with infection by other bacteria, taking advantage of the membranes' weakened condition. In that case the discharge becomes thick and yellow, and quite often the condition is followed by sinusitis (p. 186).

Nasal infection is a displeasing nuisance, often perpetuated by the sufferer's use of his handkerchief. Kept in the pocket the warm and moist handkerchief makes a breeding ground for bacteria and for continued infection. The proper alternative is paper tissues, each of which is burnt after use.

Cerebral Palsy

see Spastics

Chest Injuries

Breathing is effected by the expansion and contraction of the chest. To expand the chest we use muscles between the ribs and also the large muscular dome called the diaphragm which separates the chest and the abdomen. With this expansion air is drawn into the lungs. Then the muscles relax, the chest narrows and air is breathed out.

Air going into the lungs passes through the windpipe, which divides into two bronchi, one to each lung. They divide many times into smaller and smaller branches, ending up minute tubes leading to microscopic clusters of air sacs. The illustration shows this very diagrammatically.

It is at the air sacs that oxygen in the air passes into the blood stream. Here also the waste matter carbon dioxide, produced all over the body by the use of oxygen for sustaining life, passes out of the blood to be released with the exhaled air.

Any damage giving large bleeding in the lungs will make the patient cough up blood which is bright red and frothy. This is an emergency demanding rapid medical help.

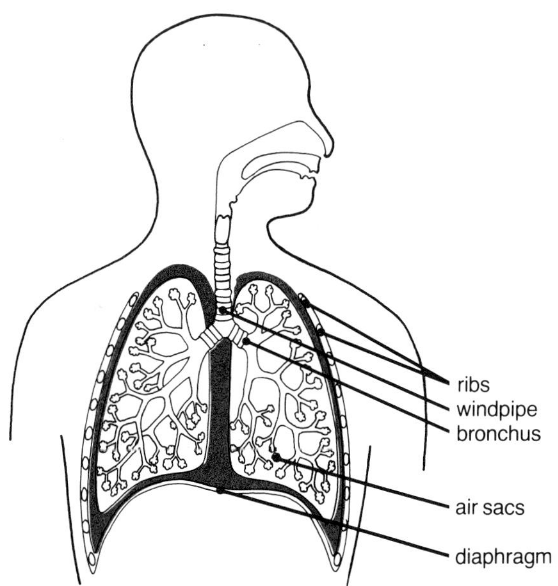

Accidental Injury to the Chest Wall
Something like a knife or a piece of flying glass or metal from an explosion may puncture the chest wall. As the patient expands his chest air is drawn in not only through his mouth and down the windpipe but also through the wound to enter the space between the lung and the chest wall. The wound may bubble as the victim breathes.

When the chest contracts air goes out through the windpipe and mouth. But often at the wound of the chest

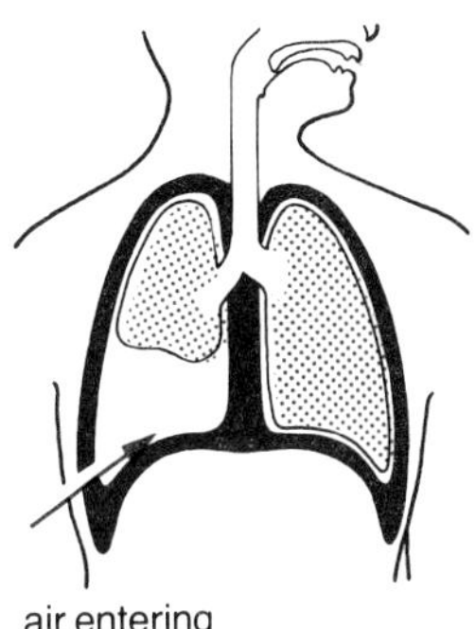
air entering

wall it may be trapped because there the tissues tend to form flaps acting like a valve, allowing the air in but not letting it out. With each full breath more and more air enters the chest cavity of the injured side. Unable to escape it builds up to compress the lung, preventing its functioning.

A severe crushing blow to the chest (as is possible in a car accident which throws the unbelted driver against his steering wheel) can give another type of injury. Several ribs and sometimes the breast bone would be fractured, grossly impairing chest movements, making breathing and the coughing out of blood painful and inefficient.

The blast of an explosion can destroy lung tissues extensively without showing outer injuries, but causing great breathing difficulties and bleeding inside the lung.

First Aid for Chest Injuries

Any patient having difficulty in breathing is easier with his chest upright for this lets him use extra muscles which do not work as well when he is lying flat. You may have to allow him a compromise between the usual lying down position after injury and the sitting position he may seek.

1. Remove any obstruction from the mouth (vomit, teeth, blood).

2. Any open wound of the chest you close immediately with firm but gentle pressure with the palm of your hand. Keep it there while you rapidly improvise a thick pad (handkerchief, towel, article of clothing). Replace your hand with the pad which you secure in position very firmly (bandages, stockings, folded towel) to make as air tight a seal as possible.

3. If you suspect severe fractures at once control that part of the chest with gentle but firm pressure by the flat of

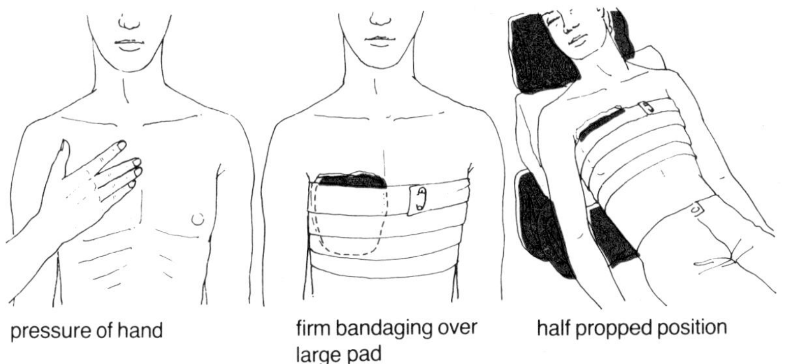
pressure of hand

firm bandaging over large pad

half propped position

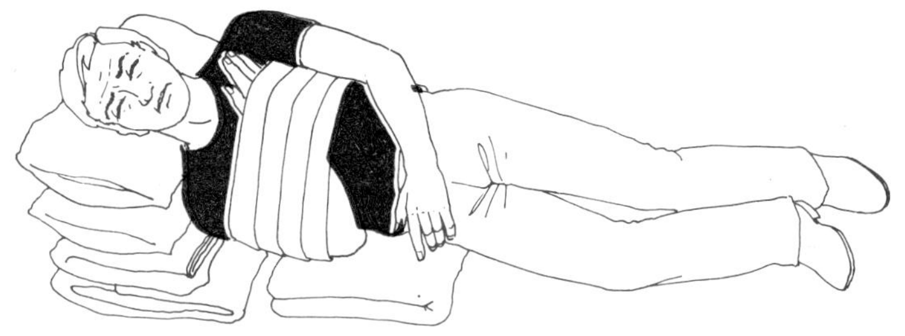

your hand. Then replace your hand by a thick pad and bandage onto the chest. If the injury is at the front use the patient's arm (unless it is injured) to lie across the chest and be incorporated under the bandages as a pressure pad. If the injury is at the back have the patient lie down on this part.

4. Loosen tight clothing.

5. Lie the patient on or towards the injured side. This prevents blood flowing from the windpipe into the uninjured lung.

6. If he is short of breath have him half propped up with head and shoulders raised to help his breathing power.

7. Loosely cover him.

8. Get him urgently to hospital by ambulance.

Chicken Pox

(Medical Name: Varicella)

(see also Fevers of Children)

Chicken pox is spread by close contact. The cause is a virus which is present in the patient for about five days before the rash appears so that he could pass on the infection (via saliva, breathing, close contact) before he is known to be ill. In fact that is the time when he is most infectious. Generally he is only mildly 'out-of-sorts'. The rash is mainly on the trunk and the upper parts of the limbs. Certainly it can be on other areas, including the face, but more thinly. It shows as a number of separate small spots which go through various stages. At first pink and flat, each spot becomes raised and then forms a little watery blister, like a tear drop, sitting on the pink base. The blister crusts over and then the crust falls off leaving a pink mark which soon clears. Often spots can be seen on the roof of the mouth or inside the cheeks.

All the spots do not develop together. They come in crops at a few day's intervals so that once the illness is well established different stages can be seen at the same time. The patient is no longer infectious about six days after the last crop appeared.

Usually he is not very ill and he need not stay long in bed. His chief worry is itching which can be relieved by aspirin or by applications to the skin prescribed by the doctor. Discourage him from scratching and cut his nails short to prevent a superadded infection of the skin from other bacteria. For the same reason keep the skin clean by gentle washing, by loose clean clothes and, if this is at all possible, by avoiding nappies on babies.

Complications of chicken pox

fortunately are quite rare: they include chest infections and, rarer still, inflammation of the brain and spinal cord.

What might be considered a very late complication many years later, is shingles (see p. 182).

Chilblains

These red or purple thickened areas of skin, seen more in children and women than men, are the result of undue contractions of blood vessels exposed to cold. They appear mostly at the extremities, the ears, fingers, heels and toes, creating very unpleasant itching and burning.

Above all do not rub them. Sometimes an easing ointment can be prescribed. There are advocates of various vitamins and minerals as treatment but there is no convincing evidence that these work. In fact most experienced clinicians announce that chilblains are far easier to prevent than to cure. Cure demands patience and the return of a warmer and more even climate.

As to prevention, those who are susceptible should wear warm covering such as gloves, double layers of socks and ear muffs. They should avoid heating themselves in front of a fire, and should recognise that smoking worsens the condition.

Childbirth

When a woman goes so suddenly into fast labour that no expert help is available, the delivery is generally simple and normal. Tell this to the mother for her reassurance.

However, your first task will be to send an urgent message for the doctor, the midwife or the ambulance. And now, waiting hopefully, you will get ready to help with the least interference. Remember it will be the *mother* who delivers the baby. You are there to encourage and control.

Get the mother to bed. Protect the bed with mackintosh sheeting or newspaper under a clean sheet. If the contractions (pains) she feels are strong, if she is straining like someone having a bowel action, do not let her go to the lavatory — this could result in a baby born in the lavatory pan. Let her empty her bladder in a chamber pot; a full bladder may impede delivery.

Wash your hands thoroughly. Boil for at least ten minutes a pair of scissors and four 9 inch long pieces of cotton or linen tape. Let them cool in the covered saucepan. Prepare clean towels for the mother, one thick one for wrapping the baby in, and gauze or cloth pads.

At some point during the labour the bag of membranes holding the fluid within which the baby lies will rupture, with a gush of fluid. This may be quite sudden and alarm the mother; reassure her that this is natural.

Delivering the Baby

When the contractions become strong and are at one to five minute intervals, or when the baby's head begins to show at and bulge the vulva let the mother lie or half sit, comfortably supported. With each contraction the head shows a little more and between contractions it may partially recede. The mother feels a natural desire to bear down with each contraction, using her abdominal muscles to push the baby out. Let her do this, but let her relax and breathe deeply between the contractions.

When the baby's head seems on the point of being pushed out fully you should try to prevent it popping out

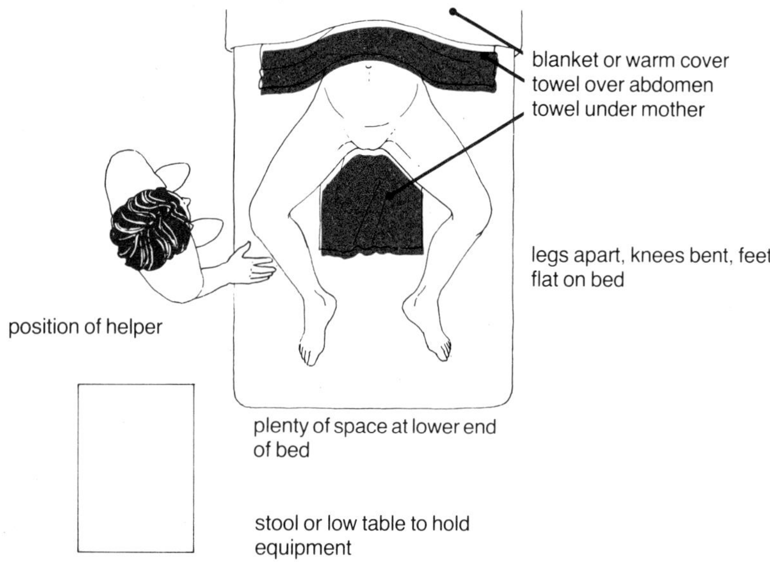

suddenly and forcefully. During the contraction cup the palm and fingers of one hand gently over it, not so much to stop it, as to control it. As this happens, with the head about to distend the vulva widely, ask the mother to stop bearing down and to pant with her mouth open: this helps to reduce the force of her pushing with her muscles. (You may well find that even though it looked certain the head was on the point of emerging it will take two or three more contractions for this to be complete.)

When the baby's head is right out it generally is facing downwards. Now gently with one finger feel round the baby's neck to see if, by mischance, the umbilical cord is wound round it. The cord feels thick and corrugated. If you find it there try to loop it gently over its upper shoulder, or even over its head, so that it does not get in the way and tighten with the next contractions.

Support the baby's head in your hand while you wait for the next contractions to deliver the shoulders. Now the abdomen and hips follow, and you can help by holding the baby firmly under its armpits and lifting (*NOT* pulling!) it out. Hold it now by the legs with its head low, so that any fluid in the mouth drains away. You must hold the baby firmly for he is very slippery.

The umbilical cord is still partly inside the mother, its other end attached to the placenta (afterbirth). It must lie lax; do not pull it taut.

It is normal for the baby to look blue at birth. Use some of the gauze very gently to clear its mouth and nose of mucus and fluid. Soon the baby gasps, breathes and cries and its complexion improves. If it does not do this within two minutes you may have to begin artificial respiration (see p.26), remembering to keep his head low and to give only gentle puffs. When

Support the baby's head in your hand while you wait for the next contractions.

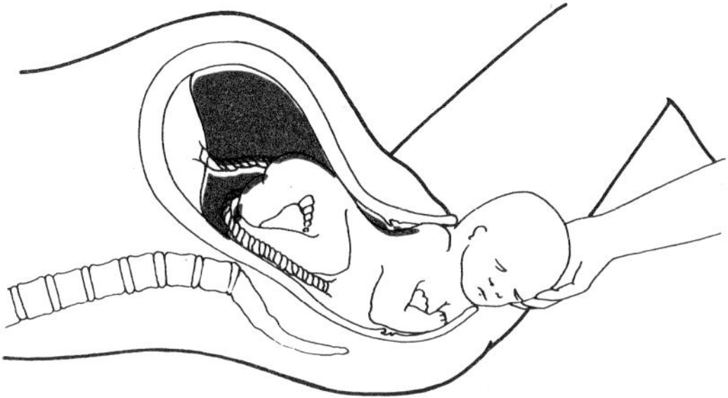

he has begun breathing lie him by his mother, on his side wrapped in the towel, with only the face showing.

Delivering the Placenta

The placenta will usually be delivered within fifteen minutes by further contractions: encourage the mother to bear down with them, to push the placenta out. A little bleeding occurs with this. If there is much bleeding it may be because the uterus is lax and not contracting firmly enough. If this happens (and only if this happens) gently but firmly rub the tip of the uterus, which you can feel through the abdominal wall at about the level of the navel.

In the rare case of blood pouring freely before or after the delivery of the placenta get the mother's head low and her legs raised, keep her covered, apply a sanitary towel and urgently renew your call for medical help. Give the mother the baby to put to the breast; this stimulation of the nipple can help make the uterus contract.

Keep the placenta for inspection by the doctor or midwife.

Coping with the Cord

If you are expecting the doctor or midwife to arrive soon, do not cut the cord. Otherwise some ten minutes after the birth of the baby (whether or

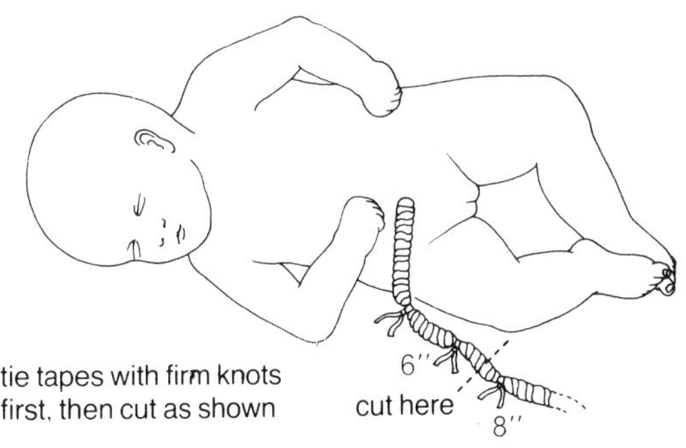

tie tapes with firm knots first, then cut as shown

not the placenta has emerged) tie the three pieces of tape on the cord, taking care *not* to pull it taut. The diagram shows the correct distances from the navel. With the scissors cut between the two further tapes, leaving two on the cord attached to the baby. Cover the cut end with a clean swab. The knots must be firmly made reef knots to avoid blood escaping from the baby. A couple of minutes later check that all is secure; if necessary tie on another tape.

Settling the Mother and Child

Keep the baby wrapped in a towel, and on his side in a warm shielded place; a small clean drawer lined with a towel will do as a cot. Do not add a pillow.

Apply a sanitary towel to the mother. Give her a warm drink and let her rest.

Choking

The airway becomes partly or completely blocked by some object which could be food, aspirated vomit, mud or part of a denture. Immediately the victim begins to cough but if obstruction is complete he cannot do this. The situation is worsened by the way muscles round the windpipe tighten up from irritation and also as a natural reaction to the victim's fright, and so hold the object more firmly. In severe cases he becomes unconscious.

If the victim can still breathe a little and can cough do not interfere. Stand by. The most you do is encourage him to give systematic big heavy coughs rather than a series of small irregular ones.

If obstruction is complete, the victim unable to cough, silent when asked to speak, follow this routine:

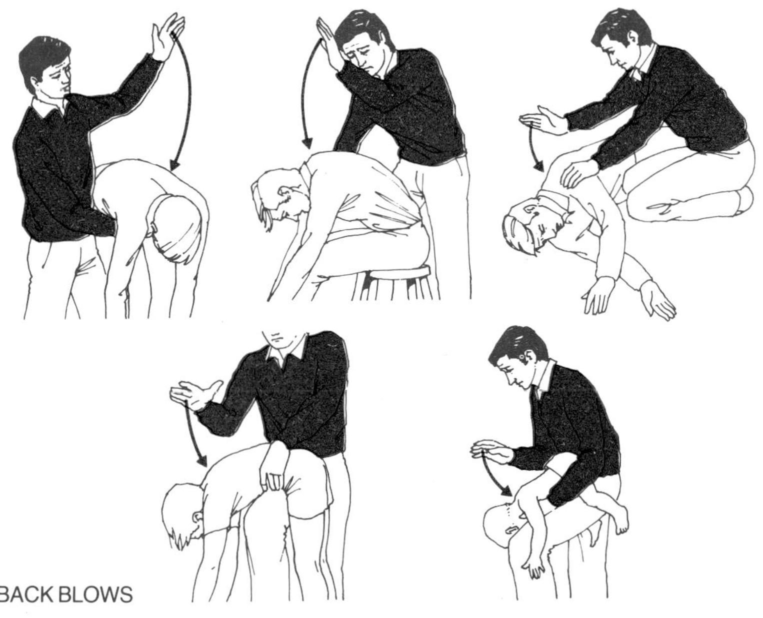

BACK BLOWS

1. *Back blows.* Standing a little behind and to one side of him give four rapid hard sharp blows between his shoulderblades with the heel of your hand. The other hand is on his chest or shoulder giving counter support.

Whatever his position try to have the victims head as low as possible.

Small children you place hanging over your bent knee, or lying over your thigh.

If the back blows fail, at once use:

2. *Abdominal thrusts* which aim to compress air in the chest and propel the blocking object into or even out of the mouth. If it gets into the mouth retrieve it with your fingers.

Stand close behind the victim, encircling him with your arms. Put the thumb end of your closed fist firmly against the soft space just below the lower end of the breastbone and just above the navel. Grasp this fist with your other hand. Give a hard quick upward thrust into the patient's abdomen. Repeat this three times if necessary. If the victim is lying have him on his back. Kneel with a leg on either side of him. Place the heel of one hand in the position between the lower end of the breastbone and the navel. Put the heel of your other hand over the first one. Bend forwards to get your shoulders directly over the hands and give the upward thrust.

A small child you hold with his head low and face upwards, on your forearm (which rests on your slightly forward bent thigh). Give the thrusts with two fingers only.

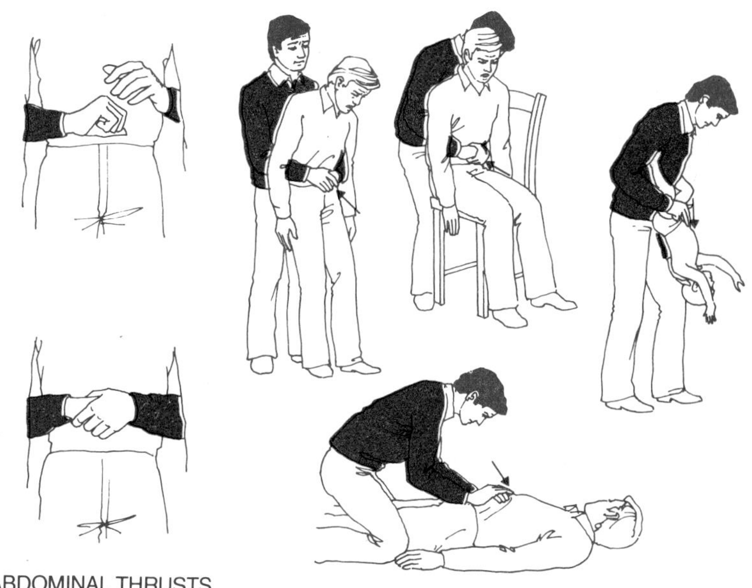

ABDOMINAL THRUSTS

3. If these measures fail repeat the back blows and the abdominal thrusts alternately until you succeed or until the patient becomes unconcious.
4. If the patient becomes unconcious and is not breathing begin artificial respiration at once (p.26). You may find that the air you breathe into the patient bypasses the obstruction to reach his lungs.

If you cannot get the air in then try probing very carefully into the back of the mouth with your finger to see if you can find the obstructing body caught up there. By a sideways hooking and taking great care not to push it in further you may be able to dislodge it and half pull and half push it out of the mouth.

In all cases get a doctor as soon as possible. The victim should be under observation even after apparently good recovery. The abdominal thrusts can rarely cause internal damage, but since the alternative would be death by asphyxia the manoeuvre is justified.

Chronic *see* Acute

Circumcision

Over the last thirty years there has been a big decline in the number of circumcisions (apart from those done for religious reasons). The operation consists of cutting away part of the foreskin, which is rather like a sleeve of thin skin covering the end of the penis. It has been said that about forty years ago one in three boys was circumcised; by now the figure is probably about one in twenty. Why so many then? Why so few now?

It used to be believed that circumcision had the following advantages: better hygiene, reduction of masturbation or of bedwetting in the child; improved sexual function but decreased likelihood of acquiring venereal disease in the man; reduction of cancer of the penis in man and of cancer of the cervix in his wife.

Recent statistical surveys have led to very considerable doubt about these tenets. Thoughtful studies of the role and nature of the foreskin and the consequences of circumcision have strengthened the anti-circumcision school.

Parents and many doctors would get concerned if the baby boy's foreskin could not be easily pushed forward or backward over its site on the penis, but now doctors recognise that the foreskin is naturally adherent to the penis until some time between the ages of nine months and three years. In fact it is usefully protective to the more delicate skin of the tip of the penis which could be exposed to moisture at a time when the child has not fully learnt to control his bladder. Circumcision should be avoided unless it becomes truly necessary for a much more definite medical reason, like abnormal tightening and inflammation of the foreskin around the penis.

Besides, no operation, however slight, is quite free from risk. It seems a great shame to subject a baby to the, admittedly small but still possible, chance of consequent inflammation and infection of the penis. Statistically thc likclihood of harm from circumcision is higher than the conjectural one of leaving the penis as nature designed it.

Cold Compress

Some injuries are helped by the application of cold. First aid to burns (p.61) is an outstanding example. Other cases are sprains and strains (p.192) where muscle or ligament fibres have been wrenched, stretched and torn. The reaction of the injured tissues is to widen their local blood vessels which become partly porous. Some of the liquid blood component, the plasma, oozes out into the area, which becomes swollen. It could be argued that this swelling is buffering and protective under natural circumstances, but in the modern world it becomes a nuisance and is best minimised.

A cold compress immediately, or within about half an hour of the injury, reduces blood flow at the site and so limits the swelling.

Take a piece of lint, flannel or a large handkerchief. Fold it to the size needed and soak it in cold water. Squeeze it out until it stops dripping. Apply it to the injured part. Do not cover it; it has to be held in position using open weave material like gauze. Keep it moist and cool by dripping on water as necessary.

Cold Effects

see also Chilblains *and* Frostbite

The human body adapts itself to varying outside temperatures to maintain its own temperature steady at around 37°C. It achieves this quite successfully by widening or narrowing the skin blood vessels, by shivering or sweating according to circumstances. But there are extremes with which it cannot cope.

Hypothermia

Hypothermia is a term which means little more than low temperature. Usage makes it refer chiefly to circumstances which lead the body gradually to becoming so abnormally cold (well below the register of an ordinary clinical thermometer) that life is in danger. It can happen to someone who is asleep, inadequately covered, in an unheated room when a sharp frost occurs. It might also hit the motorist immobilised for hours in a snowdrift and unable to keep the car warm. Domestic victims are likely to be those of the extremes of age, babies and the elderly, who have less efficient body temperature regulating processes. They are less mobile in sleep and so denied some muscle activity which creates warmth. Babies have a large skin surface, relative to their body volume, from which they can lose heat. Old people often have poor circulation; a reduced activity of glands like the thyroid which keep the body 'stoked up', and many of them are on sedatives which have a side effect of lowering their temperature.

The patient is very cold to touch, even under the bedclothes. His skin is puffy and white or blueish (but in a baby may be rosy). His pulse and breathing are very slow and weak. He is inactive, drowsy, perhaps unconscious. This can dangerously give the illusion that he is merely sleeping soundly.

Always bear hypothermia in mind and if you suspect it:

Keep the patient in bed, in the recovery position as for unconsciousness (p.210).

Allow his temperature to rise *gradually* by placing him between blankets, covering the sides and top of the head, and by warming *the room*. Do *not* warm him directly with hot water bottles or an electric blanket. His system is barely working and a rapid upwards surge of temperature with its call on the blood circulation could prove too sudden a strain on the heart.

If he is conscious and can swallow give warm sweet drinks. NEVER give alcohol.

At once notify your doctor. The condition could be an emergency.

Exposure

Exposure generally happens to members of outdoor expeditions. As they get affected they slow down mentally and physically, see and speak inefficiently, and move with clumsiness. Later they become drowsy and eventually unconscious. Such a collapse is very dangerous. Act as soon as you suspect it is developing:

Stop and rest. Prevent further heat loss. If you cannot get the patient into a warm shelter, use blankets or groundsheets as protection against wind and rain or pitch a tent over him.

If possible replace wet clothes with warm dry cover. Get him into a sleeping bag or wrap bags round him.

If he is conscious give warm sweet drinks. NEVER give alcohol.

Watch carefully in case artificial respiration (see p.26) becomes necessary.

Send for a rescue party. Move the patient by stretcher. Keep him well covered, particularly over his face and mouth.

Get medical help quickly on arrival.

Colds

The common cold is a virus illness. Without one of the very many viruses which can cause it no amount of 'chills', 'damp shoes', 'nasty draughts' or other old wively factors will give one a cold. The preponderance of the disease in winter is due less to the climate than to the way humans pack themselves together in overheated ill-ventilated places during that season.

Incubation is quite short, the sufferer showing symptoms within two days of having caught the virus from one already afflicted. The illness is an inflammation of the lining membranes of the upper respiratory tract, that is of nose, throat, larynx and beginning of the windpipe. It lasts less than a week, with an irratated throat, watery discharge from nose and eyes, cough and headache. Temperature is rarely raised, except in smaller children. These symptoms are not very specific for many more serious diseases, from measles to meningitis, begin in the same way.

Sometimes the cold extends in length and discomfort by the complication of an added 'secondary' infection from bacteria other than the original virus, and the discharges becomes thicker and yellow. This can lead to such conditions as sinusitis, tonsilitis and bronchitis.

As for treatment there is nothing which will cut the illness short. Antibiotics are of no use except to cope with any secondary bacterial infection. It is very anti-social to mix with others since the common cold is highly infectious and easily spread. It is wise to rest indoors, adequately but not heavily clad, perhaps in bed (during the first days at least), in a warm but well ventilated room. Use paper handkerchiefs and burn them quickly afterwards. Some of the discomforts can be eased by cough medicines or by pain relieving tablets, which may also hold a preparation to dry the nose discharge. However this last must not be overdone, as it could reduce the resistance of the inflamed tissues to secondary infections. Diet is simple, with plenty of fluids. The smoker must forego his cigarettes or pipe; in any case he would get no taste or pleasure from them.

Over recent years some have advocated vitamin C (ascorbic acid) as a means of cutting short, or even preventing colds. A few 'cold cure' tablets include the vitamin, but in absurdly small amounts. If ascorbic acid is of any use against colds (and careful tests have repeatedly failed to prove that it is) is should be taken at the very onset of the illness and in extremely large doses. Perhaps the kindest thing to say of the vitamin C fervour is that it does the body no harm and keeps the wheels of commerce turning.

Can one prevent oneself catching colds? Good hygiene, a good mixed diet, good ventilation, good excercise are generally helpful. Extra vitamins and preparations like cod liver oil add no benefit. Vaccines have proved disappointing. They might reduce a little the chance of secondary infections, but they will not stop the cold itself.

Colic

The average dictionary defines colic as severe abdominal pain. This is not the full story. It refers to organs which are sac-like, e.g. gall bladder or stomach, or tube-like, e.g. bowel or ureter, the tube which leads from kidney to bladder. These organs generally register no pain if they are damaged or cut, but they are sensitive to distension. They stretch if they become obstructed and their contents cannot travel on normally. It happens, for instance, if a gall stone jams at the exit of the gall bladder or if a kidney stone blocks the ureter. Then the muscle coats of these organs respond with strong intermittent contractions giving waves of pain which come and go. This is colic. Some inflammations of the bowel can give the same effect.

Colicky pain makes the sufferer writhe about rather than lie still. If severe it certainly needs medical help. Some drugs will ease the muscle contractions, but the cause of the colic has yet to be diagnosed and treated.

The word 'colic' is also used, rather loosely and inaccurately, to describe the many tummy upsets which can bother babies, and make them cry and scream. Some small babies do this regularly in the evenings for a few weeks; the cause is as uncertain as the treatment but medical advice should be sought.

Colostomy

The colon, or large intestine, is the wide part of the bowel, like a big inverted U, which takes the residue of digested food from the small intestine and brings it to the rectum, for evacuation through the anus.

There are certain diseases of the rectum and of the further part of the colon in which treatment demands that the affected part must either be at rest, free from the passage of the stools, or must be removed surgically. Some types of inflammation dictate the rest and some tumours need the excision. When the excision is made it is sometimes possible to join together the remaining ends of the cut bowel. Often however what remains is insufficient for this repair.

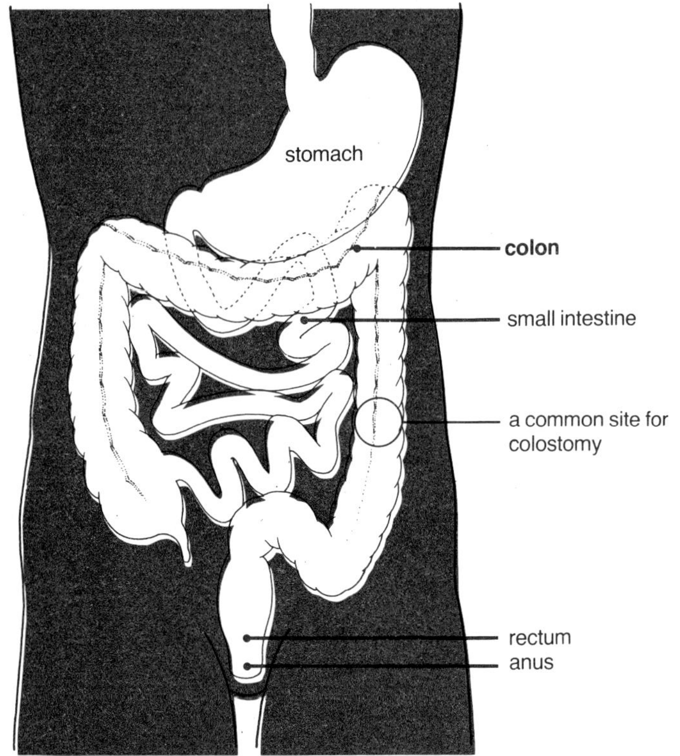

When necessary the surgeon performs a colostomy, which is the construction of an artificial opening of the colon at the abdominal wall to allow the stools to be evacuated without recourse to the rectum and anus. Sometimes this is temporary; if the disease settles down and the anatomical circumstances are right the cut ends of the colon are rejoined and the colostomy opening is closed. In many cases however the patient must keep the colostomy for the rest of his life.

Patients are appalled and embarrassed when they first face this situation. Problems of hygiene, clothing, odour and general management seem to them to be insuperable. The artificial opening is allowed to empty into a bag placed over it. The bag has to be kept firmly against the skin over the colostomy and to be replaced frequently.

Good colostomy management technique has been achieved by many years of surgical and nursing experience. Colostomy bags have been developed to a very high standard of efficiency. After the first weeks when they may believe difficulties will never clear most patients find that the colostomy empties itself with ordered regularity, that the bag can be applied, managed, discarded and renewed easily, and that they may continue with the everyday activities of life. It is safe to say that many of us have met, accompanied, spoken to and perhaps even danced with such people without knowing that they carried a colostomy.

The consistency of the stools, their regularity and the risk of 'accidents' are matters which can usually be controlled by simple measures of diet and medication. Patients find that their medical advisers can help tremendously.

Colour Blindness

see Eye Troubles

Concussion

see Head Injuries

Conjunctivitis

see Eye Troubles

Constipation

The residues from food after digestion which enter the last parts of the bowel are very liquid (see the illustration in the section on Diarrhoea, p.88). As they pass through these parts a great deal of water is absorbed from them so that the stools which reach the rectum (back passage) are semi-solid. If there is any delay in this movement too much water is absorbed and the stools tend to become abnormally hard.

A complete stoppage would be due to some total obstruction of the intestines from pressure of something outside or within them, and this is a serious condition usually attended by pain and vomiting. Partial stoppage has many likely causes and incomplete bowel obstruction is one of them. But when people speak of constipation they generally mean a slowing down of the bowel habit, or a relative difficulty in passing stools. Changes in diet, weakness following diarrhoea, lack of normal activity, pain at the anus from a fissured skin or from piles, hardening of stools not passed at the right time or spasms of the intestines are all possible reasons for bowel action to become less than usual.

But what is 'usual'? There is no absolute answer. The normal can vary from three times a day to once every three days. The notion that one bowel action a day — no more, no less — is a prerequisite for health is erroneous, but survives to worry many people unnecessarily. Normal frequency can vary from person to person and with any given person according to circumstances.

If circumstances occasion a delay, this might be a temporary nuisance but is not likely to be harmful. Distension of the rectum, slight hardening of the stool may provoke a temporary discomfort only. There is no 'poisoning' because the stools contain no poison. There is no problem of 'inner cleanliness' because to the bowel its contents are not unclean.

What is distressing to the bowel is the habit many people have of taking unnecessary laxatives when they fancy they are not being 'regular'. There are many forms of laxatives. Some are quite simply 'mechanical' in action by giving size and softness to the stool. Certain granules for instance depend on water being taken with them. This makes them swell up and the added bulk is a stimulus to bowel movement. Certain salts (e.g. Epsom salts) retain water in the bowel giving a more liquid stool. Liquid paraffin is a lubricant which eases the passage of the stool, but it may occasionally leak from the back passage and also it has a disadvantage of interfering with the absorption of some vitamins. Many laxatives, including cascara, senna and the tasteless preparation presented in mock confectionery, act on the bowel muscle by stimulating it, which is another way of saying that they irritate it.

Repeated use may end up by forming a habit, with the bowel depending on the presence of the laxative in increasing doses and no longer working quite spontaneously. Any laxatives should be taken only on medical advice. The aim would be to administer the smallest dose which gives results and then to try to train the bowel to resume its own responsibility by decreasing the dose very gradually. In this training, if there is true constipation of long standing, it seems wiser to take a quite small amount of the medicine daily, rather than wait for a larger, more explosive dose every few days.

However, there are better ways to counter constipation. Diet is important, seeking roughage in bran, fruit, raw vegetables and salads. Going to the lavatory regularly at the same time builds a habit which will eventually settle in. That the lavatory should be warm, secluded and comfortable is self-evident.

Of all steps in treatment the one most likely to be needed, and to succeed, is increasing one's fluid intake. Many of us just do not drink enough. Quite the best laxative is free, tasteless and accessible. It comes from the kitchen tap.

Doctors teach that any unexplained and sustained change in bowel habit needs medical advice. Such changes in the absence of altered diet or circumstances could result from a diseased condition in the bowel.

Convalescence

Every patient, every illness, and therefore every convalescence, have their individual differences so it is impossible to do more than generalise. But a few ideas can be thought over.

Convalescence is not the gradual lessening or tailing off of an illness. It is the planned return to full strength *after the illness is over.* Therefore it is something consciously active and not the mere passive hanging about in a dressing gown waiting for a set number of days to pass.

Here are some important points to remember (a summary of the teachings of Dr George Day).

1. Undisturbed sleep at night.

2. Plenty of fresh air.

3. Plenty of good food. The patient may have lost weight in his illness or immediately after his operation. He was doing little while lying in bed (even though some valuable exercises may have been prescribed). Once he starts moving and using more energy his nutritional demands increase.

4. Progressive activity with the injunction 'Never do less today than you did yesterday'. Aim at doing half as much again if possible, with an increase in hours up and about, distances walked and self-help until normality is reached.

5. The banishment of anxiety and the restoration of self-confidence. Exhortations by friends and relatives to 'take it easy...no lifting' are counter-productive and will keep the patient in a bottom gear of existence and self doubt. If he asks his doctor for overhaul and explanation the reassurance gained could set him on his way rejoicing.
6. Consultants like to reassure themselves about the end results of their work and add to their knowledge and experience. Patients who are asked to return to a clinic for assessment some weeks after hospital discharge may conclude thay are not yet 'all clear' and must wait before resuming normal living with confidence. Their G.P.s should be able to dispel this delusion.

Needless to say the convalescent must let himself be guided throughout by his family doctor.

Convulsions

see Epilepsy *and* Fits

Corns *see* Foot Troubles

Coronary Thrombosis

see Heart Troubles

Corticosteroids

To set the Scene

Hormones are chemical messengers produced by a number of glands; they flow in the blood stream to act on various parts of the body. On top of each kidney sits an adrenal gland, which secretes a wide range of hormones.

Steroids are a large group of compounds in the body. Corticosteroids is the name given to one set of steroid hormones produced by the adrenals. The name extends also to similar chemicals made synthetically. (This nomenclature is rather complicated as some people use the general word 'steroids' rather loosely when they mean the more specific 'corticosteroids'.)

Of the main corticosteroids made by the adrenals two are hydrocortisone and cortisone. The latter was synthesised by man in 1946 and in about 1950 became prescribable as a drug. These days a large number of similar chemicals of similar action are available; they include prednisone, prednisolone, triamcinolone, dexamethasone and betamethasone — names which appear in many formulae prescribed today.

Actions of Corticosteroids

The actions are wide and have been described as helping the body in stress. In fact high stress in one form or another activates the adrenals to increased secretions of corticosteroids. They regulate the proportions of water and certain salts in the body; they reduce inflammation and mitigate the effects of allergy (p.14). They play a part in coping with carbohydrates; they also have an effect on sexual characteristics.

Uses in Medicine

Corticosteroids can be powerful in easing many severe conditions. They do not cure, but they exercise a valuable (and sometimes life saving) control.

In asthma (p.29) they relax the tightness of the air tubes and decrease the swelling of their lining membranes. Applied as creams and ointments corticosteroids ease many irritating troubles including those caused by nettlerash.

By reducing inflammation they can show dramatic results in illnesses varying from rheumatoid arthritis to some forms of colitis. They can be taken as tablets or given by injections, sometimes directly at inflamed sites like tendons, joints or, for instance, the painful spot of a tennis elbow.

Corticosteroids are also useful in less common conditions like certain forms of leukaemia or to suppress the body's rejection of transplanted tissues and organs.

Their Limitations

With such a field of helpfulness it would seem as if corticosteroids clear a large proportion of medical difficulties. This is not so, for they also carry a big number of problematic side effects. To begin with in large doses their anti-inflammatory action could tone down symptoms and signs of some diseases such as the spread of an infection or the perforation of a stomach ulcer, and make their diagnosis difficult. They reduce the body's reaction to infection, and they interfere with the normal progress of strong scar formation and the healing of wounds.

When taken over a long period they have been known to activate diabetes or stomach ulcers, to increase the blood pressure and to thin the structure of bones. Retention of salts and of fluid in the body and changes in distribution of fat will raise the body weight and give the patient a rounded 'moon' face, or a 'buffalo hump' at the back of the neck. In children they can impede growth.

Also when they are administered for long periods the adrenal glands may adjust to this outside supply by decreasing their own corticosteroid production. Thus no patient should suddenly discontinue the taking of long prescribed corticosteroids, but should gradually tail off the dose under medical supervision. This gives the adrenals the chance to re-educate themselves and resume normal secretion. Patients on long term corticosteroids often carry a card as information to those who may suddenly have to treat them urgently.

The Pituitary and A.C.T.H.

In the brain the pituitary gland also secretes a number of hormones, and one of them is called the adreno-corticotrophic hormone or A.C.T.H. This stimulates the adrenals to produce corticosteroids. A.C.T.H. therefore can sometimes be prescribed to boost the amount of corticosteroid in the body. But it can be given only by injection. Also its sustained use may reduce the pituitary's own production of A.C.T.H., in the same way that long continued taking of corticosteroids may affect the adrenal glands.

Doctors are well aware of these features. Prescriptions give the lowest effective doses for the shortest time possible. Where sustained administration seems necessary doctors carefully weigh the disadvantages against the likely benefits. And the benefits are often very high.

Coughs and Cough Medicines

Coughing is a protective reflex by which the respiratory system advertises some damage or tries to get rid of unwanted material within it.

Tumours, inhaled foreign bodies, dust and fumes are examples. Far more common ones are secretions and discharges which are caused by infection or irritation and which we call sputum when they are coughed up. Sometimes this material does not originate in the air tubes and lungs but accumulates at the back of the throat after dripping down from the rear opening of a running nose.

In certain forms of heart troubles an inefficient circulation leads to congestion of the lungs; due to engorged blood vessels the air spaces fill up with a fluid exudate which may be coughed up as watery sputum.

Two rare and bizarre causes of coughing are irritation of the ear canal and of the stomach. These organs have nerve interconnections with the nerve governing coughing, and so set up a reflex action on the respiratory system.

Cough medicines abound. Over a dozen feature in the British National Formulary which contains the basically useful preparations. An index of proprietary medicines, that is those marketed by major drug firms, lists almost a hundred. Also many pharmacists produce their own variants.

A cough medicine can act in one of several ways. The *cough suppressant* dampens down the centre in the brain which controls the cough reflex. This can be very useful when the patient is bothered by frequent intense coughing, especially if it is due to pressure irritation as from a tumour. But most coughing is an attempt to expel unwanted secretions which are getting in the way of the passage of air; in that case coughing is useful and to be encouraged. A suppressant by itself would not help, but could perhaps worsen matters where the air tubes are bothered by thick sputum.

The name *linctus* is generally used to describe a syrupy medicine containing a suppressant. A popular one is codeine. Some suppressants have side effects, of small moment unless large doses are taken. Codeine, for instance, can cause constipation and in very big doses could depress the centre in the brain which governs respiration.

Other preparations will act by softening and thinning the sputum so making it easier to cough out. These are the *expectorants*. The very simplest (and claimed by some to be among the best) are steam inhalations and sipping a tumblerful of hot water into which half a teaspoonful of table salt has been dissolved. By liquefying the sputum, expectorants may actually increase its volume. This in turn increases the amount of cough, but improves its efficiency and makes things easier for the patient.

Bronchodilators widen the air tubes by relaxing the muscles round them. This usefully opens up the air passages to the lungs when there is any asthma-like spasm.

Demulcents, mainly as syrups or lozenges, are soothing preparations which could help when the source of the cough is an irritation at the back of the throat.

This survey teaches that no cough medicine cures. It only relieves symptoms. It is also clear how the medicine should be 'tailored' to the type of cough it treats. Many a 'cough mixture' bought at a chemist's counter contains different types of these preparations with the hope that somewhere in that lot something will do some good. It may indeed, if only psychologically.

No cough should be allowed to continue over a fortnight without medical advice. Any cough which brings up blood or bloodstained sputum should be reported to the doctor as soon as possible.

Cramps

These sudden involuntary, severe and painful contractions of muscles often come at night, especially in the legs.

Treat them not by getting up and walking about but by a far simpler method which allows you to remain in bed. Put the affected muscles on the stretch as far as they will go. In the back of the thigh: straighten the knee, raise the leg a little off the bed and bend the foot down strongly at the ankle. In the calf: straighten the knee and strongly bend the foot upwards at the ankle. These manoeuvres generally switch the trouble off at once.

Some people, especially those with a mildly defective circulation, get night cramps frequently. There are tablets, prescribable by the doctor, which can in some cases be taken at bed time to prevent their occurrence.

Cramps may suddenly develop when there has been a great loss of fluid and minerals from the body by severe sweating, by diarrhoea or by vomiting. The treatment is to drink, slowly, water or fruit juice to every pint of which half a teaspoonful of ordinary salt has been dissolved.

Cretins

The thyroid gland, which is situated at the base and front of the neck, secretes hormones (chemical messengers) which circulate in the blood and control organs in various parts of the body. The thyroid hormones are necessary for many forms of growth and development and for regulating energy exchanges in the tissues.

A cretin is a child born with deficiency or absence of thyroid hormones. (Occasionally the defect can follow an inflammation of the gland early in its life.) When he is born the baby will appear normal for he has been supplied with the mother's hormones which pass into his system. It is over the next weeks and months that the signs appear as physical and mental development are retarded.

His mother may worry because he is too good, apathetic and rarely crying. He is sleepy and, for a baby, relatively expressionless. Constipation may be a trouble.

If the condition is untreated the child eventually shows the following features: a poor weight gain; thick skin; relatively little hair; a broad face with a flattened nose; a large tongue which may protrude between thick lips; squat, puffy hands and feet; a pot belly. At the same time mental development is retarded.

Once diagnosis has been suspected and verified by blood tests treatment consists of giving thyroid preparations to correct the deficiency. This will have to continue for the whole of the patient's life. The earlier this is started the better, though the physical side generally responds well some of the mental defects may not be reversible.

Croup

Croup is not a definite disease. In medical terms it applies to inflammation at or around the larynx (voice box), often with spasm or with swelling of the tissues. When severe these reduce the space through which air can pass, creating the croaking, whistling sound as the patient tries to breathe. The chief victims are young children who have relatively narrow larynxes, with small reserves of space.

In the past diphtheria was a potent and terrible cause of croup, producing a thick membrane which blocked the airway. Happily this infection is now rare and responds to antibiotics.

But there are many bacterial and viral illnesses which will swell the linings of upper air passages of children. They may suddenly struggle for breath, with a frightening stridor. If they are blue about the face and lips and breathing is very fast, call a doctor at once. Very occasionally emergency action may have to include tracheostomy, that is an incision into the windpipe to relieve the obstruction above it.

In the large majority of cases however sedatives, antibiotics, warmth and steam are sufficient. Steam inhalations form the classic first aid treatment: subjecting the child to an atmosphere of water vapour, whether in a bathroom, from a kettle or a jug of boiling water.

One of the most common causes of croup takes the following pattern. The young patient is put to bed at the end of a day in which he had a slight cold. As he sleeps a blob of catarrhal mucus dribbles from the back of his throat down into the larynx. Irritated, the larynx goes into spasm, closes up and the child wakes up coughing and barely able to breathe. Alarm intensifies the spasm and the situation worsens into a vicious circle of fear and tension.

The parents understandably are frightened too, but they must not show it. Let them call the doctor, but also let them treat by reassurance. They should sit the child up (which helps the mechanics of breathing) and tell him he will improve with slow sips of a special drink. The drink can be anything warm like cocoa or milk; a touch of cooking dye to turn the milk pink or blue may convince the patient that this indeed is something special. As he concentrates on getting it down, perhaps through a straw, his fear and tension abate, and his larynx relaxes. The crisis is over.

Crush Injuries

In this emergency the victim's arm or leg has been pinned down by a heavy object such as falling masonry or machinery. If he has been caught there for an hour or more before it is possible to release him, special precautions are necessary. A little while after the limb has been freed it may begin to swell greatly, from fluid oozing out of contused blood vessels; this could lead to shock (p. 183) developing fast.

A further complication is kidney failure which may follow two or three days later. He stops producing urine. The mechanism of this is not certain. Kidney damage does sometimes follow severe shock. It is also possible that after the limb has been released chemicals produced in severely crushed muscles pass into the circulation and reach the kidneys to impede their action.

First Aid

1. Release the limb as rapidly as you can.

2. Keep the patient lying down, with his head low.

3. Be wary lest the limb be fractured, and should not be moved.

4. If however no fracture seems likely get the limb gently elevated, on cushions or folded blankets.

5. Cover the patient loosely and arrange for his rapid transfer to hospital, by ambulance. Let the hospital know that he has been crushed.

6. If any bandaging has to go over the limb this must not be so tight as to cause trouble if swelling forms under them.

Dandruff

Dandruff is a nuisance and displeasing but hardly an illness. More than half of the population are troubled by it at one time or another, especially in adolescence.

Our skin is constantly and normally losing small, dry scales from its surface. Rubbing from clothes and everyday activities helps them to be shed. However the scalp may be over-exuberant in the production of scales, especially in those who have greasy skin, and as friction at the scalp is not common, scales do not fall away fast and unnoticeably, tending to accumulate among the hairs.

Using a hairbrush daily helps to clear the head. So will regular shampooing, say once or twice weekly. Some medicated shampoos, such as those containing cetrimide or selenium compounds, can be useful but it is wise to get medical advice about using them.

The sufferer will be relieved to know that dandruff is not an infection and also that it does not affect the health of the hair; it does not cause baldness.

Depression

Inevitably life has its setbacks and disappointments. We may get saddened at the time. We feel depressed and this is understandable.

In the medical sphere depression has a different sense, a gloom of unreasonable depth totally out of proportion to its cause. It may also have no obvious cause. Psychiatrists describe two forms. There is the *reactive* type, in which the patient has a good reason for sorrow; he may be bereaved, or have suffered a personal calamity such as loss of money or of status in his career. But the degree of depression and the time it lasts is greatly out of proportion to the event which set it off. *Endogenous* depression is one which seizes its victim out of the blue, with no reason discernible by him or by others. It is fair to add that the dividing line between these two types is often rather vague.

How does the depressed person feel? The simple discouragement we all experience at some time or other is no measure of what is conveyed by depression as an illness. In severe cases life offers no pleasure. The outside world is grey, remote, unrelated to him. He suffers a loss of interest which can be extreme. He is indifferent to the events of the world, of his community, his family and his own self.

Depression really means what it says: not mere sadness but the lowering of every activity and the flattening of all emotions. The patient loses initiative; he cannot make a simple decision. His everyday tasks of dressing, washing, eating or going to work he undertakes with slow apathy. Voice, action, appetite and sexual feelings are duller. Sleep is poor with waking in the early mornings when misery is at its worst. Sometimes the suffering is accompanied by unjustified feelings of guilt and unworthiness, or even by hypochondriacal imaginings of bizarre physical ills.

The tendency to suicide is high, ever to be kept in mind even if the patient makes no reference to it. He must be watched guardedly, sympathetically. From day to day the illness can vary. Apparent returns to normality or near normality may deceive. It is in the beginning of one of these upward swings that the suicide risk rises; with a degree of depression still operating an increase of initiative may then lead the patient to take his life.

Such is the severest form, but many lesser degrees exist with the sufferer carrying on his everyday tasks. Even these carry danger. The 'flattening of life' and the loss of purpose experienced are rarely understood by his friends and relatives. Exhortations to 'pull yourself together' and to 'snap out of it' are as unrealistic here as they would be in cases of appendicitis. Help from doctors should be sought without delay.

Research into the biochemistry of the brain has suggested more and more that identifiable chemical factors can be related to depression. On this basis useful drugs are available. The majority however need to be taken for about two or three weeks before they become effective.

Sometimes used is the more physical method of Electro Convulsive Therapy (E.C.T.). Controlled minor 'fits' are given, created by electrical means. This may sound terrible, but in fact the patient experiences no distress.

Whatever the treatment it will also include psychiatry and sympathetic help to guide the patient towards a better understanding of himself; it may continue for a long period.

Dermatitis *see* Eczema

Diabetes

Sugar in the Blood

We all have sugar in our blood, but its amount is cunningly regulated by the body. Carbohydrate foods (sweets or starches) after digestion are transformed into the sugar, glucose, which enters the blood stream. Here it is 'burnt up' for energy and also transformed into material for building up body tissues. Some of it is stored in the liver. These things are achieved by insulin, the hormone (or chemical messenger) secreted into the blood by the pancreas.

The amount of insulin secreted excellently balances the glucose requirements of the body. For instance after a large carbohydrate meal, when the blood glucose concentration rises, correspondingly more insulin is produced to use it up; the amount of blood glucose never rises above a certain normal upper level. If now, through fasting or energetic body action, the glucose concentration begins to fall, then insulin secretion decreases; the blood glucose will not get below a normal lower level. In this way the pancreas' hormone action steers the blood's glucose between the upper and lower levels of health.

Too Much Sugar

It can happen that insulin is inadequately produced by the pancreas or that it no longer operates properly. In that case glucose is not 'burnt up' or stored and high concentrations of it accumulate in the blood. Its level rises well above the normal. This is diabetes. (The full name is *diabetes mellitus*. There is a quite unrelated illness called *diabetes insipidus,* due to abnormality of the pituitary gland in the brain).

If untreated and increasing the condition has several consequences. Since glucose is no longer being used for energy or for body building the patient becomes tired and loses weight. As the blood circulates through the kidneys some of its glucose overload passes into the urine (which normally is practically free of sugar). This carries with it extra water so that the patient is passing a great deal of urine. He may become very thirsty. Other possible long term consequences are narrowing of small arteries, with damage to the kidneys and eyes. Occasionally gangrene supervenes in toes due to poor circulation in them. The diabetic must take great care of his feet.

In addition chemical changes can occur creating unusual and toxic products in the blood which will make the diabetic person slow and drowsy. Eventually, if the diabetes is severe enough, he may become dangerously unconscious.

These are the extreme results and the general sense of feeling ill should have brought the sufferer to the consulting room long before these slowly developing tragedies have occured.

There are many who are so mildly diabetic that this is not discovered until the urine is tested for glucose, perhaps in a routine health examination. As a generalisation one can say that the older a person is when be becomes diabetic the less severe the condition is likely to be.

Treatment

If diabetes is suspected it can be confirmed by special blood tests. Under carefully controlled conditions the patient is given a measured glucose drink, and samples of blood taken at intervals over the next few hours show how his body is reacting to it.

Quite mild diabetes responds to simple restrictions of carbohydrate in the diet. More pronounced cases need drugs, either to replace absent insulin or to reinforce the action of what the body still produces. For the fortunate ones tablets are prescribed. Others have to take insulin, which works only by injection; they learn how to give themselves the regular doses.

Of course these are no 'cures'. The diabetic fact cannot be reversed by medicine, but it can be overcome and controlled. If they follow prescriptions faithfully most diabetics lead an otherwise straight-forward life.

Tablets and injections are prescribed for the patients own case, for his degree of diabetes, and for his average activity. Before he became diabetic the body organised its insulin in step with its daily or hourly glucose changes, how much had been eaten and what energy had been expended. No prescription can emulate that smooth automatic response to unpredictable variations.

Too Much Sugar

Even under treatment the patient may have rises of blood sugar above the normal upper level, especially if he eats too much or does less muscle work than usual. The situation is not serious unless it continues uncorrected for a long time.

Too Little Sugar

Now the very opposite may happen. If he is on insulin injections and (a) mistakenly gives himself too big a dose, (b) eats less than usual or (c) does much more work than usual, then the patient's blood sugar could well fall to *below* the normal lower level. The results can be dramatic and dangerous.

Unlike the very slow moving effects of excess blood sugar, those of *too little sugar* happen fast. The patient feels tremulous and weak. In some cases he may realise what is happening but has lost initiative to do anything about it. He sweats, is pale and shaking. He may become uncoordinated so that his thick speech and clumsy walk suggest drunkeness, which would be a tragic mistake in diagnosis. Then he could lose consciousness and be at risk of losing his life.

First Aid

If he recognises his condition the patient takes sugar or glucose tablets (which he is careful to keep about him). Two lumps (or two teaspoonfuls) of sugar in a glass of water act rapidly and soon restore him to normal. It is sensible about quarter of an hour later to take a second, maintenance, dose. In the absence of sugar any sweet food (chocolate, pastry) will serve.

It is far better to overdo the treatment here than to neglect it. If he has taken too much sugar no damage has been done; if he continues with too little he may die.

The attack may make him unreasonable, quarrelsome and fighting, refusing to take the sugar. If he cannot be coaxed then handfuls of granulated sugar flung into the mouth as he opens it may solve the problem.

If he has passed into unconsciousness (p.210) he urgently needs an injection by a doctor. *Never try to give anything by mouth to an unconscious or comatose person.*

Diarrhoea *see also* Constipation *and* Food Poisoning

Diarrhoea is a term which implies two points: (1) that stools are passed frequently and (2) that they are loose and watery.

The passage of food down the alimentary tract gives a clue to many causes of diarrhoea.

Anything which produces excess fluid in the stool or activity in the bowel can create diarrhoea. Irritant foods will stimulate the bowel to propel its contents faster. Also soft bulk may be added as intestinal glands protectively secrete an abnormally large amount of mucus.

As the overactive large bowel hurries its contents along, there is far less time for water to be absorbed from the stool, which arrives at the back passage in a liquid condition.

A number of things can precipitate this. *Gastro-enteritis* is a rather wide term for an inflammation of stomach and intestines for which there are many causes, the principal ones being bacterial and virus infections. Some of these are temporary and trivial, though highly incommoding and painful. The so-called 'traveller's diarrhoea' may reflect the visitor's reaction to a foreign country, meeting a number of microbes unfamiliar to his system. This type of trouble lasts only two or three days.

The word *dysentery* is rather more specific, covering infection by definite groups of organisms which could be present in food, especially where hygiene has been faulty. A rarer cause is the excessive presence of fats due to deficiency of fat digesting juices in the intestines; the stools then are very pale and bulky.

Only too common as a cause is the haphazard use of purgatives for real

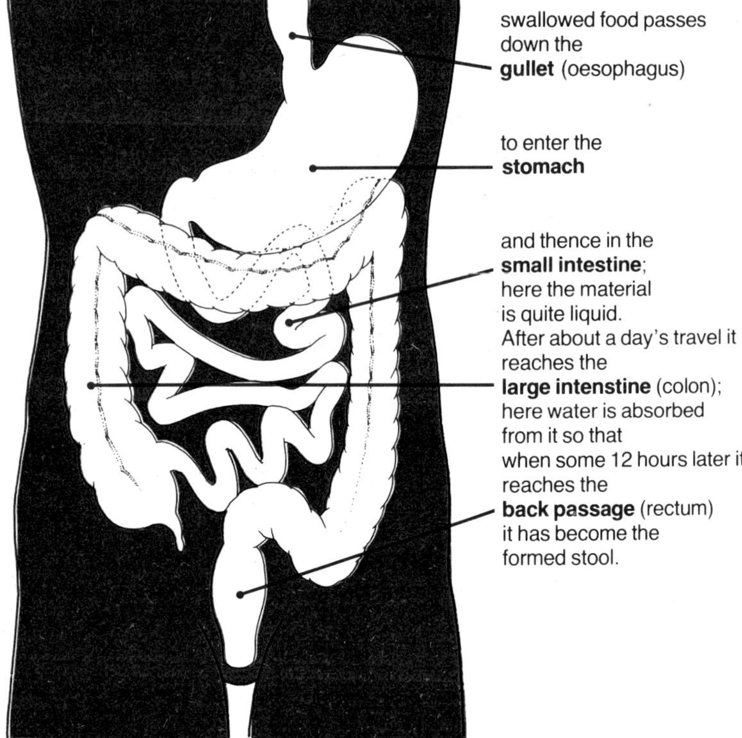

or imaginary constipation. Some drugs occasionally can cause diarrhoea. Magnesium preparations taken as stomach soothers may act as purgatives. There are antibiotics which sometimes decrease the number of those microbes which are normal inhabitants of the healthy bowel, and allow an uncontrolled upsurge of any other harmful one which might be present. Sometimes children attacked by infections in other parts of the body (ear, throat, kidneys) will begin with misleading symptoms of very loose stools.

Not only excess water is passed by diarrhoea: the liquid carries with it a quantity of salts important to the body's well being. If this becomes severe, prostration and also muscle cramps can follow. With babies and small children this loss can be really dangerous for their fluid and mineral reserves are low. Do not hesistate to get medical advice when the diarrhoea persists for two days and the child appears ill. The same problem applies to elderly and debilitated adults.

Treatment of diarrhoea obviously is that of its cause. It is quite unwise to fly to antibiotics before a medical check up has been made. But symptoms can be eased by drugs which reduce the overactivity of bowel muscles and allow the poor patient a return to some peace and comfort. Replacing fluid and salts is important. In simple cases adults can do this with drinks of meat and yeast extracts (Bovril, Oxo, Marmite). However these should be taken tepid and in slow sips; quick gulps of hot drinks could reflexly stimulate bowel movements.

Any sudden unexplained change of bowel habit which persists always needs a medical opinion. So does passing blood with the stools.

Diphtheria *see also* Fevers of Children *and* Immunisation

Very happily diphtheria is, for many countries, almost of historical interest only. In the past a sadistic killer of children it is now practically powerless under the double restraints of antibiotics and of immunisation. All health workers consider that it is essential for children to follow the full immunisation programme which has now made this fever a rarity.

Whether or not anyone has acquired immunity to diphtheria can be checked by a simple injection procedure into the skin called the Schick Test. It is useful in cases of uncertainty but not necessary where immunisation has been adequately carried out.

In the non-immunised the infection has an incubation period of some three days. The patient has a severe fever and sore throat. Poisons from the bacteria are extremely weakening; they can damage the heart, the kidneys and the nervous system. At the back of the throat a thick white discharge can form a membrane large enough to make not only swallowing but also breathing very difficult. Sometimes the airway is blocked entirely.

Treatment needs antibiotics and the urgent injecting of antitoxin to neutralise the bacterial poisons. Recovery is slow, needing careful nursing.

The Disabled

see The Handicapped

Dislocation

In dislocation one bone is displaced away from contact with the other bone (or bones) which form a joint. Most commonly this happens from injury, but it may also be due to disease affecting the shape or structure of the bones and ligaments which make up the joint. Occasionally it may be a malformation present at birth (congenital).

Dislocation from injury very often show features similar to fractures (p. 117), and from a first aid point of view are treated in exactly the same way. In fact sometimes there is some break of bone as well. X-ray examination may be needed for the doctor to decide whether a fracture is present.

Generally he is able to correct a straightforward dislocation by simple manipulations, perhaps with the patient under anaesthetic. However, a severe dislocation may tend to recur later if the inner joint surfaces and the stabilising surrounding ligaments were damaged at the time of the accident. Sometimes an operation is needed.

One or other end of the *collar bone* can be dislocated as result of injury. This rarely needs active treatment and resting the arm in a sling for a short time is usually effective. A *kneecap* can slip outwards from its position while the leg is being used

Common Sites of Dislocation

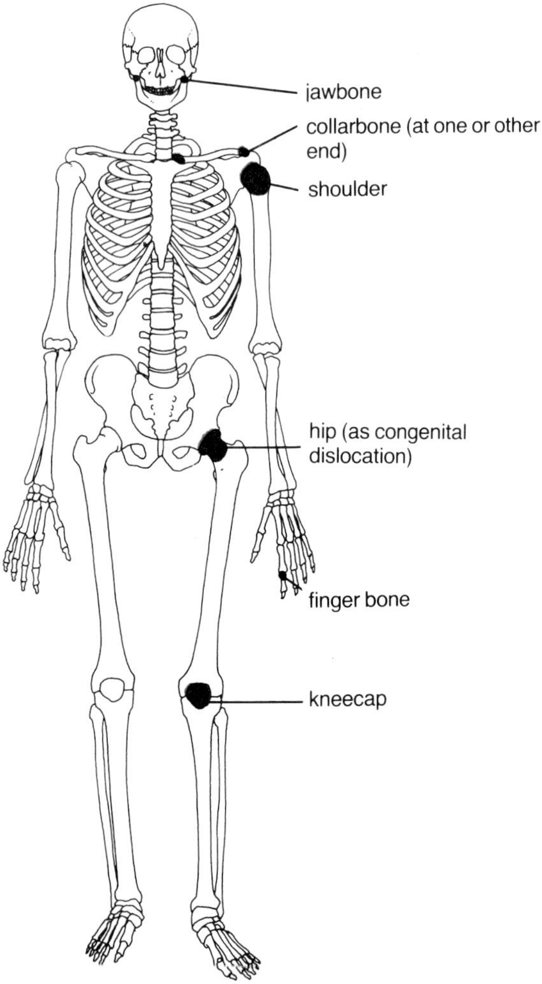

energetically in a half bent position. There is painful inability to straighten the knee which rapidly becomes swollen. The *jawbone* sometimes dislocates when the mouth is widely opened, as in a mighty yawn. Its upper tip, on which it hinges with the skull, just below the ear, slips forward. When this happens to both sides the victim is left with mouth agape and lower teeth prominent. Fortunately a simple manoeuvre by the doctor can

The shoulder blade (shaded) lies behind the upper ribs.

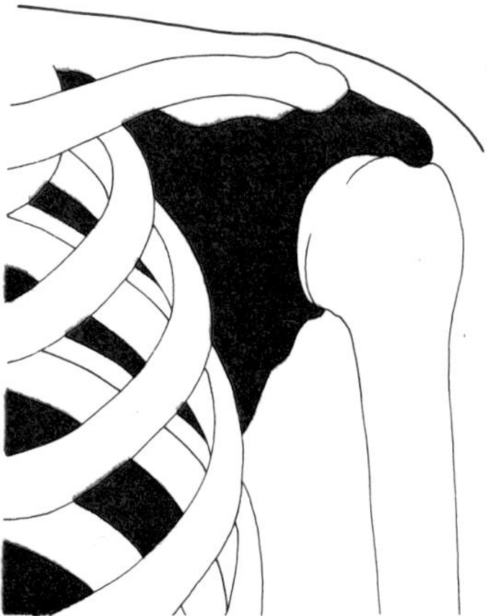

NORMAL: the rounded end of the upper arm bone fits into the shallow cup of the shoulder blade

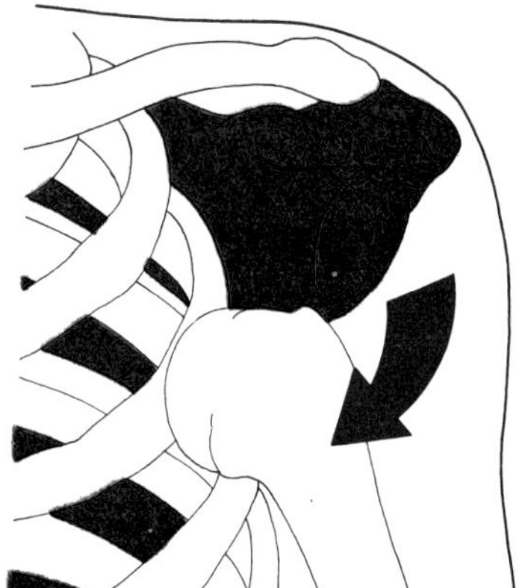

DISLOCATION: the upper arm bone has slipped down and forward out of the cup

correct it. *Finger joints* can be knocked out of position by a blow, as when the hand is hit by a hard ball. The *shoulder joint* is a well-known dislocation site. This too can be corrected by the doctor's manipulation, but he will first be careful to check whether any damage has been done to neighbouring bones, ligaments and nerves.

Dislocation of the hips in adults are rare, for the rounded head of the thighbone sits snugly in a deep bony cup, well stabilised by strong muscles. In a baby however the very young bones have a different shape; the fit is slight. *Congenital dislocation of the hip* is not uncommon, in fact one survey showed it to happen to one in every 800 girls born (it is far less frequent with boys). The condition seems to be caused by laxity of the ligaments about the hip, developing in the last weeks of pregnancy.

Most babies are screened for this dislocation soon after birth by a simple test which swings the thighs up and outwards. Even so some cases may not show.

Diagnosis is not always easy: the affected leg may look shorter between groin and knee with, therefore, some increase in the folds of the thigh. Discerning this in a chubby baby can be difficult without X-ray. If no treatment is given the baby may kick about less with the affected side, and she may walk late and with a limp. A few cases will correct themselves spontaneously. In the others the sooner the condition is diagnosed the easier and more effective the treatment. For small babies positioning the leg for some months in a special splint is generally very successful.

Diuretics *see* Dropsy

Dizziness *see* Vertigo

Doctors: How to Choose and Use

Doctors — and their receptionists — are popular subjects for criticisms, as if they dwelt in medical fortresses, whose drawbridges are only reluctantly lowered. It is fair to say that both are only too willing to be of service, but they do try to sift the minor from the major cases and to give priority to the latter. When the receptionist enquires about the nature of the illness for which you seek help she is only trying to be useful to you and to all the others who wish to consult the doctor.

You have moved to a new area. How do you set about finding a new doctor? Do not wait until you actually need one. Make your choice at leisure before any emergency has come. Also consider the N.H.S. service in which the doctor gets paid not for each act of service, but for each patient registered with him. It is a form of insurance. Waiting to have pneumonia or appendicitis before you register is rather like delaying to insure your house until it is on fire.

How do you chose? You could ask your neighbour or your landlady for advice. The truth is that their recommendations are not necessarily valid. People are conservative; they rarely change their doctor, and rarely have thought out a choice. Because the medical person is *their* doctor they tend, in a twist of psychological justification, to say that this is *the* doctor to consult. They may be right; they may be wrong.

Go into the area's busiest looking chemist's shop and check that the dispenser is in. Buy something noticeably costly, such as cosmetics or shaving kit, but something you would have to buy anyhow so that you do not waste money. Be an affable customer. Then politely ask if you could speak to the dispenser. Be prepared to wait a bit; he is a busy person. Explain to him that you are new to the district and request his help . . . Please could he suggest a doctor for you and your family . . . You would be really grateful for his guidance.

Ethical caution may prevent his giving one name outright. If he does you know where you are. But even if he offers several his way of doing it may suggest a preference.

This dispenser is an expert. He hears comments from patients and judges who is kind and efficient. He sees prescriptions coming in and learns who tends to administer the same old medicines, who is ever jumping to the latest uncertain wonder drug and who nicely blends traditional with modern science.

How and when to consult doctors is a different matter. Repeatedly they are asked to elucidate at what degree of raised temperature or under which sickness conditions their advice should be sought. There is no answer to such questions for there is no absolute measure of symptoms and safe dogmatism is not possible. Common sense (yours!) is the only guide. Many doctors set aside a time when they can be reached by telephone, and are happy to listen and advise. Do not expect to be able to get through to them directly at other hours, for this might mean repeated interruptions to them *and to their patients* during consultations.

If in doubt approach the nurse or receptionist. She is an experienced person; if requested for her opinion (and not just dictated to) she will be your helpful ally. Explain your worries; she will understand.

Some simple guidelines can assist you in asking for a visit. When the patient has a long standing condition which prevents going to the surgery ask the doctor to call when he is next in the area. If the illness is new and does not appear urgent but merits a visit the same day make sure your request gets in before 10 a.m. so that the doctor's round can be properly planned.

In the case of a rapidly rising temperature or bad pain make sure the details of the symptoms are understood and the doctor could call within a couple of hours. But if the patient has something like a fit, a collapse, a heart attack, poisoning or a severe bleed send an urgent call.

Ambulances as a rule will not respond to a purely medical condition unless the doctor has already seen the patient. However where there has been severe accident like asphyxia, electrocution or burning they are generally prepared to respond to a 999 emergency call.

One of the difficulties faced in such emergencies is finding a house in an unfamiliar area, especially out in the country or in some large new housing estate. Does the door or the garden gate bear the number very clearly? In doubtful cases post a guide in the street. At night time have the front door open, the curtains pulled back and the lights all on to act as a beacon.

Down's Syndrome

This name replaces the old term of Mongolism. (A syndrome is a group of features which characterises a medical condition.)

About once in every six hundred births a child is born with a special type of error in the disposition of his or her chromosomes: these are the microscopic particles from cell division which carry the characteristics of the body. This error dictates the abnormalities found in Down's Syndrome. It is quite unrelated to any event during the pregnancy.

These children are relatively small, with a short neck, a squat face and a flattened nose. Their eyes slant upwards and outwards and the mouth is small, giving the impression that the tongue is too big. Hands are short and stubby; often each little finger is incurved and the palms may show but one crease across them instead of the usual two.

Mentally they are retarded, but the degree to which this happens is very variable. A number will grow up with a mind comparable to that of a small child: they may manage some reading and writing and simple speech, and they may learn an easy craft. Others will not attain any of these and will need constant guidance, constant supervision. Yet they are very pleasant, amenable and kindly children, with their own personalities. Though this congenital defect is a tragedy which creates understandable stresses, many of them are easily incorporated, with affection, in the family's life.

Dressings and Bandages

see also Wounds

The Dressing

White gauze — from a freshly opened pack — is the usual dressing. Very handy are the Perforated Film Absorbent (P.F.A.) dressings, sterile and packed individually in protective envelopes. They are available in sizes 5 cm and 10 cm square and 10 x 20 cm. They can be removed and placed on without being touched by hand.

The shiny surface goes on the wound, and will not stick. Dressings can be improvised from clean handkerchiefs, small towels or pillowcases. Hold the article by two corners, let it fall open and, still holding only the corners, refold it to the correct size so that what was the inside surface now becomes the outer one which, untouched by hand, goes on the wound. A pillow case is useful for encasing a whole limb.

The Pad

This is put over the dressing as a comfortable buffer between it and the bandage. Cotton wool is customary from a freshly opened pack if possible, but it should not be used as a dressing to go directly on the wound, since its thready fibres tend to stick. Pads can be improvised by thick folding together of any suitable clean, soft objects: handkerchiefs, socks, towels.

The Bandage

Plain white bandages are the usual, but conforming bandages, crepe bandages and elastic bandages have more 'give' and are easier to adapt round uneven contours. They also help to give a firmer pressure. With these you must take great care not to apply them so tightly that they interfere with the circulation.

The Prepared Sterile Dressing

This ready for use combination of dressing, pad and bandage comes in three different sizes and is well worth while stocking in your first aid kit. Layers of gauze, backed by cotton wool, are attached near the end of the roller bandage. After you have broken open the protective wrapping you touch only the bandage part.

Adhesive Dressings

Either as continuous strips to be cut to size, or as single dressings of different sizes, these are very suitable for small wounds. The protective layer is partly peeled off the front so that the gauze pad now exposed can be applied without being touched by the fingers.

Applying a Roller Bandage

Face the patient, and have the injured part comfortably supported. Bandage from below the injury upwards. Have the beginning of the bandage pointing obliquely a little upwards; fix it by taking a firm turn round the part. Fold down the protecting tip. Now with a

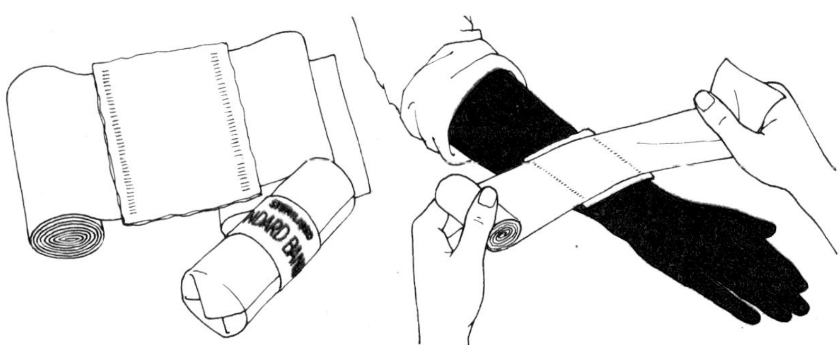

A prepared sterile dressing.

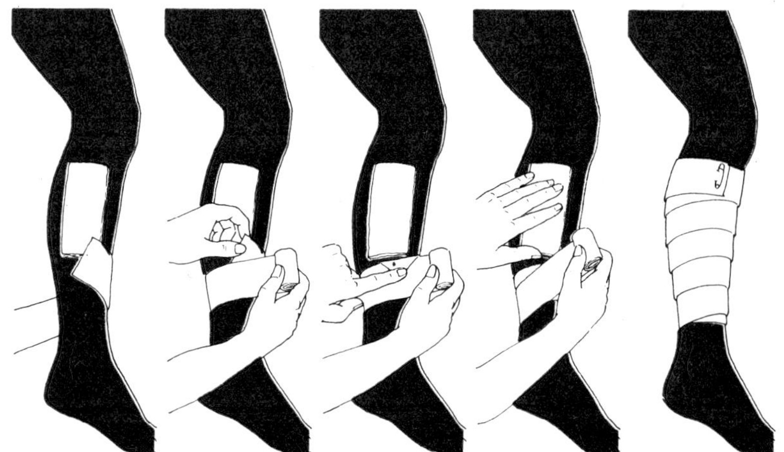

firm and even pressure, bandage from within outwards over the front of the part, with each turn covering two-thirds of the previous one. Finish above the injury, fastening the end with a safety pin. Improvised roller bandages are made from socks, stockings, towels, belts, scarves, neckties.

Dropsy

This is a nice old fashioned word for a nasty state of affairs. It means an abnormal accumulation of watery fluid in any tissue. To put it bluntly: waterlogging. The medical word is 'oedema', pronounced like its American spelling edema.

It shows up more easily in parts with rather slack skin, such as around the ankles or about the eyes, but it can affect anywhere in the body. As to why it happens there is no single reason; explanations involve simple mechanics as well as complicated biochemistry.

To begin with there may be some interference with the easy return of circulating blood to the heart via the veins. The heart may not be working efficiently, as in so-called heart failure. The veins become engorged and this in turn engorges the minute capillary vessels where chemical exchanges occur between blood and the tissues. When this happens the liquid part of the blood oozes out of the capillaries and fills the tissue spaces.

The resulting swelling to some extent is affected by gravity, showing up in the lowermost parts of the body. This would be by the base of the spine in someone who has been resting in bed for hours. For someone upright during the day it would appear around the ankles. When in doubt about it the examining doctor pushes the tip of his finger firmly against the skin; a neat dimple or pit appearing at the point of pressure confirms dropsy.

Engorged leg veins can happen without the heart being at fault. The activity of our walking muscles helps to 'milk' the blood along the veins towards the heart. Long inactive standing will cause engorgement. So will long periods of sitting, especially if the front of the chair presses against veins near the knee. Varicose veins can also interfere with the normal flow of blood from the legs, with the same results.

Rarer forms of obstruction to venous circulation could be from tumours pressing on veins or, in the abdomen, from cirrhosis of the liver (p. 153). When the part involved is inside the abdominal cavity giving a swollen belly, then the medical word used is 'ascites'.

A different set of explanations govern the dropsy associated with some forms of liver and kidney disease. Here these organs, which in health act as regulators of the body's chemical components, may fail to maintain the right balances. Excess salt or proteins in the tissues hold in water. Deficient amounts of protein in the blood allows fluid to ooze through the capillaries into the tissues.

Reduced blood proteins can also occur for the very simple reasons of a grossly defective diet: the paradoxically swollen bellies of severe starvation are due to dropsy.

Treatment of dropsy obviously means treatment of the cause. But the symptom itself can be helped by diuretics. These are drugs which incite the kidneys to excrete more water than usual as urine. They can be very effective in freeing the body from dropsical accumulations. Like most drugs they can have side effects. In many cases this extra water got out of the body carries with it useful minerals like potassium. The patient is no longer puffy, but he becomes a little deficient in this salt. Doctors are fully aware of this and may supplement the diuretic with a potassium preparation.

Some diuretics work with dramatic efficiency and doctors or nurses will advise as to the best time to take them. Another problem of this speed of action faces the very elderly or handicapped who find it difficult to reach the lavatory 'in time'. In that case they could discuss with their doctor whether a diuretic with slower, more sustained, effect would suit their particular case.

Duodenal Ulcer

see Peptic Ulcer

Drowning

see Artificial Respiration

Dysentery *see* Diarrhoea

Dysmenorrhoea

see Menstruation

Ear Troubles

The first part of the ears which sound waves reach are the outer shells. Travelling down the outer canal the waves reach the drum which is set vibrating. The movements are passed on to the three tiny linked ossicles (the smallest bones in the body) and so to fluid within the coiled cochlea. This carries the vibrations to a fine membrane within the coils. Different parts of the membrane responding to different sounds are connected to nerves going to those areas of the brain which deal with hearing.

Alongside the cochlea, three semicircular canals, fine U-shaped tubes, are set at right angles to each other in three different planes. Microscopically fine granules float in the liquid of these canals. The way they settle or move against nerve connected fibres indicates to the body its position in space.

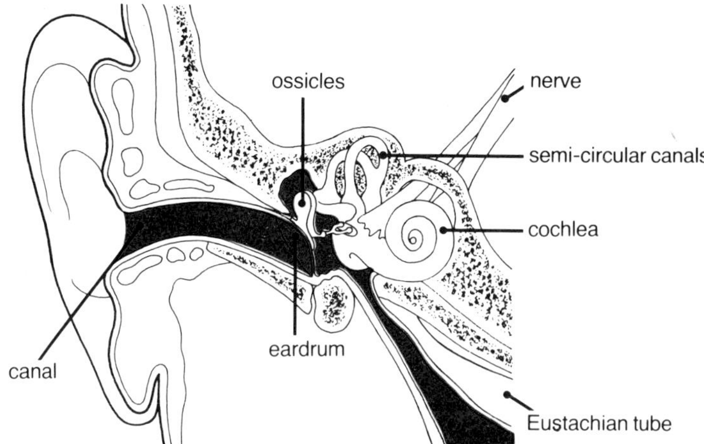

Thus serving both hearing and balance the ear has a double function.

Objects in the Ear

Small children investigating body potential in their own experimental way often push small objects into the ear. And fail to get them out. And do not tell mother. Eventually an unpleasant infected discharge may appear. No one, except a doctor or nurse, should try to clear out whatever is inside. There is no justification for D.I.Y. poking of the ear canal. Keep pins, matches, hairpins and hooks for their proper use. The ear canal is not deep, but it is narrow and slightly bent as it leads to the valuable drum. It needs medical inspection and special forceps for safety.

The insect which gets inside the canal is not dangerous but creates a really horrible irritation as it struggles. A few drops of water, medicinal liquid paraffin or olive oil poured in the ear will drown it and let its body float to the surface. (Do *not* try this if there is a chance that the drum is not intact and would let the fluid pass beyond it.)

Wax is a normal production inside the canal. Sometimes, it is excessive and becomes a plug which blocks sound. The only proper solution is syringing by the doctor or nurse. Wax often needs softening first by putting in a few drops of oil for a day or two: the softened wax may slither against the drum increasing the deafness, but this annoyance is temporary.

The Painful Ear

Earache can mislead: it might be due to a radiation of pain from throat or teeth troubles. Within the ear itself the simplest cause is inflammation of the canal which can cause a nasty swelling and irritating discharge, or tense and very painful boils. Do not try to cope with this yourself; please see a doctor who can look into the depths of the canal and decide whether drops will help.

More common, especially in children, is *otitis media,* that is infection of the middle ear. This is the part between the drum and the cochlea. A fine canal, the Eustachian tube connects it to the back of the throat. It is useful in that it allows air pressure behind the drum to equalise with that of the atmosphere, but it has the disadvantage of offering to microbes of throat infections an easy passage up into the middle ear.

Generally otitis media begins with severe earache, soon followed by deafness on that side. If the trouble worsens the temperature may rise, pus may form behind the drum, pressing against it. If the pus increases it perforates the drum and flows out of the ear. This does ease pressure and therefore pain but the relief is illusory since the infection is still active.

We really must take symptoms of otitis media seriously and seek medical opinion. Early treatment can cut an attack short very quickly. Delay may scar the drum and affect hearing permanently. And sometimes (though very rarely in our antibiotic era) the infection can spread to the nearby bone structure such as the mastoid bump behind the ear, or into other parts of the head.

Glue Ear

This is not an emergency, for it is a long developing, long lasting condition in which the middle ear fills up with a thick gummy discharge and hearing is reduced. Children are the chief victims, generally as a result of repeated virus infections around the throat and ear. Very many cases will get quite better gradually and spontaneously. In others a specialist may clear away the glue by a simple operation through the drum. Sometimes, to keep the drainage going, he will leave in the drum a very small tube, called a 'grommet'; this comes out after some months.

Tinnitus

Tinnitus is hearing something which is not there. In other words it is the sensation of sound not caused by outside noises but by some disturbance within the structure of the ear. It bothers quite a few people who have to put up continuously, or intermittently, with whistling, roaring, murmuring or buzzing sounds. Often it is accompanied by some degree of deafness.

Occasionally its origin is simple and easily remedied, like large doses of aspirin, wax in the canal or infection of the middle ear. More often than not however it is difficult or impossible to cope with the causes involving the delicate structures like the cochlea, the ossicles or the nerve of hearing. Sometimes pulsations from neighbouring arteries are the factor.

But tinnitus raises a question mark which must be met. Seek a medical opinion. The doctor, after examining, may be able to offer sympathy only. On the other hand he may find that the symptom is an early feature of a condition which merits treatment and will respond to it.

Dizziness *and* Ménière's Disease *are described under* Vertigo *p.213.*

Eczema

Is there any difference between 'eczema' and 'dermatitis'? Some doctors used to describe the former for long lasting conditions and the latter for more acute states. Sometimes the word 'dermatitis' was restricted to skin troubles due to contact with external irritants.

In fact the words are interchangeable. 'Eczema' comes from Greek terms meaning something which boils or foams up. That is not a bad description of the micro-scopical changes in the skin whose cell structure becomes swollen and puffed up, often causing 'weeping' and crusting on the surface. As for 'dermatitis', that is of Latin derivation meaning inflammation of the skin. This could apply to many skin mishaps ranging from sunburn (p. 194) to nettlerash (p. 162).

The words have so wide a connotation that by themselves mean little. Dermatologists classify eczema into many groups. Some arise from causes purely within the patient. Allergy (p. 14) is an example and so is the debilitated skin where circulation is slow and stagnant, as one finds in legs with varicose veins. Outside causes include damage by contact with irritants. The baby's napkin rash (p. 162) is an excellent example. Certain occupational eczemas arise from chemicals handled. Some people show a special hypersensitivity to what most of us can touch without trouble such as the metal of watch cases or on brassière clips, rubber in footwear, or plants, like primulas.

Itching is a major feature, and all too often the condition gets worse because, short of prescribing handcuffs, the doctor cannot persuade the patient to stop scratching. Unfortunately a lot of sufferers in the early stages of eczema buy all sorts of unsuitable ointments, including those bearing antiseptics, which are likely to increase the irritation. The only answer is to consult the doctor. Even then elucidating the true cause of eczema can present quite a big problem.

The Elderly

Almost twenty per cent of the population is of pensionable age. This was not always so. Two or three generations ago the figure was only about six per cent. This great increase in the number of the aged is not due to a basic change in the biology of men and women. Their possible life span has remained unchanged over the centuries. Increasingly however improvements in science and hygiene have allowed this life span to be achieved and not cut short by illness or violence. In the sixteenth century the average length of life was as low as thirty years. Now it is between seventy and eighty years.

We should therefore develop a greater regard for the elderly as active contributors to the social and economic scene. Although, compared to their juniors they may have handicaps and difficulties, the majority are capable of achieving a very great deal. Unfortunately it has become traditional to regard age as synonymous with disability. The elderly themselves can be worst offenders; if physical troubles appear many murmur 'what else can one expect at my age' and leave it at that.

No symptom of trouble or abnormality should be disregarded in old people any more than it is in the young. So much can be corrected, or at least improved, that anything which seems wrong deserves medical advice. Do not let problems like breathlessness, stiff or weak limbs, weight loss or inefficient vision and hearing be accepted with sombre fatalism. Give the elderly person, and his doctor, the chance to investigate and challenge the causes.

What are the most notable changes of growing old? With advancing years the arteries may harden and narrow, leading to a lessened blood flow to the tissues. This matters particularly to the brain which is extremely sensitive to the amount of blood, and thereby of oxygen, which it receives. To cope with increased resistance in the arteries the heart works harder and blood pressure may rise. Other common changes include a lowered production by some glands of the chemical 'messengers' called hormones. The thyroid gland, for instance, may secrete less of its hormone which governs the pace of activity of many body functions. Another change is decreased calcium in the bones, which become relatively more brittle. Muscles become slacker, gums may recede, hearing and eyesight may decrease. A very long list of commonplaces can be made, but we might ask how many of these changes we accept as inevitable are really the result of years of mistaken diet and of insufficient body exercise.

In illness the elderly can present new problems, of which doctors are well aware. They can be very sensitive to medicines, reacting strongly, sometimes with uncomfortable side effects to the ordinary doses suited to younger adults. They also may react less strongly to the illness process itself: an old man with appendicitis, for instance, may have deceptively mild symptoms and signs while being seriously ill.

For the many who look after the elderly in their homes a sympathetic and comprehensively useful book is Eleanor Deeping's *Caring for Elderly Parents* (Constable).

For the very many elderly people who are active there are plenty of occupations to be pursued. Some employers mistakenly overlook the value of their work in business and industry. In behaviour the elderly may seem slower than younger people, yet in general they are no less acute or percipient and they are more methodical. They may not be able to compete where fast timing is needed, but they win where accuracy and doggedness are factors.

Advice to those about to retire can be summarised as follows: retirement is not just the end of a means of existence, it is the beginning of a new form of life, allowing time to express personality and the development of interests and hobbies. It is not moving into a backwater. Do not lessen attention to appearance. Use every opportunity to exercise within your powers; walking, gardening, even games and sports. Seek too mental exercises and use the new leisure to branch out among groups of people in clubs and associations. Keep informed and up to date.

Electric Shock

Most domestic currents make muscles contract firmly so that a victim might not be able to let go of some electrified apparatus, such as a faulty drill or iron.

Do not touch a patient who is still in contact with electricity or you will risk becoming electrocuted yourself.

Stop the current at once by: (a) switching off; or (b) pulling out the plug; or (c) pulling on the cord to wrench the plug out or the apparatus away from the patient. If these are impossible knock the patients limbs clear of contact with something which is dry and will not conduct electricity: wood, rug, coat, folded newspaper or rubber. Do NOT use metal which is a conductor. When you do this stand on a dry surface. The victim's breathing may have stopped. You may now have to start artificial respiration at once (p.26).

Bear in mind that if he fell he could have broken a bone. Before moving

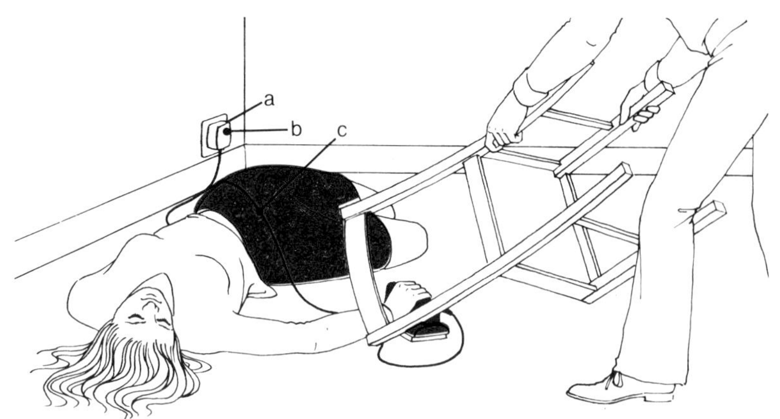

him further check as best you can for fractures (p.117). The problem is greater if you are faced as well with his unconsciousness (p.210). Also you may have to treat parts on the skin where he shows burns (p.61) from the current.

Even if he appears to have recovered you must be guarded and keep him under observation. A few victims of severe electrocution have a delayed collapse. Get a doctor or have the patient taken to hospital by ambulance.

IMPORTANT WARNING

The above concerns domestic electricity. That from overhead cables or from some high voltage factory installations are far more powerful. It could for example only make another victim if you were to get close to the wires of electric pylons in a rescue attempt. Do not try until the authorities have fully stopped the current. Until then keep back at least twenty yards.

Avoiding Accidents

Here is a brief summary of precautions.

Plugs. Modern type. Discard plugs if they are cracked, broken or become warm in use. Fit fuses appropriate to the appliance served. Ensure plugs are correctly wired and earthed. Do not put a 2-pin plug into a 3-pin socket. Never replace a plug with makeshift open wires pushed into socket holes.

Sockets and Switches. If they become warm in use, call an electrician. Never use an adaptor which does not accept all the pins of a plug. Fit with the minimum of adaptors: never overload. Never remove the cover plate. Outside fittings should only be set up by an electrician.

Flexes. Flexes should be as short as possible. Discard if frayed. Never patch or join with insulating tape. Do not run flexes under the carpet.

Lamps. Change bulbs only after switching off the current. Metal table and standard lamps to be earthed.

Kitchen. No electric fittings or apparatus touched with wet hands. Switch off and unplug apparatus (kettle, cooker, iron, toaster, mixer) before adjusting, pouring, filling, cleaning or checking.

Electric Blankets. Never used folded, rucked or damp. Checked and serviced three-yearly.

Bathroom. No sockets, no portable electric apparatus in the room (except the special ones for shavers only). Switches on pull cords or outside.

Garden and Workshop. Apparatus selected after consulting electrician. Cables suited for outside; kept clear of machine. Never link separate cables: use single continuous one.

D.I.Y. Don't (unless you are expert).

Emphysema *see* Bronchitis

Enteritis *see* Diarrhoea

Epilepsy

The brain is constantly subject to various orderly small electric impulses which can be recorded by the machine known as the electroencephelograph. In an epileptic fit the recording shows a surge of huge impulses which spread across parts of the brain.

Why does epilepsy happen? In the large majority of cases there is no clear cause. There is a slight factor of inheritance in that the child of an epileptic could have a 1 in 40 mischance of becoming epileptic himself. Known physical causes are some brain tumours, and rare after effects of strokes or brain injury. But any illness which seriously bothers the brain tissues could give an epileptic type attack during its course; this includes meningitis, abnormally high fevers, some poisons and conditions giving severe oxygen lack.

The Fit

The epileptic fit varies very much from individual to individual. The average one follows a pattern rather like this:

1. The attack is sudden and unheralded, except for a few who have a brief 'funny feeling' or awareness that one is immediately imminent. This is graced by the name of 'aura'.

2. The victim falls unconscious and silent. Some however give one cry as they fall. The situation is dangerous if the fit happens at the edge of a height or near moving machinery.

3. For half to one minute he lies still, but with tense, rigid muscles.

4. This is followed by about 30 seconds of jerking movements. They sometimes begin in one limb and rapidly extend to involve all the body. In stages 3 and 4 the patient is not breathing properly and his complexion darkens. He may froth at the mouth. He may be incontinent of urine. During the jerking he may bite his tongue.

5. Now he passes into relaxed unconsciousness which may last a few minutes (generally) or several hours (uncommonly). Breathing and normal colour return.

6. He wakes. He may be alert or temporarily confused.

First Aid

You cannot help at stages 1 and 2. If the patient has an aura he could use this moment to lie down in safety.

During stages 3 and 4, help the patient as for unconsciousness (p.210) by ensuring a clear airway. Wipe away any froth at the mouth lest he inhale it when he begins breathing again.

Do not try to restrain the jerking. But move away any furniture against which he might knock and injure his limbs. When the patient lies near an immoveable object (a wall or a heavy desk) rapidly interpose something soft like a cushion or rolled up coat between it and his jerking limb.

What about the risk of tongue biting? Many now teach that this possibility is overstated and that more harm than good can be done in trying to prevent the jaws clamping down by forcing something between them. However it might be possible to slip in the side of the mouth *something soft* (bunched edge of handkerchief, or scarf or the patient's coat lapel). Do not however leave at the mouth edge any free object which the patient might aspirate to the back of the throat when he resumes breathing.

At stage 5 continue to protect the patient as described in the section on unconsciousness. Guard the airway. Also at this point you begin to search for possible injuries, such as cuts or fractures sustained in the fall, and deal with these. You will consider putting the patient into the recovery position.

Stage 6 can cause difficulty in a public place. The patient, distressed at having had the attack, may wish to go away, out of sight of bystanders who may have collected. If the attack has happened to someone unknown, your responsibility is to have him medically checked, even if this means sending him by ambulance to hospital.

The Epileptic State

Very occasionally a patient has a number of fits coming on at short and decreasing intervals of hours or minutes. This could build up into the dangerous epileptic state of attack succeeding on attack without proper return of consciousness. He needs medical attention at once.

The Minor Attack

There is a minor form of epilepsy in which the patient does not necessarily fall and jerk (or jerks only very slightly). He just stops whatever he was doing and goes blank for a few seconds. The attack may not even be noticed by those present. When he recovers the patient may feel a little bewildered, but try to resume his activity.

Epileptics in the Community

Epileptics are not usually dangerously handicapped but they are bothered by the nuisance of intermittent attacks. Modern drugs are very helpful in reducing or even preventing these. It has been estimated that as many as 1 in every 200 are, in one form or other, epileptic. Until and unless attacks are fully medically controlled they must not drive cars or work potent machines. Otherwise most are normal citizens capable of responsibile activity and as employable as the rest of us.

The Epilepsy Association exists to help and advise.

Exposure

see Cold Effects

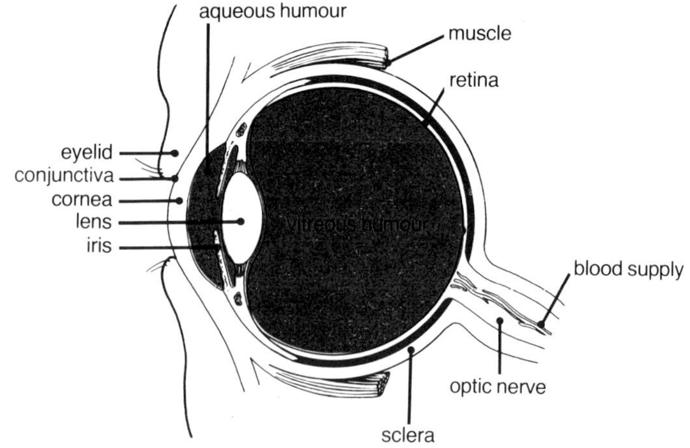

Eye Troubles

We can consider the working of the eye and its illnesses by following a ray of light which forms part of the visual scene. It passes between the eyelids to penetrate the eye first through its thin transparent cover, the conjunctiva, and then through the thicker domed cornea. This cornea is the front of the shell of the eye, which in the other parts is not transparent, and is called the sclera. Part of the sclera we see as the 'white of the eye'.

The light travels to the lens, through the pupil, the round dark opening of the iris which is the coloured ring of the eye. It widens and contracts according to the amount of light available.

The lens receiving the light rays bends them so that they focus on the retina, which lines the eyeball. It is here that specialised nerve cells pick up the light impulses and transmit them through the optic nerve, which leaves the back of the eyeball for a complicated journey to the brain.

The spaces within the eye are filled. In front the watery aqueous humour lies between lens and cornea. The jelly-like vitreous humour lies behind the lens.

The eyeball is tilted in different directions to aim at the object looked at by a set of six thin strap-like muscles which are attached at one end to the bone of the orbit and at the other to different points of the sclera.

The Black Eye

This is not trouble in the eye but bruising beneath the skin around it. The eye gets protection by being recessed within a hollow of the face. If the bruising is accompanied by a deterioration of vision then it is possible that damage has been done to the inside of the eye; a doctor should be seen as soon as possible. A black eye which appears after a blow to the head, not necessarily near the eye, should put one on one's guard for it might be due to a fracture at the base of the skull (see Head Injuries, p.129).

Wounds of the Eye

Cover these at once with a clean dry dressing and let the patient be seen as soon as possible by a doctor. If movement of the injured eye is painful then cover also the other one, for the two eyes move together. Of course you will explain to the patient why you do this.

Chemicals in the Eye

These are washed out with copious streams of water (see Burns, p.61).

Objects in the Eye

These can be extremely irritating and you must tell the patient to stop rubbing which he probably has been doing.

Sit him down in a good light. Stand behind and look down on him. More often than not the particle has moved under a lid.

Try the lower lid first. With the patient looking up, pull the lid downwards. Have ready a clean cloth, like a handkerchief moistened in one corner which you have rolled to a point. It serves well to pick up the particle.

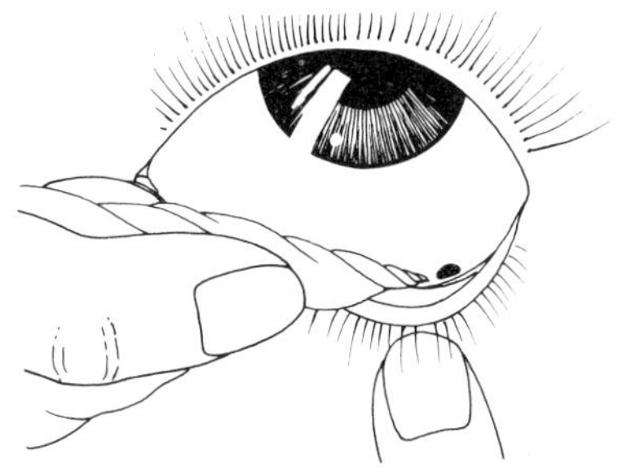

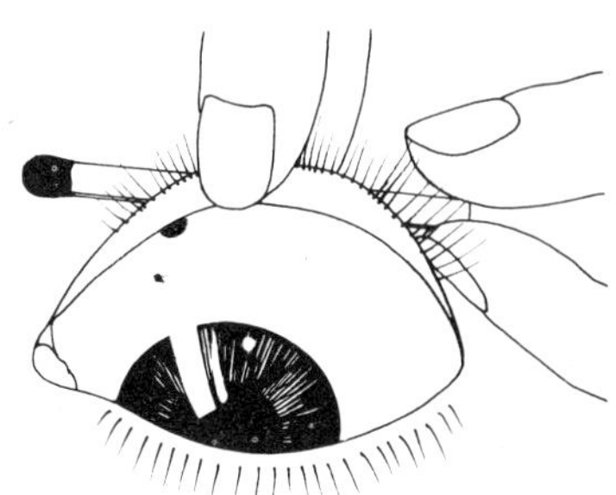

You may have to search under the upper lid. This time the patient looks down. Hold a matchstick along the 'hinge' of the lid. Grasp the edge of the lid between finger and thumb and bend it up over the matchstick. A soft hold of the lid, which may be wet with tear fluid, is likely to slip and be far less comfortable to the patient than a firm grasp.

If the particle is visible not under a lid but on the front of the eye, be cautious. Its position suggests that it is embedded.

Styes

These are infections and abscess formations in one of the skin glands at the base of the eyelashes. In fact they are small boils. Most styes if left alone will discharge and clear in time, but they can be quite painful. The patient must discipline himself not to rub the eye.

Ointments are not much help since they will not reach down to the depths of the glands, but they could protect the front of the eye from being infected in turn. Pulling out the relevant eyelash or applying hot compresses can help, but it is really wiser to get a medical opinion.

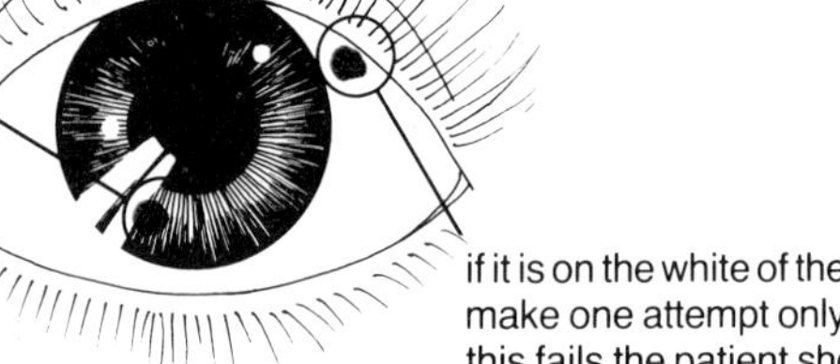

Conjunctivitis

The thin cover at the front of the eyeball is fairly vulnerable to irritation and infection. In spite of our protective blinking and of the washing and antiseptic action of tear fluid it may become red, infected and may discharge pus.

The medical profession has reserves about various eye lotions and washes to be bought across the chemist's counter. They are probably marginally less efficient than the tear fluid which constantly and gently courses over the eyeball, and has the advantages of being automatically available when needed and of costing nothing.

Mild forms of conjunctivitis clear within one week. Any attack which lasts longer, which produces pus, which is markedly painful or which interferes with vision should be seen by a doctor.

Subconjunctival Haemorrhage

This is a name for what really is a bruise under the front of the eyeball. A small blood vessel may rupture under the transparent conjunctiva, either spontaneously or after a blow. A little blood spills out and forms a bright red patch on some area of the white of the eye.

It looks quite startling but it does no harm and will slowly resolve. However, the doctor may wish to check whether a raised blood pressure had been responsible for the bleed. If the eye has received a blow he will check to see if there is any other damage.

Corneal Ulcers

It is possible to think one has conjuntivitis when in fact the real trouble is one layer deeper, in the cornea. Small scratches, the brushing of some object against the eyeball, can create a little injury capable of becoming infected and of spreading both deeply and widely. Corneal scarring could result and if the area involved is within the ring of the iris, vision would be impaired. In fact, under treatment the majority do heal without trouble, but the risk of an opaque scar does justify an early medical opinion if you have any doubts.

Glaucoma

The aqueous fluid between the cornea and the lens is constantly, if slowly, being formed and drained away through minute channels. If drainage becomes impeded or if secretion is excessive then the amount and pressure of the aqueous fluid rises. As the pressure within the eye builds up it reduces the transparency of the cornea. Much more serious is the effect at the back, interfering with the blood supply to the retina and damaging fibres of the nerves of sight. Eventually it will produce blind patches in the field of vision. This can happen very gradually, so that the patient may not be aware until late of the insidious, but serious, deterioration of his eyesight.

Glaucoma is fairly common beyond middle age. About one person in every hundred over forty has some degree of glaucoma. Over the age of sixty-five it affects one in every twenty. Early symptoms might be occasional blurring of vision for some minutes, and sometimes the effect of coloured haloes around lights.

There is also an acute (i.e. sudden) form of glaucoma which strikes with dramatic symptoms. Vision may fade, pain in the eye region spreads over the face. Often general symptoms of collapse and vomiting accompany this, giving a misleading impression of some abdominal illness. This is an emergency demanding immediate specialised attention.

Treatment of glaucoma consists in drops to help the drainage or to reduce the pressure: these must be continued strictly according to the prescription. Sometimes a quite simple operation is performed. The key to success is early detection of the trouble, and the patient's reporting suspicious symptoms without delay.

Cataract

The cataract is a barrier to light. Part or all of the lens becomes opaque, interfering with vision. Spectacles will not correct this.

It may happen as a consequence of some conditions like diabetes, but in the main it is a degeneration of the lens associated with increasing age. The opacity can begin in the middle, or at the sides, affecting central or peripheral vision respectively, but in time can spread across the lens.

Treatment is surgical by removing the lens, and there are many techniques of doing this, but the very presence of a cataract is in itself no definite reason for the operation. Often the patient can see adequately with the better eye and it may be wise to delay surgery. With some techniques the specialist waits for the cararact itself to have developed enough to allow a simpler, safer, removal. Other factors to be considered are the patient's general health, whether the other eye also (as frequently is the case) has a cataract, and what facilities for sight follow removing the lens. Some specialists have replaced it with an artificial plastic lens in the eye, but this is not considered to be generally appropriate.

The period immediately after the removal can be confusing to patients. Very thick glasses may be needed but can give some distortion. Patients able to manage contact lenses may get better results. In any case they relearn vision with new aids which have fixed focussing distances instead of the natural variable adjusting one of the eye.

Floaters

This is the name given to a few fine grey specks some people occasionally notice swimming across their vision — especially if they happen to be looking at a white surface. They are of no import, being caused by harmless spots of thickening in the vitreous humour.

Detached Retina

The retina can become partly unstuck from the inside of the eyeball. This can happen spontaneously or after a blow to the eye.

To the patient it appears as if a grey or dark curtain has floated over part of his field of vision. It may seem to ease as he lies down if this position allows the detached part to settle temporarily.

Sometimes two symptoms can warn as the detachment occurs: the patient perceives flashes of light or (quite unrelated to the 'floaters' mentioned above) a sudden shower of moving dark dots. The latter are due to slight bleeding in the eye.

Early diagnosis and early treatment are needed. Various techniques get the retina to secure itself again, at the point of detachment. This can, for instance, be done by shining onto it briefly a very intense light, or by applying an extremely cold probe to the appropriate part of the eyeball.

Colour Blindness

This is not really blindness but a deficiency in interpreting or judging one or more colours. The frequency is surprising; about every two hundredth woman and every twelfth man has some degree of colour deficiency. The retina has special nerve elements for receiving messages in colour. They are of three types, dealing respectively with blue, green and red. The other colours we see are made up by mixtures of these three.

Colour deficiency generally affects only one type and the most common is that which cannot distinguish red from green. It is an inherited defect which does no harm in itself, but causes difficulties in our sophisticated world which relies on coloured signals and colour coding. Inability to interpret any colour at all, and having to see everything as black, grey or white does happen but is extremely rare.

Squinting

Any child who squints must have a medical check. But at what age? A baby who has a constantly present squint needs immediate attention. Squinting which is inconstant and intermittent is of no special significance unless it persists after the age of six months when it should be investigated. By that age children have learnt to use double vision and the eyes should be working together.

No child will 'grow out' of a squint. He may have one eye which is far-sighted and needs correction by spectacles as soon as he can be made to wear them. It is difficult, if not impossible, to correct an established squint after the age of six years. By then the squinter will have learnt to depend on one eye alone. The squinting eye, unused, will not fully develop its faculty of seeing.

Treatment then should begin early. Glasses may be prescribed, and a nice amount of skilled parental coaxing is often needed to persuade the young patient to wear them. Sometimes the sound eye is patched or covered so that the patient is made to bring the so called 'lazy eye' (i.e. the squinting eye) into proper action. Orthoptics is the name given to exercises which assist the eye muscles to work properly.

Finally surgery to modify the length of these muscles may be needed and children stand this very well.

A squint which develops in an adult can be caused by some other physical trouble, such as paralysis of the nerve serving an eye muscle. In this case it affects an eye which has been functioning fully. Therefore as the two eyes aim in different directions the patient will be seeing double.

Fainting

Fainting is due to a temporary decrease of blood supply to the brain. This can happen reflexly as the result of pain or emotion. A hot atmosphere or inadequate food may also be the cause. Long standing with immobile legs can contribute too.

Suspect a faint coming on when there is pallor, light headedness, dimming vision, swaying and feeling cold. The pulse rate is generally slow rather than fast. Try to forestall the faint with a lying down position, with head low and legs raised. Deep breathing and loosening any tight clothes at the waist or neck will help. If necessary treat for unconsciousness (p.210).

Anyone feeling faint in a crowded place like a concert hall may not be able to struggle past others. Let him sit down and bend right forwards with his head low between the legs.

Once the patient is beginning to feel better he is given a drink of cold water. But do not attempt to make him drink unless he is conscious and able to swallow. Let him lie down and recover for a few minutes longer than he wishes: the victim of a faint generally is unnecessarily apologetic and wants to get moving too soon.

Finally: smelling salts are a relic of the past and quite useless.

Fallopian Tube *see* Salpingitis

Falls

Falls about the house are the cause of many injuries, especially in the elderly. In particular the aged thigh bone is susceptible to fracture from a relatively small blow.

The home itself can contribute to the risk of falls. Few house interiors can proudly show the absence of *all* the following: slippery floors; loose mats; rucked carpet edges; uneven floors; steps between rooms; stools or objects lying in walking area; trailing flexes; absent handrails on stairways; inadequate illumination on stairs; light switches of difficult access; low chairs, difficult to rise from by the elderly. The reader is invited to survey his or her home and see how it fares.

Quite apart from such hazards, many of the elderly have to contend with poor vision (and maybe old spectacles needing replacement) and with general weakness (maybe aggravated by the side effects of necessary drugs like tranquilisers). Some also suffer from 'drop attacks': quite suddenly their legs give way and they fall without loss of consciousness. These are likely to be due to a transient defect of blood supply to the brain.

Lifting After a Fall

First check whether your patient has any injury. If there is likelihood of a fracture it is best to leave him on the floor. Without moving the fractured part make him comfortable and covered and get help.

Then clear from around him any obstructing objects like stools or mats. If you can move him and he can use his arms and legs begin by gently turning him face down. Stand over his legs: bend down (but keep your back straight) and ease him up on hands and knees by pulling at the hips.

Now bring a stool or chair in front of him, and stand to one side of him. One hand you put into the armpit and the

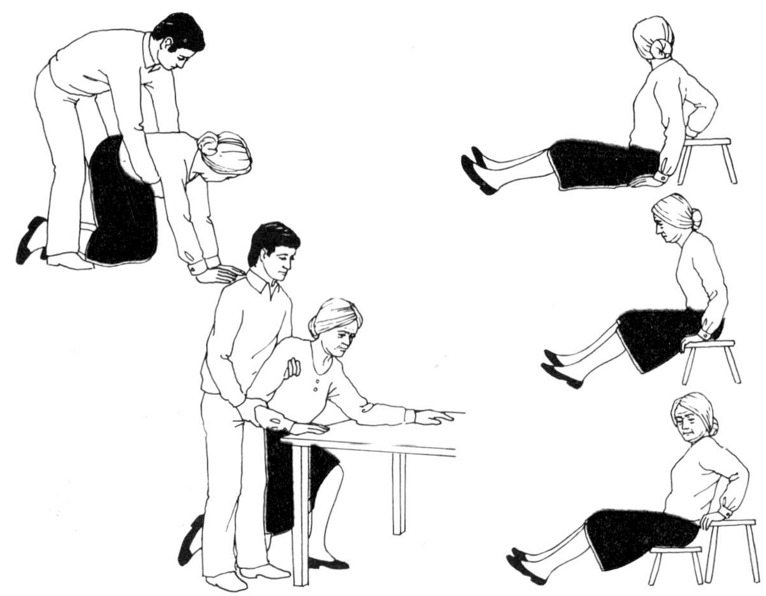

other at his elbow of the side at which you stand. Help him as he pushes himself up.

If his legs are not strong enough for the above method, get him sitting on the floor with a low stool behind him. By pushing up with hands and arms he gets himself sitting on it. The process is now repeated with a higher chair behind him.

Fevers of Children

The table summarises the average points about the 'fevers' commonly caught by children, or against which they can be protected by vaccines. The importance of such protection is described in the section on Immunisation (p.138). Each illness, including its possible complications, is also dealt with under its own heading.

The incubation period is the lapse of time between the patient catching the illness from someone else and the appearance of his first symptoms. The table gives the most likely figure; the possible variations are shown in brackets. In the same way there are variations in the period during which a patient is infective. In practically all these conditions he carries the microbes some time before he knows he is about to be ill, and can transmit them to others through the fine droplets of moisture in the air he breathes out, especially when talking.

One attack of any of these illnesses generally confers life long immunity to another attack. It is true that sometimes a second attack does show up later. This however is rare, and this second illness is likely to be very mild.

It is well worth while keeping a

Fevers of Children

Illness	Medical name	Incubation period (days)	Features	Infectiousness of patient	Immunisation possible
Chicken Pox	Varicella	14 (12-21)	Only mildly ill. Pink spots developing into small blisters, scattered over the body but specially on trunk and upper thighs. Appear in successive crops.	From 5 days before the rash to 6 days after the last crop.	No
Diptheria		2-4	Severely ill with sore throat and sometimes 'membrane' in throat handicapping breathing. Prostration and fever.	Two to three weeks from onset, less with antibiotics.	Yes
German Measles	Rubella	18 (14-21)	Mild fever and sore throat. Many small fine pink spots on body. Neck glands enlarged.	From 6 days before rash appears to 5 days after.	Yes (women of child bearing age)
Measles	Morbilli (rarely used)	10-14	Feverish 'cold' with cough and running nose. Blotchy rash of pink spots spread over body, beginning behind ears.	From onset of 'cold' to 4 days after rash appears.	Yes
Mumps	Epidemic Parotitis (rarely used)	14-28	Feverish. Painful swelling of salivary glands in front of ears and below jaw.	From 3 days before first swelling to 6 days after swellings subside.	Yes
Scarlet Fever	Scarlatina	3 (1-5)	Feverish. Very sore throat. Bright rash of fine red points over body. Peeling of skin follows.	From 10-21 days after rash appears, but 1 day only if on antibiotics.	No
Whooping Cough	Pertussis	10 (7-14)	Starts as mild cough; worsens to severe spasms of cough with whooping.	From one week after exposure to three weeks after onset, less if on antibiotics.	Yes

family record of all fevers and immunisations with their dates. This is no sign of hypochondria, but a practical move, for the question of who has had what and when, is often raised not only in school life, but also long after for business and medical reasons.

Fibroids

Fibroids are a nuisance to women, but only very rarely a danger. They are fibrous tumours in the uterus and are non-malignant (that is, they are not cancerous).

Much more common than is generally realised, they occur in some ten per cent of women over the age of forty. They can be small, or very large, they can be single or multiple. They grow very slowly and many women are unaware of possessing them and will never be bothered by the fact of their presence.

However, fibroids do sometimes give a lot of trouble. Some of them cause heavy bleeding at or between the periods. A large fibroid which projects inside the cavity of the uterus could interfere with conception, with the development of pregnancy or with the mechanics of labour. If, on the other hand, the fibroid mass were really big and pushed forward beyond the uterus into the abdominal cavity it could cause pressure symptoms there.

Occasionally the round firm fibroid hangs on a stalk like projection: and occasionally this stalk chances to twist on itself: that would give very severe pain needing immediate medical and surgical attention. More rarely a fibroid will 'degenerate', by swelling and going soft: this too will give great pain.

Treatment of a fibroid which produces no symptoms (and is discovered during examination for other things) can be summarised as follows. If it is small, leave it alone. If it is big remove it from the uterus. If it is very big or if very many are present, the uterus may have to be removed but most of the women who need this are beyond child bearing age.

Fibrositis

To some fibrositis is a very real, very painful inflammation of fibrous tissue associated with or enveloping muscles and joints; to others is almost a metaphysical concept devoid of reality. Many doctors and many textbooks deny that such a condition really exists, and seek to explain the associated symptoms in other ways. Backache (p.32) for instance is often a result of pressure on nerves from some displacement in the spinal column. Sprained ligaments or strained muscle from overuse or faulty posture could be other factors.

It is quite likely that the word will gradually slide out of the medical vocabulary, eventually to be remembered with the museum-like interest given to other discarded terms such as ptomaine poisoning.

In the meantime it is safe and reasonable to treat 'fibrositis' with the time honoured methods of heat, rest and pain relieving tablets.

First Aid

There are some European nations where it is very difficult to go through school and to grow up without having received some first aid instruction. In this country we depend on our own initiative. The sense of knowing what to do in an emergency makes the small effort extremely worth while, and that of having saved a limb or a life is beyond describing.

Classes for anyone are given regularly by the major first aid organisations. (see Useful Addresses, p.222). Your local branch is listed in the telephone book. All you have to do is enquire.

Classes are quite easy, and consist of about eight sessions of two hours each, covering both the theoretical and the practical sides. They are generally timed to make attendance easy for those who are at work.

The same curriculum is covered in concentrated courses of three days: these are specially designed for industry so that firms can send selected employees, but other members of the public may attend.

Fits

see also Breath Holding *and* Epilepsy

The temperatures of small children with a feverish infection tend to rocket up far higher than they would in an adult with a corresponding illness. The temperature may rise far enough to cause a sudden convulsion. The child becomes rigid and unconscious, his complexion darkens and he may jerk. It is very like epilepsy (p.102).

At this stage you do not leave the child to call for help. You stay with him. The attack will probably not last long, but it could be dangerous if the child's airway were not protected, as described in the section on unconsciousness (p.210).

Get him into the recovery position, see that his head is low. If his temperature is very high get his clothes off and cool him either by fanning or by long slow strokes over his body with a wet cold sponge. Do not try to reduce the temperature to normal. One or two degrees down should be enough to have it below the level likely to cause another fit. Then dry the child and cover him lightly.

These fits are frightening, of course, and to be taken seriously. However most clear quickly. They have to their credit that they tend to appear at the onset of the illness, so alerting parents to call the doctor early.

Fleas

The flea is about 3mm long. It is an insect without wings but makes up for this by being able to jump up about 25cm and forward 30cm. It gets around. Especially onto animals, since it is a parasite which lives on their blood. After piercing the skin with a sharp proboscis it sucks up the blood, which it prevents from clotting by means of a chemical in its saliva. Its very flat shape allows it to forage about easily among fur and feather.

There are over 2000 species of flea, and they have predelictions for certain animals. One type of flea is found on dogs, another on birds, another on cats and another on man. But most fleas are by no means confined to one animal. If circumstances dictate they will move to the nearest suitable, warm blooded, alternative host. Thus man can receive the attention of fleas from his pets.

Saliva injected by the bites of fleas can cause dermatitis with irritation, and allergic reactions, especially in children. Far worse is the ability to transmit disease.

The flea lays its eggs not on the host animal but in its habitat. An empty house may harbour eggs and fleas for months. When it is re-occupied the hungry insects will land on their new hosts. Fortunately the flea is susceptible to usual insecticides, including D.D.T.

Food Poisoning

see also Diarrhoea

The words 'food poisoning' have a very wide and therefore unsatisfactorily vague meaning. However, the usually accepted meaning covers vomiting, colicky abdominal pain and diarrhoea due to the presence of bacteria or their toxins. Bacteria can act in different ways. Some may produce their poisons in a food which, being kept at room temperature, acts as a culture medium. Typical are milk and cream products and also processed meat and fish. Cooking (or reheating) the food may kill the bacteria but leave the poisons unaffected. In this case the symptoms appear a few hours after eating.

Other bacteria may act after being swallowed with the food. There will be a time interval of a day or two while they develop in the gut before the patient becomes ill.

One very dangerous and rare bacterial infection is called botulism. It is different from other types in that it acts on the nervous system, rather than give diarrhoea and vomiting. The microbes may be present in foods, especially meats, that have been inadequately tinned or preserved. They produce a potent poison which paralyses. The earliest symptoms appear suddenly, about a day after the food was taken (though the time may vary from a few hours to a week). Double and blurred vision, facial paralysis and difficulty in speaking or swallowing may be followed by weakness of chest muscles and difficulty in breathing, which can be fatal.

One might expect all who share the same meal which gives food poisoning to be affected in the same way. In fact there are all grades of individual response, some escaping entirely and others severely stricken.

All too often those who suspect food poisoning in a household will in disgust throw away the remnants of any suspected food. They should, on the contrary, carefully and safely put it to one side. The doctor may wish to subject it to laboratory tests. This could be a very important community health measure, helping to trace the source of any infection, to prevent a recurrence and to discover any infringements of important hygiene regulations.

Foot Rot *see* Tinea

Foot Troubles

The basic function of a foot is movement, involving especially the smaller bones at the front. Secondary is bearing the weight of the body, on the big chunky bones at the back. This combination of stability and of springiness is enhanced by the natural arches of the foot.

A flat foot is one where tired muscles have relaxed their support, and the longitudinal arches tend to sink, with consequent stretching of those ligaments holding the bones together. The transverse arch is less affected. It is this stretching and pressure on nerves which can cause pain not so much of the flat foot, as of the flattening foot. Once the process of stretching is complete the foot aches no more. It may be a little less efficient than before, but will function perfectly.

Long standing daily without moving the foot is one predisposing cause. If you have to stay upright at work at least try to keep your feet in some form of movement.

The pain of flattening feet can be treated by exercise and by physiotherapy to tone up the muscles. Arch supports may help. They should not be bought haphazardly in a shop, but be selected or made for the individual foot through orthopaedic or chiropodist's advice.

Parents often are dismayed by the apparent flatness of toddler's feet. Let them be reassured. The arches are truly present but hidden beyond the pads of fat which fill the feet at that age.

No part of the human body is as ill treated as the foot of civilised man, which all too often is boxed in tight footwear quite anatomically inappropriate. *Callosities,* patches of thickened and compressed skin, are one example; their pressure on underlying nerve ending can be very painful. When situated on toes we call them *corns.* In either case the use of felt pads or rings to relieve the pressure is only an alleviation. Patient paring and specialist treatment by a chiropodist is the answer.

The bunion at the base of a big toe is a sad and very common example of deformity caused by tight shoes and pointed toe caps. Shoes should have

The longitudinal arch of the healthy foot keeps the bones raised with correspondingly shaped footprint.

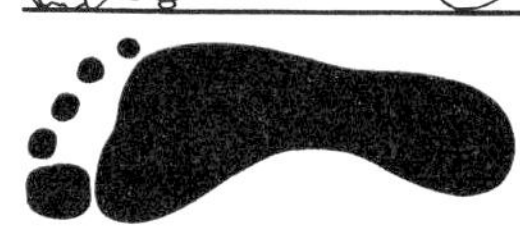

A flat foot has the arch dropped and a broadened footprint.

A good pair of feet: the inner border, including the big toe, is almost a straight line and the toes all stand free.

Feet cramped by fashionable footwear.

bunion

overlapping toes

hammer toes

displaced big toe

the inner side more or less straight to correspond with the shape of the foot. Sharp pointed shoes cramp the toes together, and the big toe is the main sufferer. The joint at its base becomes angled and prominent. Eventually it stays that way. From shoe friction it develops the bunion. The only satisfactory treatment is a simple and successful operation which reshapes the bone at the joint to recreate the straight line.

Hammer toes are the result of back to front cramping: one or more joints become stiffened in a sharply bent position. Many a set of toes shows a horror combination of twisting, overlapping and underriding through having been forced together into a tight torture chamber called a fashionable shoe. The condition can be made even worse by high and narrow heels. Not only do these give little space to the supporting heel bones, but also they let the foot slide forward into the toe cap.

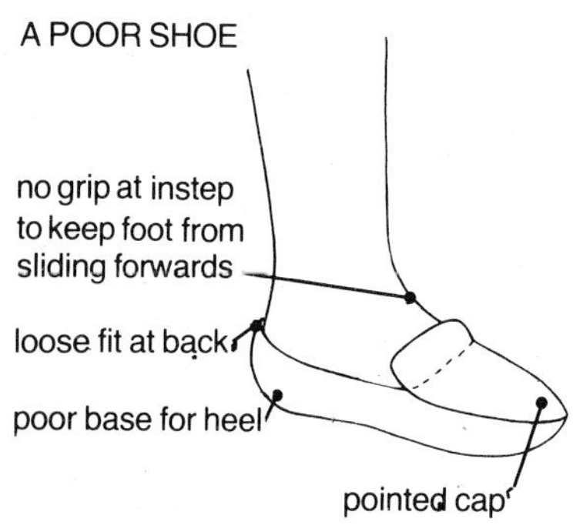

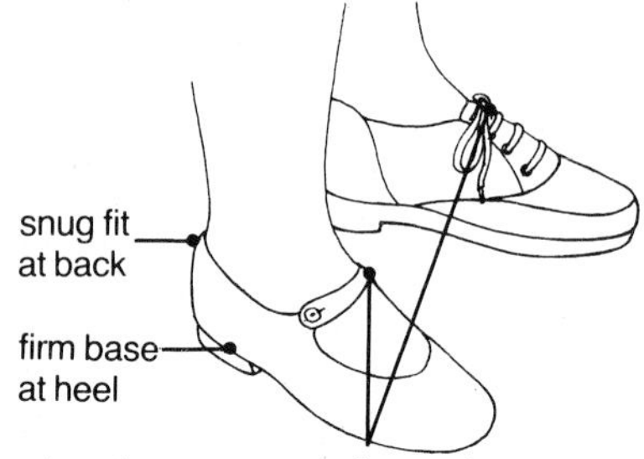

We are accustomed to associate many foot miseries with the elderly. However they are the end result of errors made when the sufferers were much younger. One cannot begin too soon to safeguard the shape of feet. Allow babies every chance to develop muscles as they kick their legs about for many foot movements depend on tendons coming from leg muscles. Keep blankets, leggings and bootees loose.

Do not let pride make you try to get a baby walking younger than did the neighbour's child. Allow him to crawl until he shows himself ready to experiment with the vertical position. Do not give him real shoes until he is walking: the bones are still soft and their early adventures or misadventures will mould them in the right or wrong ways. Small children do not register pain as their feet are being spoilt; it is later that the resultant deformity can be painful.

Buy shoes from a shop which prides itself in having an expert trained fitter, who measures the feet. That you find shoes comfortable when trying them on is not enough. Check them standing and walking before buying.

The feet of old people tend to spread: they must not be content to order shoe sizes which were right for them in years past. Another fallacy of the elderly concerns shuffling around in 'comfortable' slippers. Properly fitting shoes are less tiring and far safer for those prone to falls.

Often overlooked is the fact that tight socks and stockings can be just

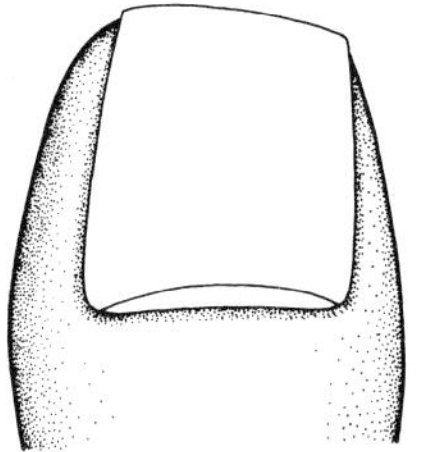

nail cut straight and beyond the toe will not give trouble

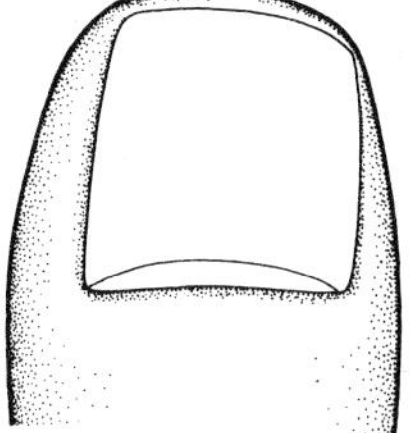

nail cut short and curved presents edges digging into the skin fold . . .

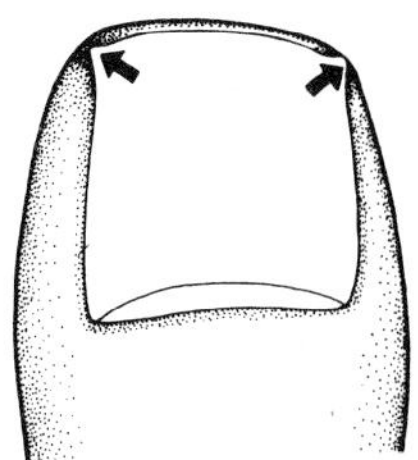

. . . and as it grows forwards these edges burrow into the folds causing pressure, pain and infection

as harmful as shoes too small. If they are stretch let them still remain relatively loose around the foot.

The ingrowing toenail is a hazard which can come from footwear pressure, but is due mainly to over-enthusiastic cutting of the big toe nail. If it develops do not keep cutting away at it; that would make it worse. Consult a doctor or chiropodist.

One last piece of advice. The State Registered Chiropodist is an extremely well trained expert. His help and his care for feet in difficulties are invaluable. Use him.

See also Tinea *and* Warts (Verucca)

Fractures

A fracture, by definition, is a broken bone. It is in fact much more than that to the victim. Our bones lie alongside muscles, blood vessels, nerves, ligaments and important organs like brain, bladder or liver. It is just not possible to fracture a bone without doing some harm to the adjacent softer tissues. Often this is not very grave, but sometimes it can be disastrous. The first aid approach must keep this in mind; well meant but inexpert help may move the broken ends and increase the damage.

First Aid

This is the first aid plan.

1. Suspect a fracture whenever a blow or crush is followed by some (not necessarily all) of the following features: pain, swelling, unnatural shape, weakness of the affected part or inability to move it properly. There is no shame in being over cautious here, but there is regret if one dismisses a real fracture as being only a 'nasty strain'. The blow which breaks a bone can be surprisingly slight, especially in the elderly. Sometimes the fracture is far from the point where the blow was received. The force of a fall on a heel may transmit itself up the leg to break the thigh bone near the hip; a very hard blow to the jaw could fracture the skull; a man who stretches out his arm as he falls on his hand can find the shoulder disabled from a snapped collar bone.

The softer and more supple bones of young children often break not across, but with a split along part of its length, rather as would a young juicy branch of a growing shrub. This is the appropriately named *greenstick fracture*. The child will show a puffy painful part, which he is unwilling to use, and the damage may look quite slight, but give it the benefit of the doubt and treat it like a fracture.

2. If you suspect a fracture, tell the patient not to move and make sure well meaning bystanders do not try to move him.

3. However, you must deal immediately with bad bleeding (p.46) and you should dress any wound (p.220). You do these trying not to disturb the part which may bear a broken bone. Do not lift up a limb to fix a bandage on it; slide the bandage beneath it. Avoid hard pressure.

4. Full first aid training teaches the correct ways to immobilise each part of the body, so as to safeguard the broken bones. If you have not had this training and if your are expecting expert help, let the patient be still and wait.

5. Take steps to minimise shock (p.183). Remember that if your patient is likely to become unconscious or drowsy or to need an anaesthetic then you should give him nothing to eat or drink: there are chances he could vomit and breathe into his air passages whatever he has brought up.

When expert help will NOT be available, you will then have to immobilise the fractured part yourself. The diagrams will help you to do this.

JAW

wide bandage

thick soft pad

Clear the mouth gently; remove dentures. If he can, patient sits up, bends forward (to let the blood flow out), supports jaw with the pad until you get the bandage on. If he is unconscious or drowsy put him in recovery position.

FOOT AND ANKLE

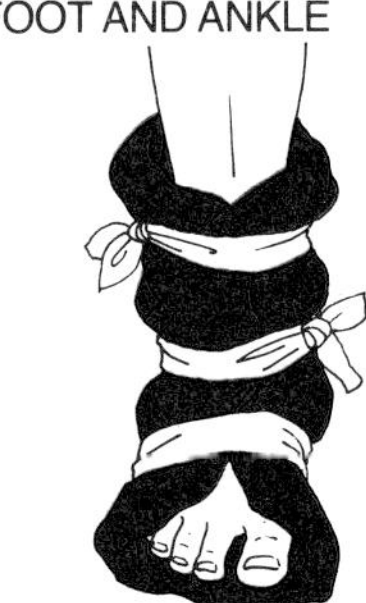

wrap round and bandage firmly a thick cushion or rolled up blanket

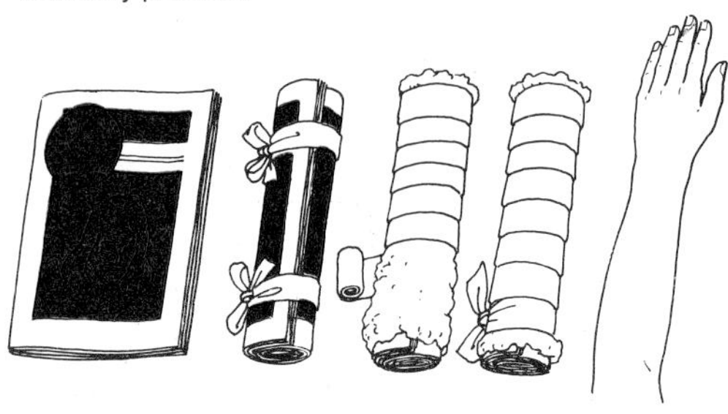

IMPROVISED SPLINT
A magazine or thick newspaper rolled and tied then lightly padded and bandaged, can be bandaged carefully against an injured forearm, wrist and hand before applying sling.

COLLAR BONE

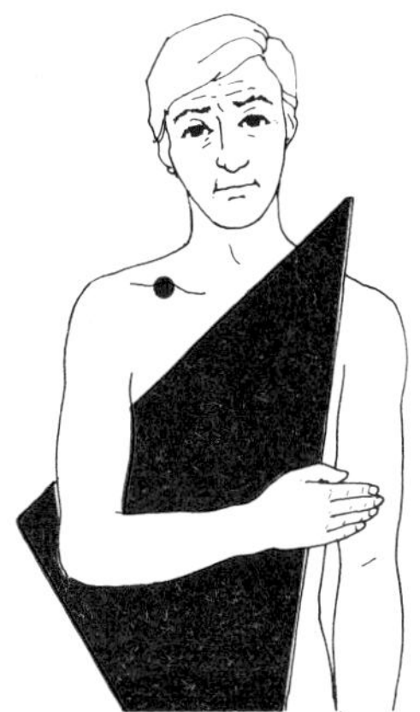
keep forearm sloping slightly

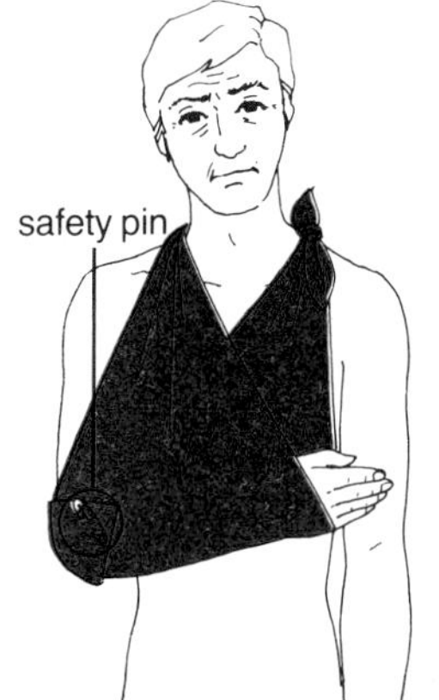

tie the knot on the good side

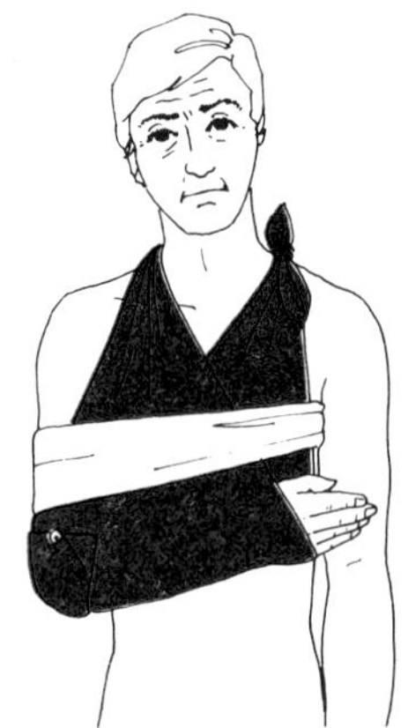
upper arm secured against chest by wide bandage

IMPROVISED SLING

Use scarf or one of these methods

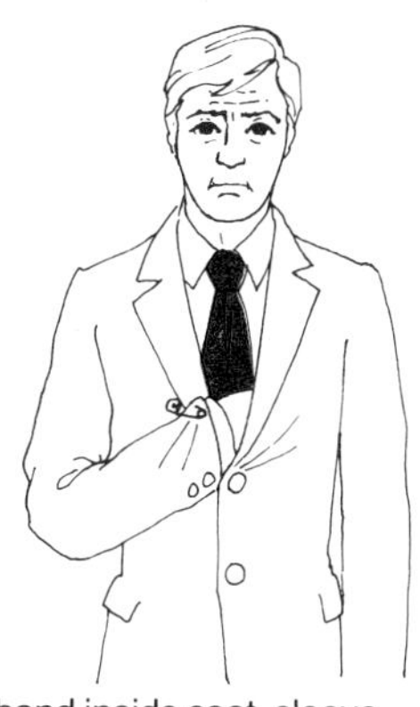
hand inside coat, sleeve pinned to lapel

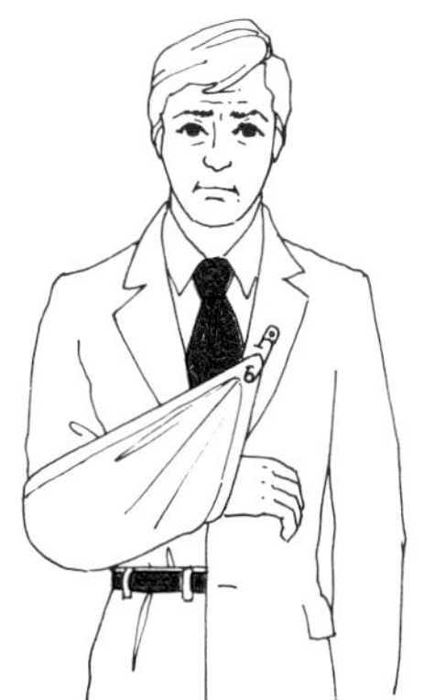
coat end turned up and its tip pinned to the opposite lapel

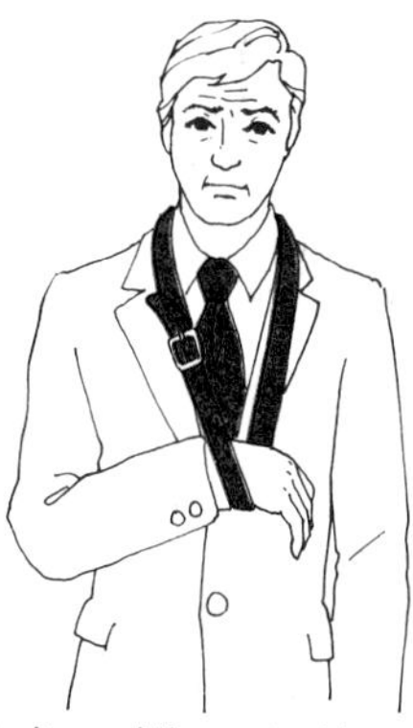
belt, necktie or stocking

LOWER LIMB

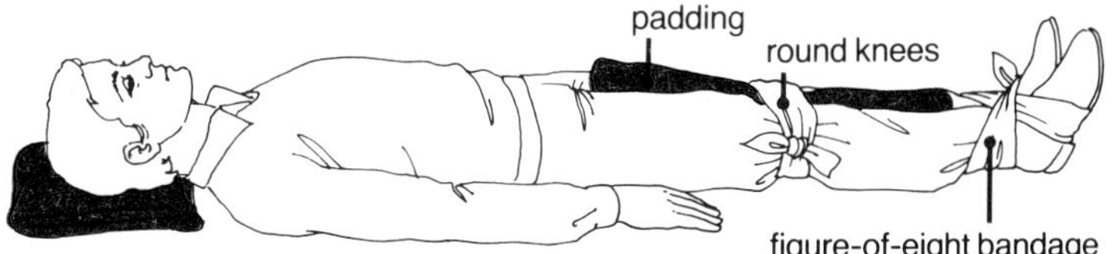

In general: use the patient's body as splint whenever possible; move the uninjured part to the injured part; put padding (e.g. wool, scarves, handkerchiefs) well tucked into spaces between the two body parts; place all bandages (scarves, towels, stockings) in position before knotting any (do not place any over where you believe the fracture to lie); tie the knots firmly (not tightly) over the uninjured part; be gentle throughout.

UPPER LIMB

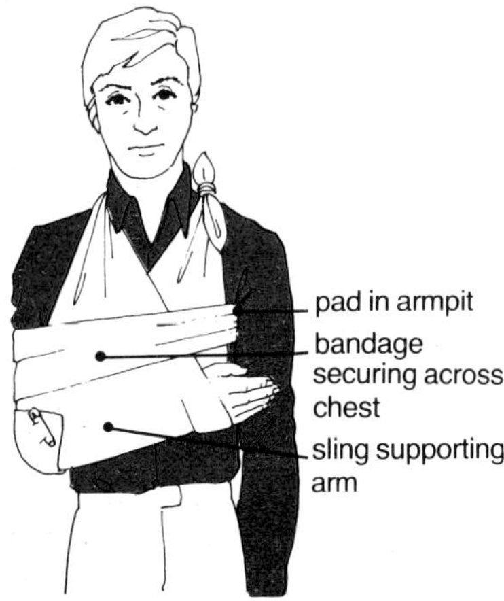

Where elbow is bent or can be bent without pain

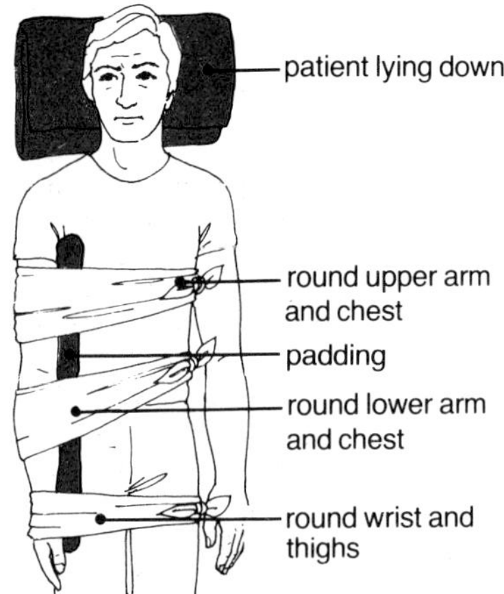

Where elbow is straight or cannot be bent

The Fractured Spine

From the neck to the lower back the vertebral column houses the spinal cord of nerves. A fracture of any vertebra might allow loosened bone to damage nerve tracts, causing paralysis or loss of feeling. This possibility is greatly increased by mishandling the patient, especially by lifting or bending him.

Always suspect a fractured spine if a severe blow or a fall from a height causes back or neck pain. *Leave the patient in the position in which you found him and wait for the experts to take over.* In the meantime you can bank rolled up coats or blankets on either side of him, and also keep him warm with a loose cover.

Frostbite

In intense cold the blood vessels narrow and the skin becomes very white and devitalised, mainly at the nose, ears, chin, fingers and toes. In severe cases there is risk of gangrene. Treat the skin gently; never rub it. Do not rewarm fast by very hot water, fire or hot water bottles. This would damage the vessels and the blood within them. It would also be painful.

Action Outdoors

At once remove anything tight near the frost bitten part; glove, ring, garter. The area may swell up. Put the affected part under dry warm cover. For example wrap frost bitten feet up in a blanket or sleeping bag; tuck a frost bitten hand under clothing in the armpit; cover the chin and nose with a dry warm hand.

Bring the patient indoors as soon as possible. You can allow him to walk short distances on frost bitten feet but not if they have been rethawed; he must then be carried.

Action Indoors

Bring the patient into a warm room. Get him into warm clothes and give him warm drinks. Rewarm the *affected part* by immersing it (if possible) in moderately warm water, just comfortable to the skin; this would be at about 103°F (40°C). Dab it dry gently, but do not rub it.

If you cannot immerse it then rewarm it slowly at room temperature. This could take some time. Now cover the part quite loosely with a clean dry dressing, and keep it elevated.

Frozen Shoulder

see Shoulder Troubles

Gall Bladder

see also Jaundice

The breakdown of fats in the intestine is achieved by digestive juices from the pancreas; these enter the first part of the intestines at a point just beyond the stomach. But (as anyone at the kitchen sink can testify) fats are not easy things to deal with. The pancreatic juices are aided by the addition of bile, which emulsifies fats — that is they break the masses up into a great number of minute globules, so that juices can get to work easily.

Bile is a thick fluid, loaded with pigments which give it a bright yellow or green colour. As it becomes concentrated in the gall bladder reservoir it becomes thicker. Any mild irritation or inflammation of this organ can start off the process where some of the bile chemicals come out of solution and solidify, in much the same way as crystals can form in a very saturated solution of salt or sugar. The first tiny solid particles act as centres around which more is deposited, so that gradually stones can develop.

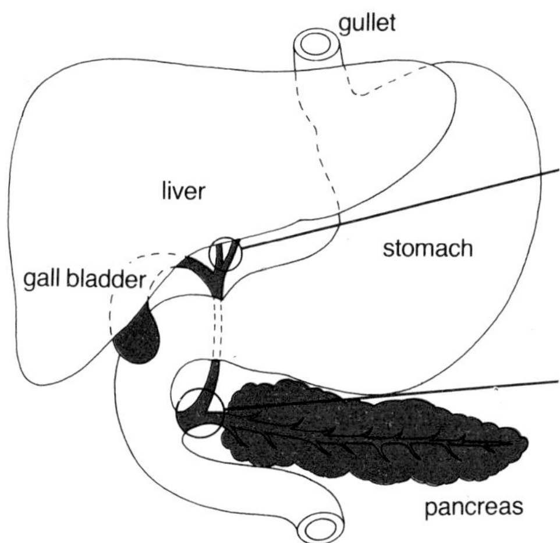

The liver, among its many functions, forms bile. Two tubes from the liver unite to lead bile into the gall bladder. Here it is stored and, by absorption of water from it, concentrated.

When fats are to be digested bile passes through another tube into the first part of the intestines just beyond the stomach. At the same point there enters the tube bringing digestive juices from the pancreas.

All medical students have heard the adage that the typical gallstone patient is 'fat, female and forty'. It is quite true that the more obese and the more beyond middle age one is, the more likely is this trouble to come, and also that women are more prone to it than men.

Many people, men and women, bear gallstones without any definite symptoms. They may have but one or they may have very many. As long as these stones are relatively small and sit quietly in the gall bladder they do not advertise themselves, but the chronic inflammation which so often accompanies them is not always so silent. The ill-defined symptoms, more likely to appear after a very fatty meal, include nausea, flatulence and upper abdominal discomfort and pain (labelled 'heartburn'). At times the pain can radiate towards the right shoulder blade.

An acutely flaring inflammation gives more intense symptoms. Very often this is due not merely to inflammation but also because a stone has moved and jammed at the exit of the gall bladder, or in the tubes leading from it. The flow of bile is obstructed; pressure in the gall bladder as well as distension of the blocked tube may create severe colicky pain.

When the diagnosis of gallstones needs confirming X-ray information can be very useful, though not always absolutely dogmatic. A few stones have the appropriate chemical composition which makes them 'seen' by X-rays. The majority however are of a quite different chemical nature and will not show up with radiography. Then the tests are repeated after giving the patient (by mouth or by injection) special preparations which concentrate in the gall bladder and which are detectable by X-rays. In the picture the shape and density of the gall bladder and its tubes can give a strong clue as to the presence and situation of stones.

Treatment is generally a straightforward operation to remove the gall bladder. The ducts from liver to intestine are left so that the supply of bile for digestion of fats continues, and patients do very well.

Inevitably one asks whether it is possible to dissolve the stone without recourse to surgery. The answer is that only some types of gallstones are susceptible to dissolution under the action of a certain drug. Even so this, at present at least, is not a perfect treatment. Sometimes the gall bladder itself is so scarred with continuing inflammation that the patient would be better without it. The dissolving process is a very slow one, so that the drug has to be taken for many months. Then, when it has achieved its purpose and is discontinued, the gall bladder might return to its bad habit of forming stones. Also the medicine sometimes has a displeasing side effect of causing diarrhoea. So even when the stones are of a chemical type which might respond, this tedious treatment is likely to be reserved for those few patients whose general condition makes them unsuited to have an operation.

Gangrene

This is the death of a tissue or an organ. It implies that it has happened through the cutting off of the blood supply, and there is implication of decomposition by bacterial action, especially when the blood supply has been stopped suddenly and has not decreased gradually. The affected tissue cannot benefit from the anti-bacterial defences of blood nor, in treatment, from antibiotics carried in the blood stream.

What could restrict blood supply? Clearly any blocking or severing of a large artery would do this, especially when the organ concerned receives its vessels from one source, and not from several. A clot which has been set free in the blood stream may suddenly jam in a vessel or the vessel may have been building up abnormal thickening or clot layers inside until the obstruction is complete. Such thickenings occur in some arterial diseases or as complications of certain illnesses, including diabetes. Smoking is known to worsen the situation considerably.

Arteries may narrow by spasm of their muscle walls. Intense cold over a long period will do this, threatening the fingers and toes. There are poisions like ergot which will cause spasm. Some chemicals absorbed through the skin will damage and close blood vessels. Phenol (carbolic acid) is one of them; it has been known for people to lose their fingers after foolishly applying strong phenol dressings as wound antiseptics.

The area concerned darkens, becomes blue and then black. A gangrenous toe, dry and mummified in appearance, may eventually separate off. When gangrene appears wet, soggy, malodourous this is a sign of much infection, with a very real danger of its spread in the body.

Defective Leg Circulation

The human leg is a common site of circulation trouble. The large artery in or leading to the thigh can become blocked or narrowed by disease or clot. Very often the patient experiences what doctors call 'intermittent claudication', long before gangrene is liable to supervene. This means that, as he uses the leg its muscles receive inadequate circulation and indicate this by pain. He can walk a short distance only before the pain makes him limp and brings him to a stop. After a rest, during which the inactive muscles recover, he can proceed only to be forced to pause again.

Such symptoms of duskiness and numbness in the foot need medical advice. An operation to disconnect nerves which contract the vessels may help. Drugs to dilate blood vessels are sometimes tried. But these measures have small effect where arteries have become too thick and inelastic. Surgeons are able to replace lengths of obstructed arteries by grafting on artificial tubes.

Where gangrene is definitely established with an infection risk, then amputation may well be needed, done at a level which still has an adequate blood supply.

In all cases the patient *must stop smoking completely*.

Gas Gangrene

This is a dangerous and special form of gangrene due to infection by certain invasive bacteria which can be found in the intestines of man and animals, in soil or in dust. They thrive in the absence of air. Contaminating deep wounds they will live on crushed or dead muscles, spreading on to adjoining tissues and destroying those in turn. Their life processes produce a foul smelling gas, which makes the infected area crackle to touch.

This is a very serious infection, whose risk can be countered by early surgery to the injured area, excising all damaged and devitalised tissues, and applying a specific antitoxin.

Gastro-enteritis

see Food Poisoning *and* Indigestion

German Measles

Medical Name: Rubella

see also Fevers of Children *and* Immunisation

This has no connection with measles which is due to another virus. Its incubation period ranges from 14 to 21 days and it is highly infectious; the patient is at his most infectious about five days before the rash appears, and ceases being infectious about the same time after.

Symptoms are mild. The rash consists of fine pink spots (less pronounced than those of measles); they appear first on the face and behind the ears, then spread downwards to the trunk and limbs. The glands about the neck and below the ears are large and knobbly. A snuffly nose or a sore throat can sometimes feature, but slightly. The child may be kept in bed until the rash and low fever have gone and that is all. However, adults who get German measles generally do rather worse and may also get headaches, sore eyes and painful joints.

Complications are rare and, though they include brain inflammation (encephalitis), they are likely to clear completely.

German Measles in Pregnancy

Mild as the illness may be to a child, to the pregnant women it is a sinister menace. If she has German measles the virus can invade the placenta and from there reach the blood and the body of the foetus. It may be severe enough to kill the baby but generally it alters the growth of some organs, particularly those which are developing at that stage of pregnancy.

Of all the lesions to the baby deafness is the commonest and this is difficult to detect at birth. Heart malformations are also likely and damage to eyes is another dreadful possibility. The worst effects occur when the mother has German measles during the first four months of the pregnancy. After that the danger is considerably less, but has not entirely gone. Any pregnant woman will avoid contact with a German measles case unless she is entirely certain she is immune which can be verified by a blood test. If she does catch the illness she should discuss with her doctor the difficult problem of whether to terminate the pregnancy. He will be able to give her some of the relevant statistics, for by no means all the babies of these women are damaged.

These disasters are avoidable. Protecting women of child-bearing age against German measles is described in the section on immunisation.

Glandular Fever

Glandular fever affects chiefly the young adult and its virus is caught characteristically by face to face contact. This being so favoured an exercise among the young it is lucky that the infectivity is relatively low. However, when it hits it is frequently debilitating and interrupts the typical patient's programmed activities of study or training.

Its incubation period varies greatly from some four to ten weeks. Symptoms in the first few days appear vaguely, insidiously, rather like influenza, until the characteristic sore throat develops. With it comes enlargement of glands all over the body, but most easily discernible in the neck, armpit and groin. They may be quite tender. Undiscernible are all those glands deeper in the body which also undergo enlargement. So much is involved in all systems that it is no wonder that most patients feel weak and depressed. They tend to perspire heavily, and a number get a rash which mimics that of German measles.

One organ always involved to some extent is the liver which may become enlarged and may sometimes be severely enough affected to cause jaundice. Characteristic are certain changes in the blood, shown by laboratory tests but not always present in the first few days of the illness. Among these is an increase in the number of white blood cells called 'mononuclears', which gives glandular fever its medical name of infectious mononucleosis.

Treatment is limited mainly to resting the patient and to easing his symptoms. In some cases corticosteroids (p.79) are prescribed to reduce inflammation but their use is not general. The patient recovers within one week to one month, but even then he is not his normal self for some time yet. Because of the liver involvement he is well advised to abstain from alcohol for a month after, or longer if he actually had jaundice; his doctor will guide on this. Sometimes weakness, sweating and general misery can persist a long time, troubling a patient who considers he should by now be fully convalescent.

Glaucoma

see Eye Troubles

Glue Ear

see Ear Troubles

Gout

Anyone can have gout. Anyone, that is, whose kidneys do not filter out enough uric acid into the urine. Uric acid is a breakdown product of many substances eaten and also from naturally worn out body cells. It is therefore normally found in the blood and the kidneys excrete it. If too much uric acid is produced and if the kidneys fail to pass it out adequately then excess accumulates and is deposited in various parts of the body in crystal form. In particular it may settle in joints, in skin and in kidneys.

Men, especially over middle age, are more likely to suffer than women. There is also a family tendency to the disease. A greedy, lustful life has nothing to do with it.

The acute attack often hits in the night, waking the patient with intense pain in one joint over which the skin becomes swollen, red and shiny. This pain has been described as if the joint were being gnawed by a dog. A common site is the big toe, but gout can affect any other place like knee, elbow or finger.

Why it should happen so suddenly is uncertain, but a minor injury (even an ill fitting shoe) could be a factor. A heavily alcoholic episode might play its part by temporarily reducing the kidney's power to excrete uric acid.

Another, and odd, form of deposit is the tophus. This is a nodule of uric acid salts just under the skin. Some of its favourite perches are on the edge of ears and by the knees or elbows.

Untreated gout may eventually deposit enough crystals into joints to deform and to handicap them severely. Inside the kidneys they can even build up into stones; these may become large enough to cause kidney failure.

Treatment of the sudden attack is by one of several rapidly acting anti-inflammatory drugs. With ease of pain and return to activity the patient is apt to heave a sigh of relief and to try to forget the whole thing. Not so the doctor who will continue to observe and prescribe. Gout is a permanent condition of abnormal body chemistry which could work against the patient's joints and kidneys even between accute attacks. The patient must indefinitely try to control it. Monitored by tests on the blood's uric acid level, further treatment will be by medicines which either reduce the formation of uric acid or encourage the kidneys to excrete it.

These drugs are very successful and obviate any need of diet restriction. Some foods contain heavy amounts of substances which create uric acid. In the past patients were told to exclude from their gastronomic pleasures things like goose, duck, venison, meat extracts, liver, brain, fish roes, sardines, rhubarb, spinach and strawberries. Today as long as they do not overdo it and their doctors do not disapprove they may continue to enjoy these . . . provided they do not default on their tablets.

The Handicapped

At first sight many of those hit by paralysis after strokes, by arthritis or by nerve diseases appear condemned to inactivity. A great deal of independence is restored by the use of special gadgets. Some are costly, but many are simple and inexpensive. Patients and their families will get advice and help from doctors and from the social services. Organisations like the Red Cross can provide items. The Disabled Living Foundation has a show of gadgets and a catalogue of very helpful books. But in every case let the patient make the first approach to his or her general practitioner.

A Few Examples of Gadgets that can Help the Disabled

In the bathroom: for the single handed, nail brush with suction pads to anchor the brush, bristles up; brushes, combs and sponges on long handles to overcome the problem of arms that cannot be fully lifted; raised lavatory seats and support bars for around lavatories.

For dressing; for those who cannot bend, gadgets for pulling on stockings and tights; long handled shoe horns; elastic shoe laces to avoid having to tie the knot each time; clip-on neckties; rug hooks for single-handed button fastening; velcro fastenings instead of buttons.

Furniture: high-seated chairs and blocks to fit on the legs of furniture to raise it; chairs with lifting seats to make rising easier.

For walking: specially shaped walking stick handles for arthritic hands; tripod sticks of adjustable height for greater stability; walking frames that can be fitted with baskets for carrying small objects.

For domestic work: gadgets to fit over stiff taps to turn them; easy turn taps for gas and electric cookers; trays with a handle and a rubber surface to prevent slipping for the single handed; bread slicers, non-slip mixing bowls, combined potato peelers and slicers for the single handed: long handled brushes and dust pans; safe kettle pourers; rocker-type electric switches which can be worked by light touch; electric plugs with special grips that can be pulled out easily.

For eating: thick handled cutlery for easy gripping; angled cutlery for when arm and shoulder movements are limited; one implement combining knife, fork and spoon for the single handed; plastic 'bunker' to be clipped onto plates to help the single handed collect food.

These and many other aids can help the physically handicapped to lead an independent life.

Haemorrhage *see* Bleeding

Haemorrhoids

These very common nuisances (also called piles) are abnormal dilatations of veins around and inside the rectum (back passage). Since they tend to appear in families heredity may play a part, but their anatomy already predisposes to trouble. These veins lie relatively unsupported in rather loose tissue which makes it only too easy for them to bulge. They are subject to squeezing pressures during bowel action, especially in any straining from constipation. Another factor can be the irritation of diarrhoea, whether from illness or from reckless use of purgatives.

Some abdominal conditions (including pregnancy) which give overfilling of the larger vessels higher up into which the veins lead will also cause bulging. But we must not overlook posture; by leaving his past evolutionary quadrupedal position to stand erect man has caused extra gravitational pressure on the veins.

Once abnormally distended these veins may remain within the rectum or they may worsen to project out either temporarily or permanently. They may burst: it is quite unusual for the blood loss to be heavy, but if it goes on day after day even the slightest bleeding can cause severe anaemia.

Never assume that bleeding from the back passage is due to piles and dismiss it as a bother which might correct itself. Haemorrhoids certainly are the most likely cause, but ulcers and tumours also bleed, so you must get a medical examination and opinion.

Pain is the one symptom which does not accompany haemorrhoids, unless some complication hits them. This could be inflammation or clotting. It could be a nipping or twisting which blocks the blood flow so that they swell to a sore, red, cushiony mass.

The simplest treatment for the simplest form of piles is to ensure a nice easy bowel action either by stopping unnecessary purgatives, or to manage constipation by adding roughage to the diet and (under the doctor's supervision) taking very mild laxatives. Suppositories are medicated semi-solid substances to be pushed into the rectum: some forms may help to reduce congestion. Certain injections can close up the base of the veins. If these measures are insufficient an operation will remove obstinate piles.

Hay Fever *see also* Allergy

It rarely causes fever, and it has little to do with hay. Here we deal with sensitivity to pollen, the fine powdery male fertilising substance produced by plants. The more specific, but rarely used, medical term is *pollinosis.*

It is an allergy which shows up seasonally when pollen is airborne, and is worse in hot dry weather. Rainy conditions reduce the amount of pollen flying about. From about February to May pollens from trees are present. Those from grasses are let loose from May to July, though certain forms persist to September.

Hay fever is rare in small children, but can show up after the age of five and adolescents are the chief sufferers. They may find comfort in the theory that hay fever is more frequent in the 'cultivated classes'.

Attacks begin with itching of the nose, mouth and eyes. The eyes become reddened, tear laden and sensitive to light. A watery discharge, with sneezing, flows from the nose. The severely stricken victim presents a sad and anti-social picture, and in some cases may develop asthmatic wheezing.

Treatment consists in seeking relief from antihistamines (p.19) with their occasional disadvantages, or from other preparations, taken by mouth or as nose and eye applications. However, overuse of nose drops will increase inflammation of its swollen membranes. Wearing dark glasses may reduce the eye discomfort.

Desensitisation outside the hay fever season, and in preparation for it, is sometimes, but only sometimes, successful as a preventative. A series of carefully graduated injections of pollen extracts is given to make the body build up defences.

Beekeepers offer a different way of desensitisation. Honey and especially the wax capping on honeycombs, contains pollen. For two to four months before he expects his hay fever the patient takes a tablespoonful of cappings (or, failing this, of honey) with each meal. He should try to obtain this from local hives, bearing the pollen to which he is likely to be exposed. This pleasant and simple method is often effective.

Headache *see also* Migraine

Headache is an extremely difficult subject to describe with dogmatism and accuracy. It is one of the commonest symptoms of being unwell, and quite certainly one of the most difficult to explain.

Only rarely does it mean anything serious. To be sure it could be due to meningitis or to a brain tumour, but headaches are due to very ordinary conditions, from measles to anxiety, from colds to hangovers . . . the list seems endless.

The brain itself is insensitive and does not feel pain; it only registers pain from elsewhere. However, its membranous coverings are very sensitive to pressure, or to stretching, and its blood vessels to dilatation or contraction.

Constipation is sometimes falsely blamed for headache. Raised blood pressure, unless very severe, is not a likely cause either. Nor are eyes which need new spectacles, though abnormally heavy work of eyeball muscles might be a factor.

Occasional headaches are not a cause for worry. Fortunately the huge majority respond to simple measures like lying down and taking asprin or paracetamol. If, however, they appear with extreme intensity, if they recur often or if they are persistent, then the doctor should be consulted.

He will be helped if the patient comes prepared to answer the following points. When did the headache first appear? Is it constant? If not how frequently does it happen? What is its site? Is it associated with any event? Do other symptoms (such as nausea, pain elsewhere, difficult balance, poor vision or fever) accompany it? Does position affect it? Does anything aggravate or ease it?

Head Injuries

At the risk of causing moments of unnecessary concern and perhaps of adding to the burdens of general practitioners, a wise piece of advice is not to take head injuries lightly. Their complications, though rare, tend to develop insidiously and unpleasantly.

The Cut Scalp

Richly served by blood vessels and structured with elastic fibres which pull wounds open, the scalp bleeds copiously when it is cut. You need to apply firm pressure with a thick pad (handkerchief, gauze) for at least ten uninterrupted minutes to control it.

If a sharp blow gave this wound it is just possible that the nearby bone was cracked. Then there arises the risk of infection spreading through this from the cut area into the underlying brain. You are well justified in seeking a medical opinion.

The Fractured Skull

In spite of its reputation the skull is very vulnerable. It is only a fair, and by no means a perfect, protector of the brain within and not designed to parry heavy blows. In potentially dangerous activities like riding a motorcycle or working on a building site, failing to wear the appropriate helmet is no mark of toughness, but displays both weakness and stupidity.

A blow on the top or side of the head can fracture the skull (see illustration). This could show up as bruising around the eye, bleeding from the nose or bleeding from the ear. Such features should make you suspect the possibility of fracture and get medical advice at once. If there is blood from the ear it is not likely to be dangerous in amount, but another

The skull may be fractured where the blow was received

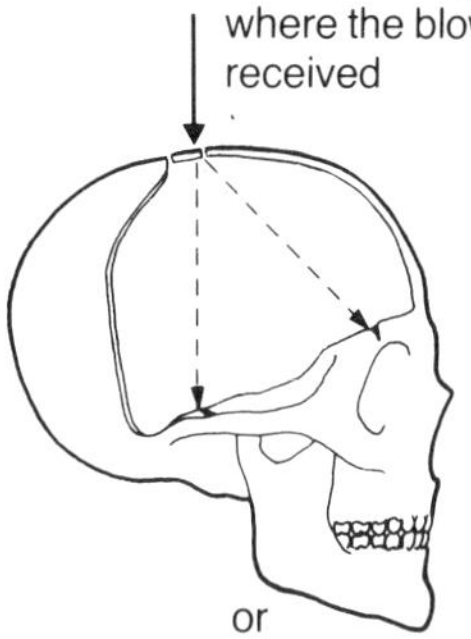

or

at its base inside, the force having travelled to where the bone is thin
this could show up as bruising around the eye or bleeding from the nose or bleeding from the ear

danger exists — that of any clot left in the ear canal forming a juicy culture medium for microbes, which could then multiply and migrate through the fracture towards the brain. Therefore this is blood which you encourage to escape, and you do not plug the ear. Instead lie the patient towards the bleeding side, and loosely cover the outer ear, to protect it from dirt without preventing blood from flowing out.

Concussion

This is the 'shaking up' of the brain from a blow, without any obvious structural damage, in other words the 'knock-out'. The victim becomes unconscious immediately (p.210) and he may remain so for any length of time from a few seconds to several hours. When he comes to he will be rather 'muzzy' and probably have a headache. Recovery should be complete unless some complication like compression supervenes, but keep him at rest and under your eye, and do not let him return to work or play until he has had medical advice.

Compression

This is quite a different affair, one of pressure on the brain itself. Fitting very closely within its bony container the brain has no margin of space to withstand pressures. These could come from a depressed piece of fractured bone, from bleeding inside the skull, or from its own general swelling after injury. Very sensitive nerve areas which control such things as circulation of blood, breathing and other life activities will suffer and the patient gradually becomes drowsy, perhaps unconscious and perhaps even at risk of dying. Thus it does not show immediately, but will develop within minutes or hours after the blow. This is why the patient, even after recovery from concussion, must be at rest, and under observation, ideally with medical supervision.

Do not overlook that: (a) a head blow may give the patient both concussion and compression. He may recover consciousness and then after a lucid interval (minutes or hours) sink back into unconsciousness from compression; (b) all patients with head injuries may have other injuries elsewhere and you should look carefully for these.

Heart Troubles

Basically the heart is a double set of two muscular chambers, the upper opening into the lower. The valves are of great importance, opening out to let blood pass in one direction only as auricles and ventricles contract. They close sharply against any back flow in the wrong direction.

Of course the heart is nothing like as simple as the diagram. Its components are folded against one another so that the big vessels enter and leave it at the top. One large vein brings the oxygen-low blood from the head and arms, and another from the rest of the body. Four veins bring the oxygen rich blood from the lungs. (A vein is a vessel in which the blood flows towards the heart; an artery takes the blood flow away from the heart.)

The eddies and vibrations of blood through the valves produce the typical noises of heart beat one can hear with an ear against someone's chest or through the doctor's stethoscope.

Disease and malformation of the valves mean inefficiency of heart beat. A valve whose flaps have become hardened or thickened may not open out easily as the chamber wall contracts. Conversely the valve flaps may loosen and close inadequately, so that there is some reflux of blood in the wrong direction at each heart beat. These valve inadequacies mean that the heart muscle has to work harder to overcome the difficulty and that blood circulation may be below par. The nature of any valve defect can be detected by characteristic changes it gives to the heart sounds, creating what are called 'murmurs'. However, there are many heart murmurs of no harmful significance at all. Also a valve anomaly can range from a very minor change, giving no handicap, to a major defect which does slow the patient considerably.

The Heart Beat

In health the heart contracts and pumps out blood between 60 and 80 times a minute. At rest or during sleep the rate is lower; during exercise or emotional stress it will be faster. The vibration given to the aorta by each

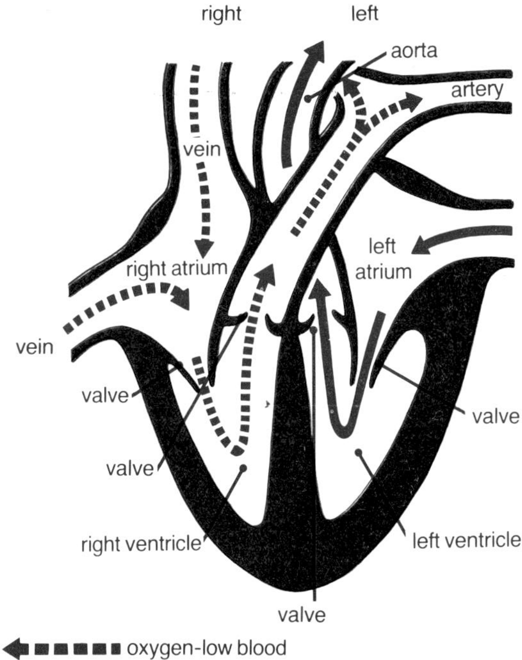

Veins bring blood to the heart
On the right: oxygen-low blood from the body tissues
On the left: oxygen-replenished blood from the lungs

The blood enters the **atrium** or collecting chamber. When the atrium contracts it sends blood through a **valve** formed of flaps into the main pumping chamber, the **ventricle**

With the contraction of the ventricle blood is forced out through another **valve** into the first large **artery.**

From the right it goes to the lungs to take up more oxygen. From the left the artery is the large **aorta** which branches to supply the whole body.

beat runs down the system of arteries. At some points, such as near the wrist, this can be felt and counted as the pulse (p. 176).

Within the muscles forming the chamber wall is a system of nerves governing the orderly contractions of atria and ventricles. The impulse begins by the atria and is conducted to the ventricles.

Sometimes this system goes wrong. In *atrial fibrillation* the muscles at the atria beat in a fast uncoordinated way, and their impulses then make the ventricles respond with irregular and weakened beats. In *heart block* the ventricles fail to respond to and to follow the normal beats of the auricles. They then beat at their own slower rate, say 40 times a minute. Both conditions can be helped by medical treatment.

Heart Failure

This is not a very good term, but it is here to stay and will continue to be used to describe circumstances where the heart is no longer an efficient pump and cannot maintain blood circulation adequately for the needs of the body. The patient may be breathless, perhaps blue around the lips, and he may find ankles and feet becoming puffy. In many cases heart failure is mild and causes symptoms only when the patient exerts himself or becomes emotionally worked up. He has to learn to restrict his activities. If overweight he will have to diet and if he is a smoker he will have to forego his cigarettes. There are efficient drugs which improve the efficiency of the heart muscle.

Angina

Like every muscle that of the heart needs a good supply of blood to keep working. Unlike other muscles it never rests but keeps going constantly. Its blood supply comes not from the contents of the heart's chambers but from arteries within the chamber walls.

Age, disease (and heavy smoking!) may narrow these arteries so that the blood flow decreases. If the narrowing is slight this may not produce symptoms in someone leading a sedentary life, but activity or excitement may call upon the heart to work harder, and the blood flow may prove inadequate.

Muscle deprived of adequate blood for its tasks experiences pain. In the case of the heart this is felt behind the breastbone and the patient may become breathless. He has angina. The sufferer will generally free himself from pain by putting himself at rest. There are also tablets he can take to help widen out the blood vessels and so increase the blood flow.

Badly affected hearts can give anginal attacks so frequently that the patient finds his daily activities severely limited.

Coronary Thrombosis

The blood vessels of the heart muscles are called coronary arteries. Thrombosis is a clot within the vessel, and this could block it entirely. If this happens then the area of muscle served by the vessel is denied its blood supply and the situation is that of an extreme, and dangerous, attack of angina. Intensely severe pain in the chest, may spread to the neck and jaw or to the arms. Rest will not relieve it. The patient is pale and breathless, extremely distressed, and may be sweating. His pulse rate is fast, weak and, perhaps, irregular.

This needs urgent medical help, even if the symptoms appear milder than those described. While awaiting the doctor have the patient at rest, with clothes loosened and lying down lightly covered. If he is having great difficulty breathing he may be easier sitting against banked up pillows.

The patient's very natural anxiety can worsen the effect on the heart, and any first aid measure should include the important double component of 'sympathy and confidence'. Let him realise you understand how much he is in pain and that you are doing all you can to help him. At the same time by your calm attitude and firm behaviour, avoiding fussing or signs of your own dismay and fears, convey an impression of confidence that once treatment begins the situation will ease very fast.

Acute Heart Failure

In this case there is no pain. Suddenly the heart muscle becomes inefficient. Blood is not pumped adequately out of the chambers, which become congested. Congestion spreads backwards along the veins from the lungs and into the lungs themselves.

This situation causes fluid from the blood to seep into the lungs' air spaces. The patient is very breathless with fast pulse. His breathing sounds wet and bubbly. Sometimes he coughs up watery sputum which may be blood tinged.

Not infrequently these attacks happen at night, waking the victim up.

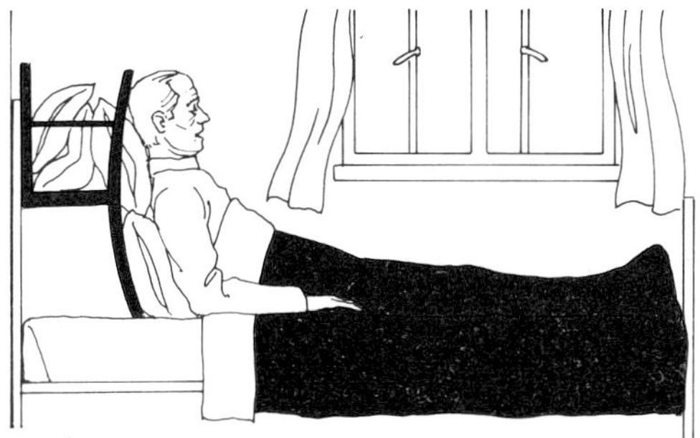

ACUTE HEART FAILURE
In his breathlessness the patient is best sitting up in bed.

It is an emergency needing and generally responding well to immediate medical help. The principles of 'sympathy and confidence' apply again here. In his breathlessness the patient is best sitting up, in bed, as this is easier for the chest muscles. Loosen his clothing, keep him warmly covered and allow fresh air to the room.

Heartburn

This is a foolish name for something that has nothing at all to do with the heart. It is a pain in the lower part of the chest due to some digestive disturbance. In a similar way the popular expression of 'wind round the heart' is completely without validity. There is no such condition.

On the other hand a number of patients disregard pain truly of heart origin, dismissing it as 'indigestion'. Heart pain tends to be felt higher up the chest; it may be related to exertion or to strong emotion; it may spread to the neck or to the arms; it may be severe and feel like a tight vice. The only safe measure in doubt is to get a medical opinion.

Heat Exhaustion

On a very hot and sunny day a healthy man sets out to dig his garden. Perspiration runs down his face and gives a salty taste as he moves the tongue between his lips. Ignoring the heavy sweating he continues to work hard. For a time all goes well, but eventually he begins to feel faint and then suddenly collapses.

In hot circumstances perspiration is an extremely useful thing. From the skin glands sweat reaches the surface. It then evaporates off the skin into the air. To change from liquid form to vapour it needs a great deal of heat, taking this up from the skin and the tissues beneath it. In this way sweating is a fine protection, helping to keep the body cool under abnormally hot circumstances. Were we to examine the collapsed man we would in fact find that his temperature is normal or only very slightly raised. Why then did he collapse? He is pale, with a fast and weakened pulse.

To begin with he has lost fluid in large amounts over a relatively short time. The body, especially the brain and the circulatory system, try to adapt and compensate but there is a limit to what they can achieve. It is not only water which he has lost. The sweat carries with it, out of the body, a great deal of salty material. These 'minerals' are essential to general well being. The weakened collapsed state is greatly due to their depletion. Another hazard is that to muscles lack of salt can precipitate tight spasm of muscle fibres, causing severe, painful cramps.

First aid to heat exhaustion is clear. Put the patient to rest lying in the shade. Loosen his clothes. Give him drinks containing salt. Suitable ones will be meat and yeast extracts. Or you can use fresh fruit juices, to each tumbler of which you add half a teaspoonful of salt.

The Most Common Sites of Hernia

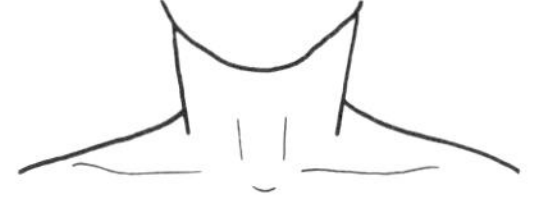

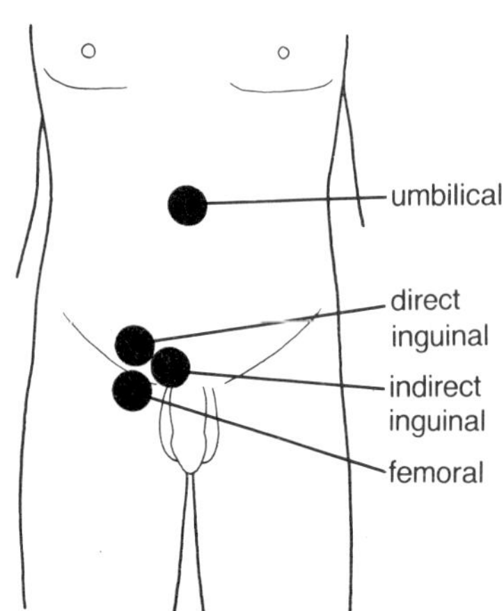

Hepatitis *see* Liver

Hernia

see also Hiatus Hernia

A hernia is the same thing as a rupture. It is the protrusion of an organ (or part of it) through the wall of the space within which it normally lies.

What has happened is that some strain has forced the herniating part through a weak point between the fibres of that wall. For example a person lifting a heavy weight may use more than his arm and leg muscles; he tenses those of the abdominal wall and greatly increases the pressure in the abdominal cavity. Something inside the abdomen is then forced through between fibrous or muscle bands and pushes against the inner surface of the skin.

The great majority of hernias are at the groin, and generally it is part of the bowel which protrudes, and which comes to lie as a soft swelling under the skin. It brings with it some of the peritoneum, the fine membrane which lines the abdominal cavity and its contents. Sometimes the protrusion contains part of a fatty apron-like fold of peritoneum, called the omentum, which hangs down inside the abdomen in front of the intestines.

At the region of the groin there are, under the skin, some anatomical canals where structures pass from the abdominal cavity to nearby parts of the body. These are weak points inviting hernias. Just above the line of the groin the inguinal canal runs obliquely towards the vulva in a woman and towards the scrotum in a man. The male inguinal canal is more receptive to a hernia than that of the female. It has been the site of travel of the foetus' testicle migrating from the abdomen, where it began development, to its position in the scrotum. The canal now contains the spermatic cord. In the female it holds only a ligament which is part of the remote attachment of the uterus.

In what is called the *direct inguinal hernia* the lump appears by the upper outer end of the canal, and does not move down it. An *indirect inguinal hernia* on the other hand has the projecting part move into the canal, and sometimes right down it into the scrotum itself.

Just below the groin line in the femoral canal bringing a large vein from the thigh into the abdomen. It is here that a *femoral hernia* can occur, and this is more common in women than in men.

At the navel an *umbilical hernia* can bulge through the weakness of a muscle gap, especially in the new born baby. In an adult a hernia in this region is more likely to be just alongside rather than at the navel itself, and is then graced with the name of para-umbilical hernia. They may look much the same but in fact are different since the baby's hernia is likely to mend itself without treatment.

Sometimes a hernia may develop where the abdominal wall has been weakened by an operation or injury scar; this would be called an *incisional hernia*.

When the rupture happens its victim generally feels a sudden pain and then, or soon after, finds a soft swelling at the site. He may find that if he lies down the bulge, obeying the law of gravity, disappears, only to return if he stands and stresses his muscles.

Many of these bulges can be made to return to their original cavity this way, or by simple gentle pressure of the hand. Force must never be tried. But the risk of leaving a hernia untreated is high, even if it is small and soft and amenable. It may gradually increase in size. Its structure may suddenly twist on itself and get trapped: the blood vessels serving that bit of bowel are nipped and closed; the whole thing swells and becomes very painful. It is now impossible for it to slip back into the abdomen. It is very likely that it will become gangrenous, and urgent surgery is needed.

Much better therefore, when a hernia has been diagnosed, to arrange for the earliest convenient planned surgical repair before any emergency could arise. The operation is simple, and (with rare exceptions) completely successful,

In the absence of an operation, or while waiting for one, a truss may be worn. This is a belt-like gadget, sometimes with a metal band incorporated, bearing a pad which presses down over the hernia area — over the *area,* not over the hernia itself. A truss never cures. Its purpose is to make it impossible for the hernia contents to slip out through the wall weakness and therefore the patient must have obtained the truss only after medical advice. He must first lie down and let the hernia correct itself, and then, still lying, get it round him. He must be aware of exactly where to site the pad, and how to fix the belt part. He must be prepared to find the truss slipping and needing readjustments. He must keep the skin clean and powdered against chafing. He must put up with an ungainly harness-like thing under his clothing.

In other words he would be far better off with an operation. Trusses should be reserved for those whose health or other circumstances make them quite unsuited for surgery.

Hiatus Hernia

The diaphragm is a large domed muscular 'shelf' which separates the chest from the abdominal cavity. The gullet (oesophagus) pierces it just before it joins the stomach. At this point the arrangements of muscle fibres act as a valve which, under ordinary circumstances, allows swallowed food to pass down into the stomach, but prevents the stomach contents from flowing back into the gullet.

In a large number of people there arises here a weakness which lets part of the upper end of the stomach slip out through the diaphragmatic aperture alongside the lower end of the gullet.

This condition, known as hiatus hernia, is more likely to happen in the elderly and in those who are overweight. Often it gives no trouble and is discovered by chance as in X-ray examinations.

In some cases however it can produce distressing symptoms. The stomach contains acid digestive juices and is designed to withstand them. The gullet is not; it resents the presence of acid and reacts with spasm and with a distressing pain felt in the lower part of the chest.

Obviously any flow from stomach to gullet is encouraged by the position of the patient. When he is upright the chances of its happening are lessened. If he lies flat or if he stoops, he may then feel the characteristic pain. Going to bed may be a very unpleasant experience. In unusually severe cases it can be accompanied by the regurgitation of acid tasting fluid; such cases need specialised surgical treatment.

However, the huge majority of those with hiatus hernia symptoms can be eased by quite simple measures. They avoid bending whenever possible. They take their meals sitting well upright, and do not lie down within two hours of eating. The head of the bed can be raised several inches by wooden blocks under its feet; sleeping in a sloping position is an art quickly acquired. Fat patients would do well to lose weight. Meals should be light, especially before bedtime. A simple 'nightcap' of a soothing milky drink can be very useful.

Doctors can help these patients very effectively. Some can benefit by

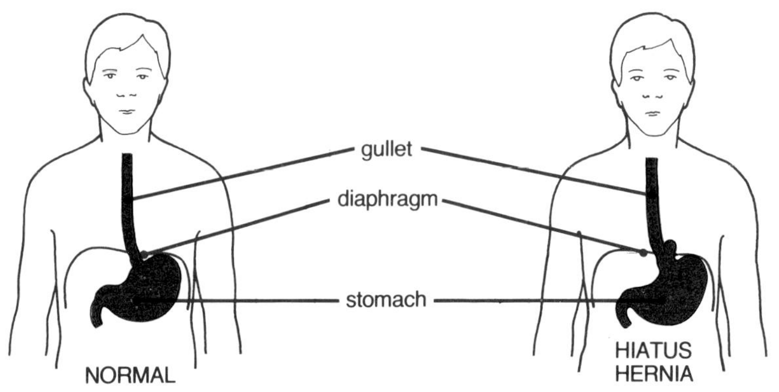

medicines which reduce the acidity in the stomach or which give the lower end of the gullet a protective coat to its lining.

The irritated gullet may bleed a little. This blood passes into the stomach and therefore is not obvious, especially as it is very small in amount, but if continued for a long time even slight bleeding may eventually produce anaemia. Fortunately when this happens its treatment also is easy.

"Hole in the Heart"

see Blue Baby

Hot Water Bottles

There is a right and a wrong way to do even the simplest thing.

Begin by examining the bottle to make sure it looks intact. Lie it, with the stopper off on a flat surface to get air out.

Use very hot, but not boiling water to fill it, by tilting the upper half towards you; only half fill it. Were you to keep it upright while filling you might get scalded by a sudden bubbling up of the contents.

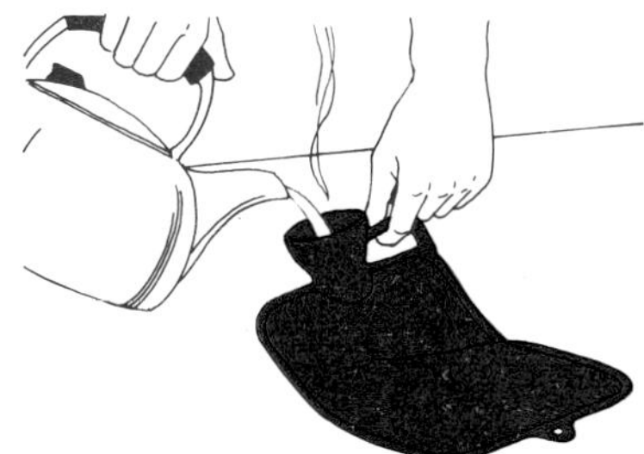

Carefully compress the upper half to get air out and screw on the stopper. Hold bottle upside down to check there is no leak. Put a cloth cover round it, and place it in the bed, but not against the patient. You aim to warm the bed, and not to heat one part of its occupant.

Do not put the bottle in a bed near an unconscious or paralysed person, or an infant — it might burn him should it slip and touch his skin.

Housemaid's Knee

Dotted round the body, alongside anatomical surfaces which move or glide against each other are small closed sacs of fibrous tissue containing a very little fluid. Their task is to smooth and cushion the movements. Each is called a bursa.

The knee has quite a number of such bursae. One of them in particular lying between the kneecap and the skin is likely to give trouble to those who kneel a great deal. Repeated pressure and rubbing, irritating the sac, will make it inflamed and distended with excess fluid. Sometimes it gets infected and contains pus, but the knee joint itself is unaffected.

Some decades ago this was a relatively common affliction of housemaids not yet assisted by electric appliances like vacuum cleaners. Today they are less likely to be bothered by 'prepatellar bursitis' (the medical name) than others, such as carpet layers, who work on their knees. Miners name it 'beat knee' and clergymen do not tell us what they call it.

Treatment consists in rest or avoiding pressure (by using a thick mat), by firm bandaging and sometimes by the doctor aspirating the fluid with a syringe. In the rare tough and intractable case the bursa can be surgically excised.

Hydrocoele *see* Testis

Hysteria

Hysteria is an illness often wrongly and unfairly assessed by the layman. Beset by anxiety or unhappiness the patient presents bodily symptoms as an expression of mental disturbance. It is customary to think of this as the prerogative of women. Its name is derived from the Greek for 'womb', for this once was thought to be the seat of the trouble. In fact males can be as hysterical as females.

Long standing frustrations or uncertainty can lead a person to a situation he does not know how to overcome. Sympathy from others is much easier to obtain in cases of physical illness than for mental problems. With no evil intent the victim unconsciously signals for help by simulating a bodily ailment. He disguises profound emotional difficulties as a failure of some organ, and the very first person to be taken in is the sufferer himself.

Scared stiff, he may believe he cannot breath, or that he has a paralysed limb. He may even develop a severe 'pain' or a 'collapse' or any other symptom.

The doctor faces a big problem. He must do his best to make sure there is in fact no physical lesion. Sometimes this is fairly easy as when the patient shows a paralysis or a loss of sensation which contradicts the anatomical patterns of nerve and muscle. In most cases however diagnosis is difficult, and needs a series of tests and investigations. That all these are being made may only convince the patient all the more that he has a serious physical trouble.

To cope with a sudden and obvious attack of hysteria give the patient very clear and rapid reassurance, but at the same time avoid soothing sympathy which might increase his symptoms. Since the greater his audience the more the hysteric tends to worsen, get rid of any bystanders as quickly as possible. You may have to explain to anxious watchers that what may seem an unfeeling approach is for the patient's good. Instead of requests or suggestions give him firm orders with reassurance. Tell him to rest, or to lie down and that he will improve with a drink of anything suitable like water or tea. Do not order the victim to 'pull himself together'. This is a silly phrase which means and achieves nothing. Do not tell him that there is nothing wrong. There certainly is something wrong, but not what the patient thinks. He is no malingerer but a sick person who will need all the psychological and social help which his family, his friends and his doctor can offer.

Hypothermia *see* Cold Effects

Immunisation

In many cases of infection the body produces in the blood a chemical which will neutralize or inactivate the microbes concerned or their poisons. This chemical we call an antibody. After the patient has recovered from the illness the antibody remains in his system to protect against further attacks of that particular infection. It may last a limited time, or it may be present for the rest of his life.

We can create immunity to certain diseases by administering (by mouth or by injection) the microbes, or their poisons, which have been so altered

Age given	Diptheria*	Tetanus*	Whooping Cough*	Polio-myelitis	Measles	German Measles	Tuber-culosis
3 months	●	●	●	●			
5 months	●	●	●	●			
9 months	●	●	●	●			
15 months					●		
4½ years (School entry)	●	●		●			
10-13 years							●
13 years (Girls)						●	
15-19 years		●		●			

**Diptheria, Tetanus and Whooping Cough Vaccines can be given in one combined injection.*

and weakened that though they will not produce the illness, they will stimulate the body to develop antibodies. For some illnesses, such as measles, a single dose is enough. For others, like poliomyelitis or whooping cough, several extra spaced 'booster' doses are needed to build up an effective antibody concentration.

The usual scheme advised to protect children against common infections is shown in the table above. In detail it may vary somewhat from area to area, or according to the recommendation of individual doctors.

Babies begin their immunisation programmes at about three or four months. Some advocate waiting until they are six months old for by then their bodies are far more efficient at producing antibodies. However, an illness like whooping cough can have so devastating an effect on those under six months that it is deemed wise to begin earlier.

In general immunisation is delayed or avoided if the recipient has a feverish illness (but not a simple snuffy 'cold'), is pregnant, has a malignant disease like cancer or, in the case of a few vaccines containing antibiotics, if the patient has a sensitivity to those antibiotics.

Diptheria and *tetanus* immunisations have no known serious adverse effects.

Whooping cough vaccine has been the subject of recent controversy. A few hours after being given it can produce slight feverishness, but this clears within a day. More serious is its reputation for occasionally causing fits or screaming attacks. However, over the ages at which this vaccination is given so many children do have fits of one form or another, whether or not they get immunisation, that there is real doubt that the vaccine is responsible. Whooping cough vaccination has also been blamed for causing brain damage.

Those who have carefully studied the statistics agree that rarely, very rarely indeed, this could be possible. But they point out that the risk of brain damage (or death) from the *illness* of whooping cough in a non-immunised child, though still a rarity, is relatively far greater.

Whooping cough can be a horrible disease with possible severe complications especially in children under a year old. The vaccine gives a high degree of protection. However, to be on the safe side, it should be withheld if the child has a medical history of fits or of some nervous system disease, or if one of the parents or a close relative has had epilepsy.

Poliomyelitis vaccine comes in two forms, one by injection and the other by mouth as tasteless drops in syrup or on sugar. The latter is preferred. It should not however be given while the recipient has diarrhoea for then it would not be properly absorbed. Very rarely the dose may be followed by some muscle weakness and even more rarely does this weakness become permanent. There is no need to stress that in the non-immunised the poliomyelitis *illness* itself carries a high risk of permanent paralysis.

Measles vaccine does not 'take' satisfactorily in the young baby and the child should be at least fifteen months old when he receives it. One dose is probably enough for life immunity. Approximately one in ten who get it have, about eight days later, a slight fever and perhaps even a mild rash; these are short lived. Other complications do include, rarely, fits and very rarely some brain inflammation. The risk of brain trouble as a complication of the measles *illness* is rare too, but not as rare as that from the vaccine.

The reasons for withholding measles vaccine from unsuitable cases are the same as those for whooping cough vaccine.

German measles is generally a mild illness. Often one cannot remember for certain whether one has had it. The reason for vaccinating is the damage German measles can give the unborn child if a pregnant woman catches the disease. Doctors recommend vaccinating girls of about thirteen. This involves a single dose. How long the immunity thus given lasts is not yet established, and vaccination if offered also to any woman who has just had a baby and on whom a blood check shows she is not immune. Complications are very rare and include a mild transient arthritis two or three weeks afterwards. The vaccine is not given to any woman who might become pregnant in the following three months.

Children between ten and thirteen years old are offered *tuberculosis* immunisation. A skin test can show whether they have previously had that common minor form of the infection which gives no obvious trouble yet leaves the body protected. Those who have not acquired this protection are immunised. Today the incidence of tuberculosis is very low, and it is not certain just how necessary it is to immunise. However, it is wise to do this where the risks are higher, as in some geographical areas or with occupations involving medical and social work.

Smallpox is considered to be eradicated and vaccination is not now done as a routine but, for safety, health service personnel and travellers to certain parts of the world may still be vaccinated. It is not given to anyone suffering from conditions like eczema, as this could lead to severe skin complications.

Travellers may need immunising against typhoid and paratyphoid fevers (two doses one month apart and, if necessary, a booster in three or four years), cholera (two doses one month apart and, if necessary, a repeat in six months) or yellow fever (a single dose, repeated if necessary in ten years).

Vaccination against influenza is described in the section on that disease. Mumps immunisation has recently become available but in the United Kingdom it is not often given. The protection it gives may be limited to ten or twelve years. Would someone vaccinated in childhood remember to get re-vaccinated later? Having mumps as an adult carries a greater risk of complications than catching the disease and getting done with it as a child.

Impetigo

This infection on the surface of the skin was a disfiguring calamity in the recent past — especially to children. It is very contagious and attacks, mainly on the face, spread easily from child to child at school. To be sure it generally got better without leaving scars, but treatment consisted in painting with gentian violet, with hideous clown-like effect.

Nowadays, happily, antibiotics (as ointment or tablets) do the trick fast and pupils are no longer kept away from school until declared clear.

The rash often appears around the mouth. Infection in the nose can be the starting point. Small itchy blisters soon become blobs of pus. They then break leaving damp sores which will crust over. Meanwhile the child is likely to have been rubbing and scratching and therefore spreading the trouble.

So one important part of treatment is hygienic caution. Keep hands off the face; use disposable tissues rather than handkerchiefs; cover pillow-cases; let them and towels be for the patient only, and washed separately; get the patient to wash his hands with almost exaggerated care and frequency.

Incontinence *(concerning children: see* Bedwetting*)*

Embarrassing and troublesome to all, this is a great affliction, yet it is an extremely common one. A survey estimates that in the United Kingdom there are nearly two million sufferers from incontinence, the inability to control bowel or bladder action.

The many causes can be divided into three basic groups.

a. Local troubles. This includes weakness of controlling muscles, bladder stones, hardened stools in the bowel and infections. Often medical treatment can give great improvements.

b. Malfunction of the nerves which regulate bowel or bladder. This could result from strokes, or from illnesses or accidents affecting the spinal cord; sometimes it is due to congenital defects.

c. Mental confusion which accompanies certain illnesses or some states of the elderly.

Society has trained us since early childhood to feel shame if we cannot properly manage what we euphemistically call our 'body functions'. Thus conditioned the incontinent may try to hide or to deny their disability. This is as unhelpful as seeking to disguise a limp. They and their families should, without embarrassment, frankly face the problems as they would those of any other handicap. A great number of aids are available.

Above all one must seek the doctor's advice at all points. There are so many types of patient, so many types of incontinence, that recommendations cannot apply to all. General practitioners, assisted by community nurses, health visitors and members of the social services must be consulted before any measures are taken.

Stress Incontinence

There is a form of bladder weakness which lets some urine escape when the patient makes any strain increasing pressure within the abdominal cavity. Lifting a heavy weight, coughing, sneezing or even laughing might do it. It is more likely to happen in women, and sometimes is a temporary nuisance after childbirth.

In their useful *Notes on Incontinence* the Disabled Living Foundation describes simple exercises which can help tone up the muscles concerned. One should persevere with the exercise for at least three months.

Firstly sit or stand comfortably, without tensing the muscles of the legs, seat or abdomen. Imagine that you are trying to control diarrhoea by consciously tightening the ring of muscle round the back passage. Do this several times until you feel certain that you have indentified the area and can make the correct movement. Now sit on the lavatory or commode and commence passing water; while doing so make an attempt to stop the flow in mid-stream by contracting the muscles round the front passage. Do this also several times until you feel sure of the movement, and the sensation of applying conscious control.

The exercise can be carried out sitting or standing. Tighten first one and then the other (back and front) and then both together. Count four slowly, then release the muscles. Do this four times, repeating the whole sequence once every hour if possible. With practice the movements should be quite easy to master, and they can be carried out at any time — while waiting for a bus, standing at the sink or watching television.

Lavatories and Commodes

Incontinent people may avoid 'accidents' by going frequently to the lavatory. Here a raised seat or support rails could help those who cannot sit down easily. The lavatory should be of easy access. Where there is difficulty a commode can be kept in the bedroom. This should be carefully chosen with professional advice. It should, for instance, be easy to move, but firm on its base; its height should be just right for the patient (usually 45cm). There are designs on the market which disguise (almost) its nature and make it look like an easy chair.

Quite a number of people are on diuretics, medicines to stimulate the kidneys to greater activity. If they have a condition like arthritis or weak limbs which make them move slowly and if the diuretics are quick and sharp acting, then they may have trouble getting to the lavatory or the commode in time. Sometimes the doctor will be able to change the diuretic prescribed for another with a slower, sustained, but as effective, action.

Clothing

Rapidly adjustable clothing may

prove very useful. Women will wear full skirts, easy to pull up and knickers easy to pull down. Men's trousers can have a long fly opening, with zip or Velcro fastening. Materials should be easily washable.

Urinals

Urinal bottles which the patient can quickly reach are available in many designs, for men and for women. They are made in easy-to-clean materials like plastic or stainless steel. There are also some small disposable forms which are discreetly portable. Men can easily wear under the clothing urine collecting appliances which are very efficient. There are also designs for women, but these are more difficult to use.

Personal Protection

There is a great number of protective pads and pants to choose from. The doctor or nurse will advise as to the best for each patient. Some pants combine their own pads and some are suitable not only for bladder but also for bowel incontinence.

The Bed

A bed may need protection too. There is a whole range of disposable or washable bedpads and mattress covers. Some are excellent in their power of absorbing fluid. A great number of them are available through the nursing and the social services.

Laundering

Home washing may build up to big problems. Sometimes the social services make financial allowances to cover this. Put soiled material in special buckets with lids, with some disinfectant. Disposable material can be temporarily wrapped in newspaper and put in plastic bags. Deodorants can help and so can antiseptics, but one should try to avoid a home atmosphere reeking of an antiseptic with a powerful tell-tale odour. Windows are to be kept open as much as possible.

Health Points

Restricting fluids drunk does not really reduce incontinence. A heavily concentrated urine may make matters worse by irritating the bladder. Let the patient drink freely, except to avoid fluids in the two or three hours before bedtime.

Nurses and doctors will advise on the all important matter of looking after a skin which repeatedly becomes wet or soiled.

Constipation can make things worse and should be treated. Avoid haphazard taking of purgatives, and act only on medical advice. Plenty of fluids, fruit and vegetables in the diet may be all that is needed.

An extremely helpful work detailing the points touched on is *Incontinence* by Dorothy Mandelstam (Heinemann Medical). She also has edited a comprehensive book of multiple expert authorship: *Incontinence and its Management* (Croom Helm). These, and a number of information lists, are available from the Disabled Living Foundation.

Indigestion *see also* Hiatus Hernia *and* Peptic Ulcer

Indigestion is the same thing as dyspepsia and both words mean nothing very definite. They have been applied to any stomach discomfort which in the mind of the sufferer is more or less associated with eating. He is not always right, for he may attribute symptoms of some lung, heart, circulatory or kidney troubles to his digestion.

Even when there is something amiss in the stomach or intestines, the list of possibilities is quite big. It can range from peptic ulcer to a blockage of the bowels, from appendicitis to hiatus hernia.

The word sounds reassuringly harmless so that often some unfortunate person has given himself a treatment not only inappropriate but also harmful. An important rule, for instance, is never to take a purgative for an undiagnosed abdominal complaint: it could rupture an inflamed appendix or worsen some cases of accidental poisoning.

Where there is true indigestion (that is, a difficulty in digesting food), then the patient, in retrospect, might recognise himself as responsible. Let him consider the list of likely causes: irregular meals, hasty eating and insufficient chewing, eating too much, imperfectly cooked foods, excess fried, hot and spicy dishes, mental stress at mealtimes, too much alcohol or smoking, or irritation from preparations like aspirin and iron tablets.

But do not let this list deter him from seeing his doctor if indigestion keeps on bothering him. There might be something more seriously amiss than twentieth-century living.

Influenza

The trouble with influenza is that so many people equate it with the common cold. The latter is a mild nuisance, the former is a serious illness. Epidemics of influenza tend to happen in the winter or early spring.

It is an easily caught virus infection with an incubation period of about two days. Symptoms appear suddenly with headache, fever, sweating and chills. There is aching in the back and limbs and a hard dry cough. There can be nausea and vomiting; almost always there is loss of appetite.

There is no special drug which will help. Let the patient be at rest, let him have a light diet with much to drink. He can relieve his symptoms with aspirin or paracetamol.

Generally it is a week's illness. Sensibly the patient spends two to three days in bed, and the rest of the time gradually getting up and resuming activity. Attempts to cut this short could lead to a miserable convalescence and perhaps to complications like a lung infection from bacteria.

The elderly and those with bad chests and hearts seem especially at risk of complications, so that for them the doctor may prescribe antibiotics. These have no effect on the influenza itself, but can protect against complicating infections.

Vaccination against influenza is possible and is best given in the autumn, but each time it is a small gamble. The influenza virus is constantly changing its biological structure and its nature. Vaccination against today's virus may have little or no effect against the type which will strike in a few months time. Research scientists work very hard to predict the virus strains to come and to prepare the appropriate vaccine. Each year the World Health Organisation recommends from what strains of virus the vaccine should be prepared.

Insect Stings

The bee is a good example. Its sting penetrates and pumps in venom. The bee then tries to withdraw the sting. When the victim is man it does not succeed, for the sting is barbed and human skin is too tough to let it out easily. The sting remains set and gets torn off the bee, which will die of its wounds within a couple of days.

The detached sting continues to pump venom in, so the quicker it is extracted the better. Trying to grasp it from the top, where it protrudes would only squeeze more of the venom down. The best thing to do is to pull by very fine tweezers applied to the lower part against the skin. In the absence of tweezers, scrape it out with a finger nail. In any case the sting is best out, for if left in it will irritate as would any foreign body sticking in the skin. Also it produces a scent which signals to other bees to attack and sting near it.

Applying old fashioned remedies like alkalis or a blue bag is useless. The pain and redness from the venom can be eased by a quickly applied cold compress. Better is an antihistamine cream (though some people can develop sensitivity to this). Even better is a steroid cream of the sort used for some skin inflammations. A doctor may agree to prescribe this to beekeepers. Some beekeepers try to anticipate trouble by taking an antihistamine tablet one hour before working on the hives.

A sting inside the mouth is very unpleasant and possibly dangerous, soft tissues here may swell considerably, to the extent of blocking the airway. Immediate sucking of ice will help, but a doctor is needed urgently if the swelling becomes threateningly big.

Most beekeepers in time become less and less sensitive to stings. A few, a very few, people however become extremely allergic to the venom, and can get serious reactions: a tight chest, difficulty in breathing, a rapid, weak pulse, dizziness and collapse can overtake them. Rapid medical help is essential.

If a beekeeper finds himself gradually reacting more and more to stings he ought to consider passing his hives on to someone else, or to see his doctor about a course of desensitising injections.

The same principles apply to stings from other insects, except that they (including bumble bees and wasps) have smooth stings without barbs, which pull out easily from skin.

Insomnia

There are three approaches (not mutually exclusive) to this problem. One can give sleeping tablets. One can explore why the patient is not sleeping. One can advise a form of relaxation.

Sleeping Tablets

Tablets to ensure sleep are tremendously useful and do a great service. Millions are swallowed every night and the doctor selects the type best suited to his patient. Barbiturates until a few decades ago formed the mainstay but today we can choose from a number which are far less 'doping' and much more naturally sleep-inducing. Some of them are very safe in that large overdoses will not kill but merely might make the patient remotely anti-social at breakfast. This in no way should encourage individuals to augment their stated doses, for other side effects, including confusion, hallucinations, and even over-excitement, could be very unpleasant. This applies specially to the elderly whose response to drugs is often unpredictable

Do not keep the bottle at the bedside. There have been many cases of patients waking drowsily and reaching out for more, and perhaps more again, through the night. If a doctor has recommended a possible extra dose in the middle of the night then have the exact number, and no more, handy.

Most tablets swallowed with a drink of water take about thirty to forty minutes to become effective. Use this fact to time their taking.

Do not let us forget that instead of tablets the very simple measure of a warm drink of milk or cocoa is often all that is needed to settle into sleep. A warm bath may also help.

Why Insomnia?

The answer to this question is generally far more important than the prescribing of tablets. If it is pain which keeps the patient awake, then some simple pain relievers will be the answer. Preparations like aspirin or paracetamol are useful, but their effect generally lasts only about four hours. However, some forms are marketed as 'enteric coated': this means that a special covering to the tablet has to be dissolved by the digestive juices before they begin to take action, which is thus delayed by about four hours after swallowing. If pain is likely to be an ongoing misery through the night the patient may take, before bedtime, his ordinary tablets and then, as he goes to bed, swallow whole the enteric coated variety. These will take over when the ordinary ones are ceasing to function. The doctor will advise if any case is suited to this routine.

If unavoidable noise or illumination about the bed is the problem, then block this out using ear plugs or eye shields which can be bought at the chemists.

Anxiety about self, work or family all too often delays falling asleep. Depression, on the other hand, is more likely to wake one up in the middle of the night. Clearing up the source of these mental problems is, of course, the true line of treatment. This is not always so easy but those who lie tormented in bed may find some reassurance in the fact that body and mind enterprise is at lowest between midnight and 3 a.m. Things appear very much better in the morning.

Relaxing

We have been taught that about eight hours of sleep is necessary for health; many believe themselves abnormal if they do not achieve this. Then they begin to worry and to enter a vicious circle. Old people do in general sleep less than they did when younger. And there are plenty of authenticated reports of men and women who, naturally, night after night, sleep but a very few hours and feel perfectly fit.

To those who find themselves quite awake when they believe they should be sleeping the advice is not to worry about the situation but to turn it to advantage. Let them use the time purposefully. This can be by a placid occupation like knitting, writing or planning some project ahead. Reading can be very pleasant in the quiet: certain literature is both interesting and gently soporific. (The novels of Sir Walter Scott are highly recommended for this purpose.)

Those who do not wish to busy themselves can enjoy the opportunity for relaxing completely, a luxury which most of us deny ourselves in our active everyday life. Lying in bed and, following the technique described under Relaxation (p. 177) is a soothing approach to peaceful comfort . . . and perhaps to sleep.

Itching

Its medical name is pruritus and it is a thoroughly annoying symptom, not only to the patient, but often also to the doctor who may find the discovery of its cause a difficult problem.

Skin conditions like eczema and nettlerash are the first things to think of. Some rashes, as that of chicken pox or impetigo, are other examples. The parasitic scabies has the popular name of 'the itch'. Other parasites like fleas and fungus (tinea) have their places in the list. An itch localised aroung the vulva or the back passage could make one suspect a number of irritating factors like thrush, threadworms or the sugar laden urine of diabetes.

But many causes are quite hidden. Some old people suffer from severe itching of a skin which looks quite normal except for being rather dry. Hormone changes appear to be a factor in the irritation felt by some women in late pregnancy. Certain drugs will give the symptom. And there are a number of general, rather hidden conditions which mysteriously cause itching: certain diseases of the blood, kidneys, and liver may have to be suspected and looked for if no others are found.

As to the symptom itself, it can be relieved by soothing lotions and creams, and sometimes also by sedatives. A major task is to persuade the patient to stop scratching as this can perpetuate itching well after its original cause has cleared. And scratching seems to be a much loved, ineradicable occupation of the sufferer who will even do it under the pretence of showing the doctor the site of his trouble. Aspirin has proved to be remarkably effective in relieving many cases.

Jaundice

Jaundice is not one disease. It is a symptom of many possible diseases, being the discolouration of skin and eyes by a bile pigment called bilirubin, when this is in excessive amounts in the blood.

Blood always holds some bilirubin. What would make it contain too much? The answers lie in reviewing, in an elementary way, the normal history of this substance.

Stage A: Red blood cells live for about four months in the circulation before naturally becoming aged and breaking down. When this happens they liberate bilirubin.

Stage B: The liver takes up the bilirubin and processes it, with other chemicals, to form bile. Bile passes from the liver into

Stage C: The gall bladder, which stores it until it flows through bile ducts into the intestine, where it helps to digest fats.

At each of these stages something may go wrong which would overload the blood with bilirubin.

Stage A: Certain, fairly rare, types of anaemia are due to excessive breakdown of red blood cells. The blood then contains far too much bilirubin for the liver to manage. The newborn 'rhesus baby' suffers a great destruction of its red cells. But there is also a perfectly normal jaundice of the newborn. The mature foetus has a very high number of red blood cells, and this is rectified soon after birth by a breakdown of the excess. It shows up by slight jaundice at about the third day of life, and will clear in a few days. The baby remains well.

Stage B: Some diseases and a few chemicals can damage the liver structure so as to interfere with free flow from it of bile. This then cannot reach the gall bladder and bilirubin moves back to the blood stream. The diseases include the virus infection called 'infectious hepatitis' which is one of the commonest causes of jaundice. It has a long incubation of three or more weeks, and is ushered in with nausea, loss of appetite and fever, before the jaundice shows itself.

Stage C: The gall bladder or its ducts may become blocked, so that the bile cannot flow into the intestine. Gallstones will do this commonly, so could tumours, but this is rare. Here also bilirubin would be reabsorbed into the bloodstream.

The conditions given under stages *B* and *C* are blockages of bile fluid flow, and the resulting jaundice is called 'obstructive'. Since no bile reaches the intestines, the stools will fail to show the normal dark colour given by bile pigments and will appear very light or grey. On the other hand, much of the excess pigment in the blood will be filtered out by the kidneys, so the urine will darken, often to a deep brown.

Jaundice, whatever its cause, can make the patient feel wretched, depressed and irritable — justifying the phrase of 'a jaundiced view of life'. The obstructive type often causes itching. No one should ignore jaundice. It needs investigation so that the cause can be treated. The first suspicious symptom ought to be reported to the doctor without delay.

Kidney Troubles

The kidneys are a filtering system to get rid of unwanted substances (like urea) from the blood. In addition they act as an extremely efficient control of water and of many chemicals. They remove these from the blood through a collection of very fine microscopic tubules and then return a proportion of what they have extracted to maintain the exactly right amounts needed in the body.

Of the many ways in which this delicate living machinery can go wrong, there can be two main subdivisions, inflammation and obstruction.

Inflammation

One type generally affecting only one kidney is due to bacterial infection. This is called *pyelitis,* referring to inflammation of the renal pelvis. Since infection rarely affects the renal pelvis alone, but tends to spread to the area with the filtering tubules as well, the name *pyelonephritis* is generally used, the extra term indicating that the substance of the kidney is included. The patient is feverish and has a painful back in the kidney region. Urine may look cloudy when passed. (Urine which stands some hours after being passed often becomes cloudy and this is of no significance.) It may have a fishy smell which can be described as that of seaweed at low tide, and it may contain some blood. The bladder (p.42) often shares the infection with a degree of cystitis. Antibiotic treatment is very effective.

Quite different is the non-infectious condition called *glomerulonephritis,* which is likely to affect both kidneys at the same time. When it comes on suddenly it may be a type of allergic reaction by the kidneys to a recent infection elsewhere in the body, such as scarlet fever or some forms of sore throat. This affects not the renal pelvis but the whole filtering system, which then functions badly. Water is retained in the body and may show up as puffiness of the skin. Generally all

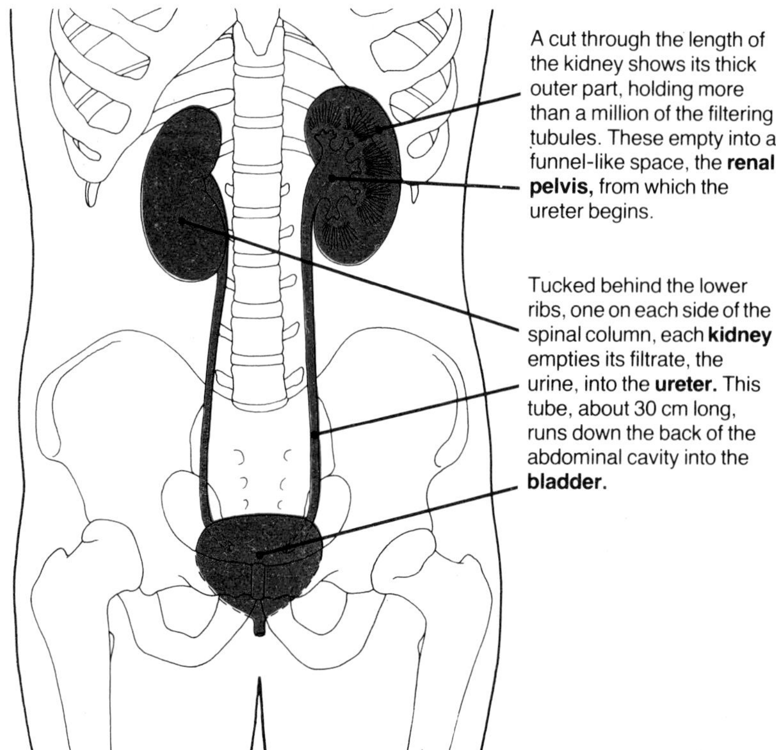

clears completely with a few weeks of treatment.

The long-standing, chronic, slowly progressive form of glomerulonephritis is another matter. Gradual deterioration of the filtering mechanism takes place over months or years and could lead to kidney failure. Why this happens is not clear.

Obstruction

Stone formation is the most likely thing to block the flow of urine in the channels of the renal pelvis and ureter. Sometimes a small stone, which has been lying quietly and giving no hint of its presence, will change position to lodge in the ureter. Intense colicky pain immediately hits the patient. The ureter is undergoing spasm. With good fortune and with treatment the stone will shift again, getting free to descend into the bladder. Perhaps it will be voided (with discomfort) some time when the patient passes urine.

Occasionally really large stones may build up in the renal pelvis, and rarely they may actually mould themselves to its shape. Quite apart from the chance that it may become big enough to cause an obstruction, any stone remaining in the urinary tract can predispose to infection. If it is not likely to pass out spontaneously it may be wise to remove it by operation.

Kidneys and Blood Pressure

Some forms of raised blood pressure are inter-related with kidney trouble. The kidney substance is believed to produce chemicals which maintain a normal pressure. Diseases of both kidneys could decrease their amount and allow a pressure rise.

Another effect comes through the kidneys' production of renin. This is a hormone (i.e. chemical messenger acting through the blood stream) which activates a rise of blood pressure. If the blood supply to the kidneys is impaired (as when arteries become narrowed) they automatically secrete more renin as if to encourage better receipt of blood by increasing the pressure of flow. This may be of immediate convenience to the kidneys themselves, but it could create trouble for the body by the overall blood pressure rise.

Kidney Failure

The filtering task of the kidneys is essential to health and life. Fortunately it has great reserves, so that if one kidney is irreversibly put out of action by injury or by disease, the other one can do the work for two. If both fail the situation is serious. Waste products accumulate in the blood, and the body's necessary chemical balance is no longer held. This can threaten life.

Dialysis is the use of a special membrane to extract from a liquid substances which will filter through it. This is the principle of the *kidney machine* which can do artificially what the failing kidneys no longer can accomplish. A tube inserted into an artery of the patient takes his blood to a filtering system which mimics that of the kidney and returns it through another tube to one of his veins. This is very time consuming: the patient may have to undergo dialysis three times a week, for some six hours each time. Some learn to do this themselves with apparatus set up in their homes; others have to attend special hospital centres. Britain has a very high proportion of dialysis patients taking advantage of home kidney machines.

Use of the kidney machine inevitably restricts patients' movements and activities. They are still beset by kidney failure, subject to complications of diet and special treatment, but it keeps them alive, and many are able to hold down a job in the intervals.

The alternative to repeated dialysis is transplantation of the kidney from a donor relative or from a body very soon after death. The successful recipient regains medical and personal freedom.

Removal of a kidney from a body for transplant cannot be done without the right permission. Time is very short and specialist surgeons, anxious to help their patients, are concerned over what might be called lost opportunities. Many far thinking people carry a donor card, which authorises the use of their kidneys after death. Anyone can obtain the card from doctors, hospitals or some chemists . . . and should.

Laryngitis

The 'voice box' or larynx sits at the top of the windpipe and at the lower end of the big cartilage in the neck which we call Adam's apple. Bands of tissue, the vocal cords, stretch from front to back. Their varying tensions and vibrations as air is breathed past them

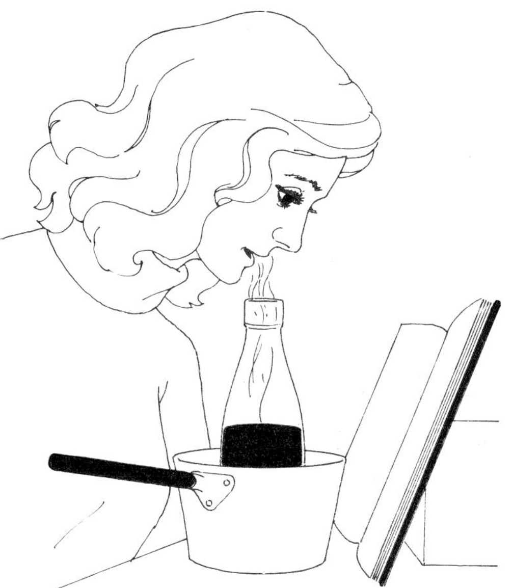

The pleasant way to inhale, not under a towel but openly with your favourite book or T.V. programme. One teaspoon of Friar's Balsam added to a warmed milk bottle filled with steaming water to a level just before it begins to narrow at the neck. The bottle stands in a pan lest it cracks.

make the basic sounds of speech.

Inflammation of the larynx generally comes from the spread of some infection in the mouth or in the nose. Mucus dripping down from the discharges of the common cold can be responsible. Irritation from dust, smoking or too much speaking and shouting may also contribute.

The larynx feels raw, and the voice is hoarse. There may be a dry cough. Speaking can be painful. The simplest form of treatment is also the most difficult. It is very hard to persuade patients that because complete rest will cure most inflammations, they should therefore stop talking — and that includes whispering. It is not the activity of the vocal cords but the force of the air passing over them which determines the loudness of sound. In clear cut bacterial infections antibiotics may help.

Gargling is a waste of time; the fluid gets to the back of the throat, but it will not reach the larynx. Steam inhaling is unlikely to cure, but it can give great relief. A couple of menthol crystals or some Friar's Balsam (Compound Tincture of Benzoin) added to the steaming water has no therapeutic effect, but makes the inhalation pleasant and adds the psychological touch of a pharmaceutical aroma. Naturally the patient will be persuaded to stop smoking, if not for ever at least until he is better.

Inflammation can be irritated by other troubles in the larynx. These are little protruberances, called polyps or nodules, developing on tired vocal cords. They are not dangerous but a nuisance and can arise from long overuse of the voice, as in professional singing. A throat specialist will cope with these.

Rarely one finds more dangerous tumours on the vocal cords. Most respond very well to treatment if seen early. They have the grace to advertise their presence by a persistent and painless hoarseness, which should alert the patient to consult his doctor without delay.

Laxatives *see* Constipation

Lice

Three varieties of louse affect man: the head louse, the body louse and the pubic or crab louse. Each can move from host to host by simple personal contact. Long hair styles, untended, could predispose to the trouble.

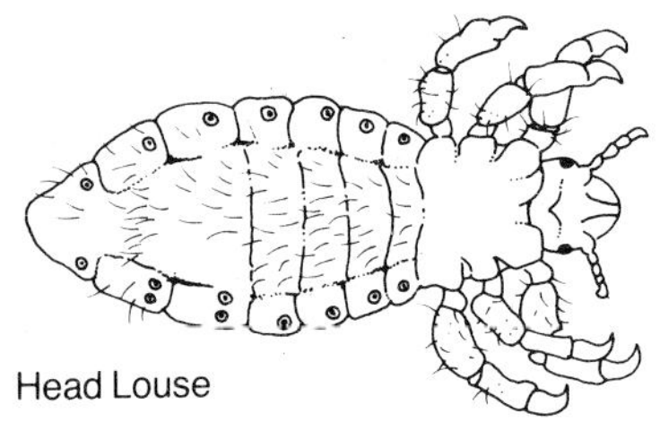

Head Louse

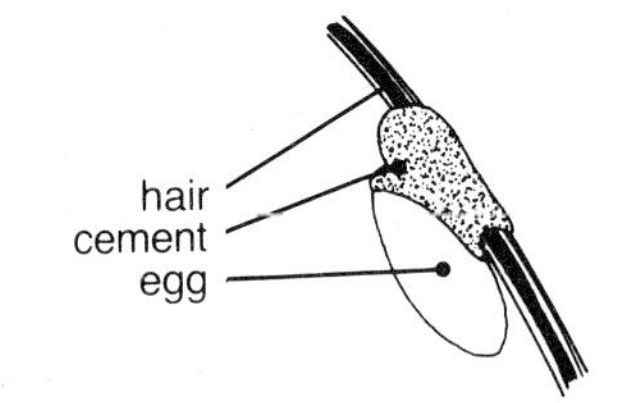

Egg of Head Louse

The head louse is about 3 mm long and pale grey in colour. It lurks within the protection of the hair and is best looked for at the back of the scalp. The female lays about eight eggs a day, fixing firmly to a hair by a tough 'cement'. The egg, a minute white oval, hatches out in eight days. In another eight days the new beast is sexually mature, and will live a further four weeks. Two or three times a day every louse pierces the skin of its host with a needle-like mouth part and makes a meal by sucking blood, leaving a small red and irritating spot.

The body louse prefers attaching itself to clothing and feeds from its attachment, therefore causing irritation specially where clothes lie firmly against skin, i.e. shoulders, waist or upper parts of back or buttocks. In dealing with this infestation, clothes and bedding need treating.

The crab louse lives in the pubic hair, but is not averse to migrating to eyelashes or beards. It is a little smaller, with a more rounded shape than the other lice. It can live a few hours if fallen off its host, so that although it is often said that it is transmitted by sexual contact, it could just as easily have been acquired from a lavatory seat.

What to do if your children seem to have head lice? In the first place reassure yourself that this is regrettable, but no stigma. It can happen to the best people, the cleanest people and to adults. Notify the school, as a matter of courtesy and care, lest others there be involved. The Community Health Nurse on the staff will help in confidence. Also check other members of the family.

Treatment today is easy and safe with special lotions which kill not only the lice but also loosen and kill the nits. One application is made at bed time. It is left to dry naturally (using a hair dryer could cause irritation). The next morning a full normal shampoo is given.

Liver *see also* Gall Bladder *and* Jaundice

The liver is a chemical monitor, factory, laboratory and storehouse of almost unbelievable versatility. It has over four hundred functions. No wonder it is the largest and warmest organ in the body.

Tucked closely under the diaphragm its wedge shaped bulk lies by the lower ribs at the right, but some of it spreads over to the left side. The gall bladder is underneath, with its tip just appearing below the liver's lower edge. To begin with it manufactures bile — three or four pints every day. The bile passes by ducts to the gall bladder which, in turn, sends it to the intestines to assist in the digestion of fats.

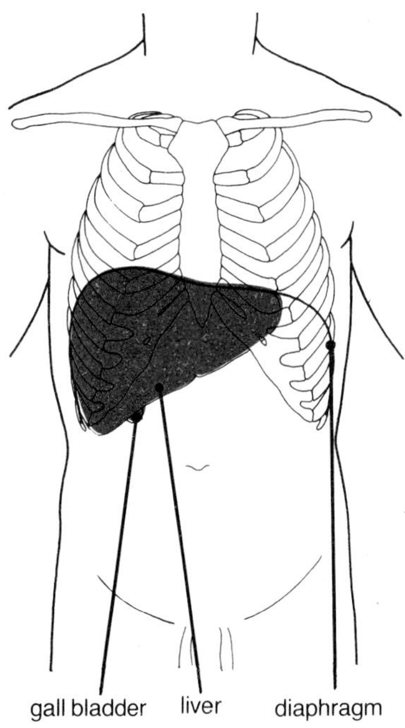

The liver intercepts, checks and processes the products of digestion. The results of all we eat (except the waste matter which moves on to form the stools) go first to the liver. Instead of being absorbed into the general bloodstream, the breakdown products pass into special blood vessels forming a 'hot line' between bowel and liver, and which is named the portal system. None of it will be let loose into the body until the liver has looked at and looked after it.

Many things taken into the liver are stored there, having been turned into compounds usable by the body's cells. Sugars, fats and certain vitamins are examples. The liver deals with a number of chemicals which could be harmful to tissues. Neutralising poisons it changes them into less toxic substances. It also has its specialised elements which catch and destroy unwanted things like cell debris, bacteria or microscopic particles brought in by the portal system. Its busiest function is the synthesis of a great number of complicated compounds essential to life, such as the blood clotting materials as well as anticoagulants, and the protein constituents of blood plasma.

One can understand that with such a lot of tasks a diseased liver will have a widespread effect on general health. Fortunately liver tissue has great reserves and its damaged cells regenerate so that the average liver complaint has only temporary symptoms. The symptoms are not very specific: weakness, loss of weight, poor appetite, nausea, and vague abdominal discomfort do not point directly to the liver.

The liver is liable to receive parasites like amoebae or those of malaria. Far less common is the virus infection known as infectious or viral hepatitis, with its long incubation period of several weeks. There are two types of virus involved. One is likely to come from contaminated food. The other is transmittable, in spite of routine precautions, from injected material; particular care is taken to avoid it where blood for transfusion is collected.

After a few days of indefinite symptoms with fever, the patient shows the characteristic features of a dark urine and pale stools, followed by jaundice (p. 147). A few cases can be very serious but the majority recover completely in a few weeks. The main point of treatment and convalescence is to be as considerate to the liver as possible. One avoids all drugs or foods which would put an extra strain on the biochemical tasks of this busy but weakened 'factory-laboratory'.

By its generous processing and neutralising of so many poisons the liver tissue is open to damage from what might be called overwork. Poisons in this context include a great many things which we swallow in the ordinary way of life. Alcohol is one of them and every drop of it is a job for the liver. It will manage alcohol well in moderation, but the very heavy and chronic drinker may prove too much for his liver, which accumulates damage to its cells faster than it can regenerate them. In the long run its tissue becomes scarred and fibrous, creating a hard knobbly texture. This is *cirrhosis* and the liver's normal functions are impaired. Any repeated damage or infection of the liver can give cirrhosis, but we must face the fact that in our civilisation a sustained excess of alcohol is the main cause.

Tumours rarely begin in the liver, but it is likely to receive spread of tumour cells from other organs, especially those of the digestive tract.

In fairness to the liver one has to add that this marvellously clever, almost indefatigable and certainly essential part of the body, rarely bothers its owner with symptoms. It generally overrides and forgives the dietetic insults to which it is subjected. The expression of 'feeling liverish' is slanderous. What the speaker is experiencing generally arises in his stomach or bowels. The liver is coping silently.

Lumbago *see* Backache

Measles *see also* Fevers of Children *and* Immunisation

Measles is a virus infection with an incubation period of ten to fourteen days. The blotchy rash is preceded by two or three days of severe 'cold' symptoms. At this stage the right diagnosis can sometimes be forecast by carfully looking at the gums or the inside of the cheeks. They bear the white Koplik's spots, which look like a few grains of coarse salt against a velvety red background, and which fade as the skin rash appears and the temperature rises a little further. The patient is rather miserable now, beset with coughing and with the inflamed eyes of conjuntivitis. It is a mistake to think that he should be in a darkened room; yet because of the eyes it is kinder to avoid too bright a light shining on the face.

The rash lasts about four days and as it develops the patient improves, to feel much better about eight days after starting his 'cold'.

There is no special treatment for measles unless it develops complications. These are relatively infrequent and are due to bacterial infection superimposed on the tissues weakened by the virus. Pneumonia and ear infections are the usual ones, but rarely inflammation of the brain (encephalitis) can occur. Antibiotics are prescribed for complications but they are of no help against the measles virus itself.

Immunisation (p.138) is now a useful routine to prevent or at least to attenuate the illness.

Medicines — Taking and Keeping

Giving detailed advice on administering medicines may appear rather pedantic. Experience shows that many people take their prescriptions in bizarre, if not risky, ways so that there is justification for a few rules.

When to Give Medicines

Obviously give medicines as instructed by the doctor. Note whether before, after or between meals is advised. If nothing is stated then work it out at your convenience. Antibiotics in general do better, being absorbed quicker, when taken on an empty stomach.

If the instructions advise taking twice, three or four times a day, then try to space out doses so that an equal number of hours come between them. However, if this is followed with mathematical exactness it might mean waking the unfortunate patient, and the administrator, in the middle of the night, so some compromise is forgiveable (unless the doctor has specified against this). An antibiotic four times a day, for instance, could be taken on waking, half an hour before the midday meal, in the mid afternoon and last thing at night.

If a variety of medicines and tablets must be given during the day, work out a timetable, write it down, and stick to it.

How to Give Them

Always read the label on the bottle each time, even if you are certain that you recognise it and know it by heart. Shake the bottle well, turning it upside down at least once. Use a plastic measuring spoon available from chemists as it measures the exact dose. If you are using a measuring glass hold it so that its marks are at eye level. Never pour out a guesswork 'dollop': you may make bad mistakes. Replace the stopper at once. Unless instructed that the medicine must be taken neat add a little water to it. This softens any unpleasant taste, even though it may lengthen swallowing time.

Tablets taken from their containers you treat with the same care. Some new pill boxes have safety caps which are difficult for children to open, having to be pushed firmly down while being unscrewed. Unfortunately they have also proved rather difficult for those with weak hands, who may need help.

Always put the medicine or tablet container away. Never leave a box of sleeping tablets alongside the bed. Patients waking through the night can lose count of what they have taken and unwittingly give themselves overdoses. If an extra tablet is to be available in the middle of the night let that one, and only that one, be accessible to the waker.

Always finish a full course of medicines; this is specially important with antibiotics (p.17). Do not stop the course without asking your doctor. If you suspect it is giving side effects tell him. A lot of patients blame antibiotics and other medicines for unpleasant feelings caused by the illness itself.

Any preparation which is left over from the course you discard, preferably down the lavatory. Do not treasure it for some other time when anyone is feeling unwell, nor accept a friend's left-overs on his recommendation. As for the empty containers, throw those away too, or wash and return to the chemist. Please do not transfer pills from one container to another which is unlabelled or which bears an incaccurate label: nasty accidents might happen.

Finally, if a lot of different pills are being taken, do not mix up a sample lot in one container for convenience: the resulting mixture may look like an attractive fruit salad but will lead to confusion.

Keeping Medicines

What you do legitimately retain and what you store, like aspirin, for emergencies must be in a safe medicine cupboard. It is safe if it is in a dry room and inaccessible to children. That at once rules out a bathroom cabinet.

The ideal medicine cabinet is compartmented and has a sloping top so that bottles cannot be left lying there. It is best without a key, openable only by special catches which need the action of two adult hands. Suitable cabinets can be found in branches of stores such as Mothercare.

Meningitis

Meningitis is dreaded but, thanks to antibiotics, the overall recovery rate is high. However, this greatly depends on early diagnosis and treatment.

The brain and spinal cord are closely covered by three fine layers of membranes, the meninges. Between two of these is the cerebrospinal fluid. The whole acts as buffer and protection. The illness consists of their inflammation brought about by infection. An injury to the head could precipitate this, but in the majority of cases bacteria or viruses have spread to the meninges through the blood stream from some other part of the body, often the nose or throat. Sometimes it is very difficult to pinpoint the origin.

Children are more commonly affected than adults. Meningitis can vary from a quite mild condition to one which is alarmingly severe. The most common type is that known as cerebrospinal fever. It has also been called 'spotted fever' because it may produce blotchy rashes. After an incubation period of one to five days its symptoms appear suddenly. Fever and headache are the beginning, often with the eyes abnormally sensitive to light. The patient may vomit, may become delirious or comatose and may have convulsions.

There is a reflex spasm of the muscles around the spine and at the back of the neck. Moving forwards against this is difficult and painful, so the patient may lie straight with a stiff neck, which resists attempts to bend the head forward. (A milder form of this stiffness however can sometimes be found in quite different fevers, with no disturbing import.)

Sometimes, as when the infecting microbe is that of tuberculosis, the symptoms develop so slowly and insidiously over several days that the likely diagnosis is not immediately evident.

In all cases the patient's cerebrospinal fluid is of great diagnostic importance. Lumbar puncture is the method of collecting this fluid for laboratory study; it is aspirated from the space between the meninges by means of a hollow needle passed between two of the lower vertebrae. Its appearance, the types of cells floating in it, its chemical composition and the check on any bacteria present indicate the type of meningitis and the antibiotic needed. Bacteriological testing, however, takes a little time, so treatment is often begun speculatively, but urgently, so that no time is lost.

At the risk of causing some false alarms and unjustified anxiety the following must be stressed. Very young children and babies may begin meningitis attacks with misleading vague symptoms suggesting, for instance, chest or abdominal troubles. This could delay hospital admission and appropriate treatment. Suspect the possibility when a child with a fever combines irritability with drowsiness, shows a distant stare, resents being handled and becomes stiff or jerky, or has a convulsion.

Menstruation and Menopause

Every month during the child-bearing years of a woman, the lining of the uterus becomes rich in blood vessels and thickens up. It has made itself cushiony and receptive to a fertilised ovum.

The two ovaries more or less take it in turn, once a month, to liberate an ovum, and send it on its way travelling down the fallopian tube towards the uterus. A whole set of hormones (chemical messengers circulating in the blood) governs what happens to the uterus. To put this complicated interrelationship of chemical signals as simply as possible, hormones from the pituitary gland in the brain control the ovary and those from the ovary adjust the uterus.

If fertilisation does not happen then the ovum degenerates. The superficial part of the uterus lining is shed together with blood. The menstrual period has begun.

If on the other hand the ovum is fertilised, this happens in the Fallopian tube, where it is met by the questing spermatozoa. The fertilised egg moves to the uterus and embeds itself in its lining which is then maintained. Pregnancy has begun.

Some Statistics

Menstruation generally begins between the ages of 11 and 13 and ends

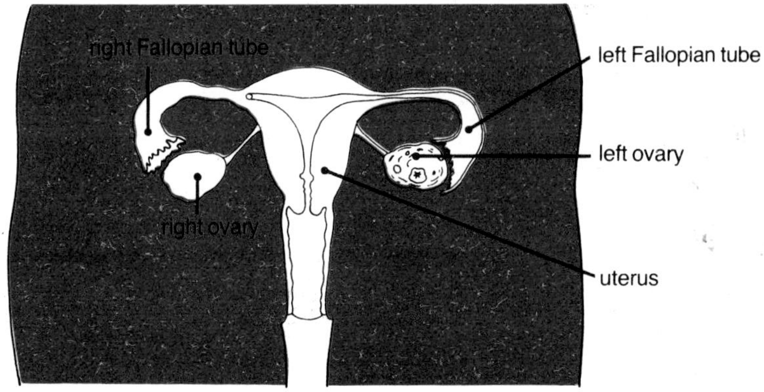

between the ages of 47 and 53 (but these are very variable); it comes every 26 to 30 days and lasts 3 to 5 days; the total blood loss ranges from two to eight ounces.

Fallacies

Even in the enlightenment of today some young women receive from their well meaning but utterly misinformed seniors extraordinary advice about periods. Women should feel quite well during menstruation, which is a normal happening. A lot of them still get crazy information that they will feel ill, and should be at rest. They are told to take no baths, not to wash their hair nor to change their underwear, or that they should wear extra clothes.

Absent Periods

If an expected period does not happen the simplest explanation is pregnancy; another is the onset of the menopause, or change of life. However, of quite a number of other valid causes the most common is a disturbance of the hormone balance which regulates the periods. Emotion can do this. Less common causes are constitutional disturbances like growths, severe anaemia, infections, malnutrition and drug-taking.

Rarely, girls as they grow into their teens do not begin to have periods, and may be helped by hormonal medicines. Very rarely they do in fact have a blood loss which does not show though they may feel a monthly discomfort. They have a congenital blockage at the lower end of the vagina, and this can be easily corrected.

Heavy, Irregular, Prolonged or Frequent Losses

Again hormonal or emotional factors may be at work, but disorders of the reproductive organs, such as inflammation or growths of the Fallopian tubes, ovaries and uterus must be ruled out. Fibroids (p.112) are common nuisances in this respect.

Any woman who has such abnormal periods *must* (not merely 'should') see her doctor early and not put up with them with the vague idea that this is just a misfortune of women. It is most likely that a simply treated cause will be found. If something serious is present it will have been found early. In any case these heavy losses are so very likely to cause anaemia that this in itself justifies medical advice.

If the patient is on the contraceptive pill, then perhaps a change of the type of pill will be all that is needed.

Painful Periods

No woman should accept more than a mild discomfort at the time of her periods. If she gets pain in the back, the lower abdomen and thighs she should do something definite about it. That pregnancy and childbirth generally cures forever has a limited application.

A generally active life with exercise is a valuable beginning. Simple pain relievers like aspirin or paracetamol often are all that are needed. Retiring to bed with a hot water bottle on the abdomen often helps, but disrupts the daily time table and is a rather inadequate approach.

A lot of the pain is due to spasm of the muscles of the uterus; recent research has found that several drugs primarily designed to relieve the pain of arthritis counter a chemical in the uterus which causes spasm. In some cases of period pains they have proved very successful. Hormonal preparations, including the contraceptive pill also can be effective.

Sometimes women who have never been troubled this way before develop painful periods. The cause then could be some illness like inflammation or infection in the reproductive system.

The moral of all this is that the doctor's consulting room, rather than the bedroom or the chemist's counter is the right place to begin seeking relief.

Premenstrual Tension

During the five or six days leading up to the beginning of a period, and sometimes for two days after, a lot of women are emotionally altered. In varying degrees they become anxious, depressed, easily upset and relatively less efficient. Some careful studies have shown how girls in school examinations, housewives at work, or women in business do less well in the premenstrual days. Crimes by women also occur with far greater frequency at those times, and the influence of premenstrual tension has been accepted as a defence by some courts of justice in France and England.

The sufferers also have to put up with retention of water in the body which gives them a bloated feeling and increase in weight. They may find their usual skirt bands and bra fittings too small.

The cause of premenstrual tension is physical, and imbalance between two of the hormones involved in the menstrual cycle. Sedatives or diuretics (which increase the kidney's action) help but are aimed at symptoms. Hormonal preparations treat more directly.

The Menopause

The menopause is due to a decrease of one hormone from the ovary. There are several normal patterns by which the periods cease at the 'change of life'. The intervals between them may lengthen; the loss may decrease; sometimes the periods stop quite suddenly. Does this mean that the woman is now unable to conceive? It would be a gamble on her part to assume it and some doctors recommend her continuing with any contraceptive precautions she might be taking for at least two years.

It is most important to realise that prolonged, frequent or heavy losses are not features of the menopause. They, and any bleeding after the periods have ceased, need medical investigation.

Some women undergo the change of life without any definite symptoms at all. So many symptoms have been ascribed to the menopause as to make it appear responsible for practically any ill to which body and mind are subject. In fact the two main symptoms irrefutably related to the hormone decrease are flushing and a dryness at the vagina. Other changes liable to occur at that time of life may not have such a direct relationship. The hair becomes thinner and coarser; the breasts lose shape and elasticity; bone begins to become less dense and, in later years, resists fracturing less easily. Headaches and muscle or joint aches are not menopausal symptoms.

Hot flushes, sudden redness of the skin with warm sweating, are due to instability in the tone of blood vessel walls. They can be very uncomfortable. In addition the poor woman is embarrassed, certain that they are obvious to all bystanders — which in fact they are not.

On the mental side difficulty in making decisions, loss of confidence or tendency to depression are features which tend to appear before the menopause. Around the age of fifty many women undergo a change-of-life unrelated to their bodies, but to their domestic and social scenes. Children, now grown and independent, no longer need their mother; a husband is perhaps immersed in his work and career and less concerned about the home than he used to be; the woman may be worried about losing her femininity, her increasing weight, or a lessened sexual libido. Some women have a tendency to blame any symptom on their age, whatever that may be, and the menopause is an obvious scapegoat.

Treatment of the true symptoms has often been reassurance and by mild sedatives. Administering small amounts of the missing hormone has been used more and more recently with very good results. It has to be given with some watchful precautions, and doctors tailor the prescriptions to their patients. Often tablets are given in interrupted courses, with a break of one week every month. Routine checks for any untoward side effects may be needed.

Ménière's Disease

see Vertigo

Migraine

A lot of people think this is any severe headache — especially if they have it themselves. The condition in fact has to show very definite characteristics before it can bear the ignoble name of migraine. The headaches are recurrent in someone who, in the intervals, is well. They may come in a series almost daily or may be separated by months. The onset is sudden, but sometimes the sufferer has felt vaguely unwell for a day before the attack. This begins with a constriction of blood vessels in the brain, giving one or more symptoms of neurological disturbance, such as numbness, tingling or weakness in a part of the body like a limb or at the lips. Trouble with vision is a common manifestation. The patient has blind spots, or is bothered by the impression of shimmering lights or bright zig-zag lines.

After a few minutes of this there is a change. Now the headache develops as blood vessels at the brain are dilating abnormally. It is very severe and may sometimes last for days. Sufferers describe it as pounding and throbbing (at the same rate as the pulse). Very often it is accompanied by sickness. Many patients welcome this for with vomiting the headache becomes easier.

Migraine generally comes first at puberty, and is likely to carry on into middle age or, in women, until the menopause. Often it runs in families. Many have described those most likely to get it as intelligent and meticulous in character; others disagree, believing that though migraine can attack any personality it is the meticulous and intelligent who will report it to the doctor.

Whatever they may be like these people seem to have a basic predisposition which can then be triggered off by some factor such as worry or overwork. Exposure to bright lights (including long sessions in front of the television) may do it. For some the trigger is fired by certain foods, particularly chocolate, wines, cheese, citrus fruits and fried dishes. On the other hand, missing a meal or fasting, which lowers the sugar in the body, can also be guilty. Women sufferers are more prone to attacks at the time of their periods, or just before if they are bothered by premenstrual tension. The oral contraceptive sometimes makes things worse.

Treatment begins with prevention. Some tablets can keep a patient relatively clear if he is bothered by frequent attacks. He may wisely keep a gastronomic diary to check if any special food appears to be a factor.

For the attack itself there are other preparations taken either as tablets or (where vomiting is severe) as suppositories. The really important thing is to begin these immediately an attack threatens, to cut it short at the beginning, and so it is sensible to keep them always handy.

Miscarriage *see* Abortion

Moles *see* Birthmarks

Mongolism
see Down's Syndrome

Mumps *see also* Fevers of Children *and* Immunisation

The diagram shows the position of the three glands, on either side, which produce our saliva; ducts from them lead to the inside of the mouth. The largest glands are called the parotids and generally are the ones most noticeably enlarged in mumps.

This is a virus infection with a rather long and variable incubation period of about two to three weeks. Before the glands become large and painful the patient may feel generally ill and feverish for a few days; his saliva already harbours the virus and so he may transmit the illness to others.

The parotids are the first to become swollen and tender, sometimes slightly only and sometimes immensely giving the unfortunate victim an absurdly puffy face, made even worse when the glands under the jaw swell up a few days later. The degree of swelling and tenderness however bears no relationship to the severity of the illness. Chewing activates the glands and therefore increases pain. In general the mouth becomes rather dry. The patient may be unwilling to

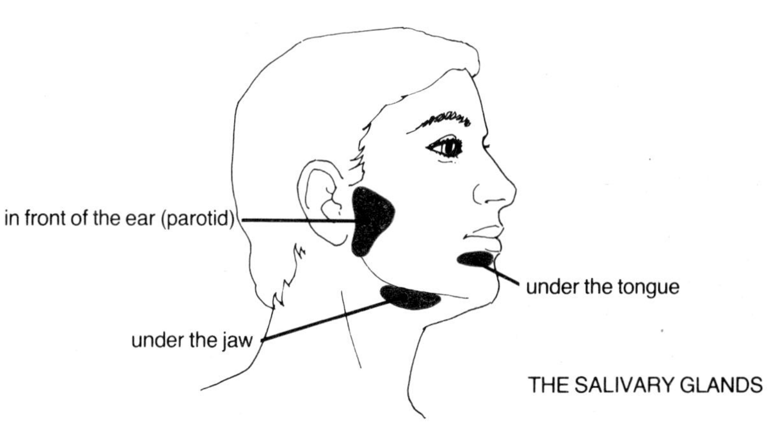

THE SALIVARY GLANDS

eat, but will face soft foods and liquid diet.

The duration of the attack is also variable from a few days (generally) to two weeks and the patient is infectious until six days after the swellings have subsided. In the meantime there is no special treatment except bed rest, pain relievers and, sometimes, mouth washes.

Complications may rarely happen, and are more likely to do so in adult patients and in those who are not at rest during the illness. They include (rarely) meningitis, inflammation of the pancreas and thyroid glands and (occasionally) inflammation of the testes or the ovaries.

Muscle Strain

see Sprains and Strains

Napkin Rash

Probably there is no single cause, but an interaction of several: chafing and rubbing; long sustained dampness; chemical irritation from urine or from inadequately rinsed napkins; infection from stools or from napkins.

The prevention of napkin rash therefore depends on straightforward care: soft napkins, not too tightly applied; washing and drying the area with each change; use of sterilant solutions in the buckets in which soiled napkins are dropped; full rinsing of napkins after washing; frequent napkin changings (this applies especially to the useful disposable type, which tend to get soggier sooner); avoiding plastic pants whenever possible.

The use of plastic pants can be regarded as applying a poultice of stools and urine. Ideally they should be reserved for visits to rich bachelor uncles. However, many domestic as well as social occasions encourage their use. Then the pants should not be tight, but the sort which freely allow air in and out at the edges. The more air which reaches the baby's bottom the better. Giving the baby daily regular sessions of free un-nappied kicking is an excellent habit.

A napkin rash can be anything from mild redness to severe infection. If the rash appears try to arrange as long periods as possible with the baby's bottom unclothed, or only very loosely covered. Do not use creams or lotions unless they are prescribed by the doctor or nurse. If the rash persists after ten days or develops any hint of infection visit the doctor. Sometimes extra troubles such as thrush (p.206) can supervene on the original rash.

Nettlerash

This is known medically as urticaria. However strange the word, we are all familiar with *Urtica Dioica,* which is the ordinary stinging nettle. It has the undeserved honour of giving its name to the hightly irritating skin trouble, popularly known as nettlerash. The nettle liberates histamine when touched. It is this which produces the typical redness and swelling of the skin, just as may happen in cases of allergy (p.14).

The body can develop sensitivity to anything, but with nettlerash we are generally concerned with foods, or at least with things swallowed. Shellfish and strawberries are common examples of items which give trouble. Some people will get a rash after certain drugs, ranging from pain relievers to antibiotics. Insect bites can provoke nettlerash and rarely cases have arisen from the presence of parasitic worms.

The rash does not always appear immediately; sometimes a few days may elapse. It begins with severe itching, and then the weals appear. These raised red areas, paler in their centres, tend to develop in crops, coming and going so the pattern changes daily or hourly. Pressure has a lot to do with it. The rash will be pronounced where the skin has been rubbed or touched, and can show where the patient has been lying or has worn belts or braces. If (or rather, when) he scratches, there will he raise further weals. By rubbing with a finger he can even shape out designs or letters on his skin. Emotion plays a part; anger and frustration will certainly worsen the condition.

Cooling applications like calamine lotion, or even water, can give relief. Aspirin is very helpful too (unless, of course, the patient is sensitive to it). Antihistamines (p.19) form the best treatment. In some cases of great severity the doctor may choose to give corticosteroids (p.79) or adrenaline injections.

Nose

see Bleeding, Catarrh *and* Sinusitis

Neurosis

Neurosis is an illness. To be neurotic is no less deserving of sense and sympathy than being 'pneumonic', 'measlic', 'appendictic', or anything else. In neurosis the sufferer has disturbing beliefs, fears or behaviour and recognises this. He does not lose a sense of reality and he is aware there is mental disturbance. He does not like the situation but cannot help it.

This is different from the less common 'psychosis' (p.175) where the victim really has lost some form of reality. (This word must not be confused with psychoneurosis which is a more technical name for neurosis.) The neurotic knows who, why and where he is, but somewhere in the past events which threatened, saddened or humiliated him have twisted his values. Forgotten, but hidden in the unconscious mind, they still influence and perhaps distort conscious judgments.

Many could be traceable to mentally traumatic experiences of childhood or adolescence. They could be related to learning about matters of living and feeling, such as responsibility, sex or personal relationships. When later in life parallel situations arise the conscious mind behaves as if afraid, guarded or hostile.

This can show itself in many ways. Tics (habitual twitches or spasms) form a gentle example. Mild or severe phobias — to birds, to closed-in spaces or to open areas, for example — are forms of neurosis, and so are anxiety state (p.20) and the reactive form of depression (p.84). Some neurotics develop obsessions with repeated unnecessary actions such as touching objects or hand washing.

Depression and anxiety can be relieved by drugs, but they are only symptoms and not the cause.

Treatment involves psychiatric investigation. It tries to guide the patient sympathetically into discovering and understanding the forces working within him. This can be difficult and time consuming, but it will work, whereas commands to 'pull yourself together' will certainly fail.

Nursing

Advice on nursing in the home risks appearing like a series of platitudes. However these can add up to a very positive contribution to the patient's well being. The same organisations which teach first aid (p.112) also run worthwhile, easy nursing courses. The Red Cross manual *Nursing* is an excellent investment, obtainable at modest cost from any of their branches.

In this section only a few general points can be mentioned, but see also the sections on Antiseptics, Baths, Bedmaking, Bed Pan, Bed Sores, Blanket Baths, Convalescence, Dressings, Falls, Handicapped, Hot Water Bottles, Incontinence, Medicines, Pulse and Temperature.

Relationship with the Patient

Some authority is necessary. In the home familiarity may have bred if not contempt then, perhaps, a certain disregard of the family member acting as nurse. Lay on a friendly but definite dogmatism.

If the doctor has given specific advice about rest, medicines, diet or special procedures, then make sure the patient knows that you are following his professional instructions. It is always worth asking the doctor for clear cut information on such points to strengthen your task.

A housewife ill in her home is much like a man in bed in his factory or office, unprepared to relinquish reins of office. She listens to every domestic noise, assessing what is going on and may be worried that no one is dealing properly with her domain. Shield her as much as possible from such concerns.

Always maintain an atmosphere of 'sympathy and confidence' — whenever possible you show fullest sympathy with the patient in his present situation, but at the same time you create an atmosphere of complete confidence about his improvement and recovery. The combined attitudes make a great contribution to his morale.

Let the adult patient realise that you assume the professionalism of not discussing his illness with anybody who is not involved.

The Bed

The patient is likely to be far easier in his own bed than if moved to another in the house, but the site of a bed as sleeping quarters is not necessarily an ideal one for nursing. It might be possible and necessary to move it from alongside a wall to an open position which makes it approachable from both sides. If it is very low

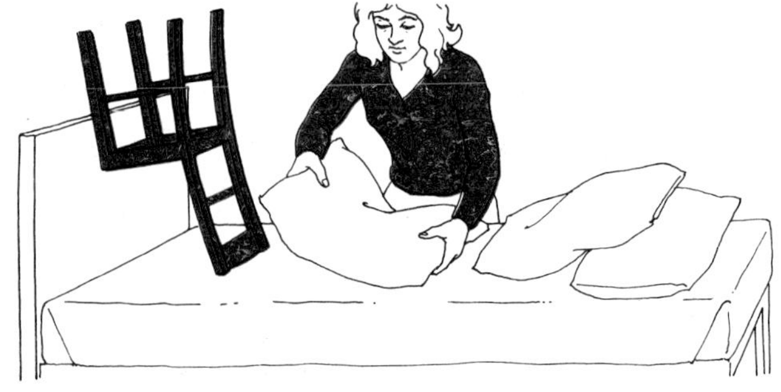

and the patient is likely to be bedfast long, then it could be raised by wooden blocks under the feet; these can be obtained through the social services or the Red Cross.

Extra pillows, and sometimes a back rest are needed for patients sitting in bed. A back rest can be provisionally improvised by a chair placed upside down at the head of the bed, and then backed with pillows. If the patient is very hot, it may be wise to give him fewer blankets than usual.

Encourage the patient to move about in bed as much as his illness allows. If he himself cannot move much, change his position every couple of hours if you can.

Get a bedside table on the right of the bed for a right handed patient. Often these little tables are far too small to hold what the patient needs and accumulates and they can be supplemented with another table. Put at the side a waste paper basket lined with a plastic bag.

Allow the patient a signalling system. Unless he is the sort likely to amuse himself by sounding it often and unnecessarily have a bell or whistle secured to the bedclothes.

The Room

Warmth and ventilation have a common priority. The room temperature should be between 60°F and 65°F (16°C and 23°C). Air should be allowed freely from outside through the window. Keep the door closed, or nearly closed; draughts are not dangerous but they can be uncomfortable.

Remove any unnecessary mats. Let the room have at least two chairs; add a comfortable one for the patient when he begins to get up and sit out. Make sure there is an extra table to give a good clear working surface for equipment likely to be needed, and for taking trays.

Avoid noise in the room, but do not overdo this. Creeping about on tiptoe can give the wrong impression to the patient.

Lighting

The room should have a good top light. The patient should have an accessible stand lamp. Both should have shades or avoid glare. The ideal lighting (including that from the window) would come from above and from the left for a right handed man. A hand torch at night is often useful if the stand lamp is not particularly easy to get at.

Food and Drink

Eating in bed can prove a surprisingly messy affair. Let the patient have a big towel across the bed and another to use as a bib. Large size paper tissues will also be useful.

Serve food up attractively. When appetite is low small portions on a large plate will be more effective than large amounts heaped up. Never hurry the eater; let him eat in his own time. Clear the tray and plates away as soon as he has finished.

A high fluid intake is generally important. If the doctor agrees encourage an adult patient to drink five pints a day. Have a jug of any pleasant and permissible drink by the bedside at a level easy to reach and pour from. It should have a lid or a clean cloth cover.

A patient who cannot sit up to use an ordinary glass or cup uses a feeding cup. Every home has one — though it might be disguised as a small teapot.

Visitors

Use your judgment and do not let

them be tiring. Welcome them to the house, but do not hesitate to use tactful excuses to prevent them going to the patient when they arrive inopportunely. Place the chair of those who are admitted so that the patient can see them easily from his pillow.

Children

How sad for the small sick child to feel uncertain and insecure tucked away isolated in his room. Most doctors would agree to have a cot brought to the living room, or the bigger child settled there on the sofa, turned into a bed.

The small patient needs a lot of toys to keep him contented, but not a whole cluster together. Bring them out one at a time so that with variety comes renewed interest.

If he has to take medicine which tastes unpleasant, let him know in advance that he might not like it, but that it will help to get him back to liberty quickly. Have a favourite drink handy to follow it up.

Obesity

Fat people are fat because they eat too much — more than their body can burn up. Obesity due to a defect in a gland does exist but is sufficiently rare for it to be a specialist's showpiece to clinical colleagues.

Why does one eat too much? Obviously because food is nice, yet it could be a matter of habit and also one of emotion. Repeated over-eating distends the stomach which eventually gets used to its distension and sends hunger signals as it empties. A vicious circle has been established.

We tend to turn to food for solace and celebration, a habit which well-meaning parents may have begun and which has continued as we grew up. The hurt or unhappy child is comforted with a 'sweetie'. The achieving child is rewarded with a cake or chocolate. In adult life the pattern has formed almost like a reflex. The bereft, the lonely, the frustrated may unconsciously turn to food for consolation. This might explain many a fat person's problem.

Why Fight Overweight?

The clearest reason is the aesthetic one of looking nicer. Vanity and fashion are powerful incentives. So are self-reproach and self-respect. The obese do not like their image of themselves and they can foresee the better personality awaiting in the thinner self.

Far more urgent is the factor of health. The ailments to which obesity predisposes include severe heart and circulation troubles, gallstones and diabetes. In addition excess weight and flabbier muscles can contribute to osteoarthritis of the leg joints, backache, hernias and varicose veins.

Motivating Oneself

A programme of encouragement to lose weight could include several manoeuvres. A realistic daily view in the bedroom mirror of oneself naked, tape measure in hand, can be very effective. So can daily weighing, again naked, on the bathroom scales. This can be followed by boldly writing the day's figures on a wall chart. Realising that others in the family will be reading them too will powerfully help one's efforts. In fact, the whole family can, and should, actively support in every way.

Some advocate joining a club of fellow reducers who meet regularly for weighing and exhortation. Certain temperaments do find encouragement thereby but it can prove an expensive method of doing what others prefer to manage on their own.

How to Lose Weight

Exercise helps. This does not necessarily mean sessions of 'physical jerks' for it can be adequately done by a deliberate bounciness in everyday activities. Avoiding the car when a bicycle will do, running instead of plodding upstairs, moving speedily in general — all can help. But this is not the full answer. It has been assessed that to lose one pound in weight the average person should walk or even run some fifty miles. And what would that do to his appetite?

Appetite reducing drugs are of little help except for the first two or three weeks of taking them. Their effects wane and the patient is back where he started. Besides, some may give unpleasant side-effects like insomnia, restlessness and dryness of the mouth.

Many other approaches exist to tempt the would-be reducer. Massage belts, plastic suits, electric vibrators and body lotions are not likely to do much more than keep the wheels of commerce turning. One is left with the only successful method: dieting.

What Diet? What Weight?

The weight to which one should aim and the diet by which one gets there are matters for medical advice. A diet can be a simple matter of guidance as to what foods are least nutritious and which most fattening. Sugars and starchy foods have a high degree of guilt here and many can lose weight by avoiding them.

Other Points for Reducers

Before each meal decide what you will eat and keep to that. Take no second helpings; do not eat or nibble between meals; do not try to fill up with too many vegetables or salads, this would keep the stomach distended; chew fully and slowly, the meal will seem bigger; get up from the table still feeling a little hungry; brushing the teeth immediately after meals helps to remove the feeling of wanting more.

Sudden pangs are likely to pass off within twenty minutes. Spend that time doing anything (except eating!) which is active and interesting.

Aim for a steady moderate loss instead of dramatic results from a crash diet. Do not expect a consistent rate of reduction. Weight loss on a diet can be quite erratic — just keep dieting.

For most of the obese dieting is not a programme set for a fixed time. It is really a way of altering eating habits for the rest of ones life. The body will change and so will the personality. A new self-confidence will be born.

Osteoarthritis

see Arthritis

Pain

Pain is extremely useful. One can make out a case for welcoming it as a warning signal of something being amiss. However, we cannot be entirely reassured that pain is a reliable guide. Sometimes it is missing when most needed. Tumours, for instance, are painless. It is only if they grow big enough to press on a sensitive organ that the signal begins. Also bowels in themselves do not beget pain in the ordinary way. If anything goes wrong with them they will not register pain unless they become distended or twisted or until any inflammation they have spreads to their covering membranes, to give peritonitis. Nor does brain tissue itself produce pain if, for instance, a sharp object penetrates it. Headache is caused by abnormal changes in brain coverings or blood vessels.

Another possibly misleading feature is that pain may not be felt directly in the area of the body concerned. The ramifications and interconnections of the nervous system are immensely complicated. Impulses travelling along a nerve may spread to adjoining nerves, giving sensations far afield. Trouble in an organ will send messages towards the brain by nerves which relay with others via the spinal cord. At the point of the spinal cord where they do this some of the messages can influence other nerves serving other parts of the body from the same spinal cord level. The brain, receiving these, may interpret the pain as arising from those parts.

Thus pneumonia in the right lung can mimic pain in the appendix region. Also every doctor knows that a patient may complain of pain in a knee which appears quite normal on examination, because the real cause lies in the hip joint above it. *Referred pain* as this is called has many examples. Inflammation at the diaphragm below the lungs may manifest as aching in the shoulder.

The appendix lies low on the right side of the abdomen. However the first pain of appendicitis, when the organ is getting distended and stretched, is referred to near the navel. Later, inflammation spreads to involve the membranes around the appendix. This now becomes the major producer of pain, which moves down and to the right marking the true site of the trouble.

The sounding of the brain's alarm bell, so to speak, can be very loud or quite low according to the amount of hurt being done. Something else may muffle it. The degree of pain felt can vary greatly if the body is experiencing other things at the same time. The brain is no passive indicator. That it spontaneously manufactures its own pain relieving chemicals has been shown by recent research. These chemicals, named endorphins, behave in some respects like morphia. They could be produced as reaction to other things stimulating the nervous system. In this way a special emergency calling for action or for concentration of effort would create a higher amount of endorphins, and a reduction in pain. This would help the hurt person to carry on until the emergency was over.

Susceptibility to pain is a highly personal thing. Perhaps this individuality is related to the ability of each brain to make endorphins.

Period Pains

see Menstruation

Peptic Ulcer

Definitions first: an *ulcer* is an open sore or erosion of the surface of the skin or (as in this case) of the lining membrane of an organ; *peptic* here refers to the stomach and to the duodenum, which is the first part of the intestines after the stomach. A third word, *gastric*, also needs explaining. It is an adjective for anything relating to the stomach.

Those who speak of a 'gastric stomach' are saying the same thing twice over and describing nothing more than a 'stomachy stomach'.

So the term peptic ulcer covers two different things: a gastric ulcer and duodenal ulcer. Medically however they are not so very different for they arise in similar ways and produce quite similar symptoms.

The main symptom is pain, felt in the upper part of the abdomen and below the ribs. This is associated with the effect of hydrochloric acid which is normally present in the stomach. Very useful and necessary it is too, since it plays a role in digesting foods. The lining membrane stands the acid well, except where an ulcer forms, and that may happen at some gap in the protective coating of mucus which covers this lining.

When the ulcer is in the stomach the pain is likely to appear within half an hour of eating. That of the more common duodenal ulcer comes as the stomach empties, about two or three hours after full meals. There may also be vomiting.

The patient will feel easier if he takes small amounts of bland foods, like milk, or medicines which reduce the stomach acidity. He will feel worse with alcohol, with spicy and fried or very hot foods. It is surprising how many people cheerfully pour down their gullets drinks of so high a temperature that they would not like to spill any on their fingers. Strong emotions of anxiety, anger, or stress and hurry aggravate the condition. The rushed and busy business executive who takes irregular and hasty meals is a likely victim.

Untreated an ulcer can, in the long run, do a lot of damage. It may extend in depth and perforate a stomach wall, leading to peritonitis and an emergency operation. It may leave scarring which narrows the stomach or duodenum. More frequently it may bleed, perhaps only slightly and unnoticeably but so consistently that the patient becomes anaemic. Heavier bleeding could show up by the way digestive juices alter the colour of blood; black stools or black vomit demand a doctor's opinion.

The presence of the ulcer can be confirmed by investigations. Though itself it is not visible in X-rays, its shape can be outlined by the patient's drinking a fluid which is opaque to X-rays. Gastroscopy is the examination of the inside of the stomach by passing down the gullet a fine tube fitted with optical equipment and a light. This gives very clear information and is not as afflicting to the patient as it sounds.

As for treatment, this should, in severe cases, begin by rest. Meals will be taken slowly in a relaxed manner. Modifying one's life style to something near a smooth routine with very frequent eating of small amounts is important. Medicines to reduce the acid in the stomach help greatly. The ulcer should heal, but this can take longer than the patient thinks; do not let him stop treatment before his doctor allows just because he has become free of pain.

Surgical measures are reserved for the ulcer which refuses to heal. It can consist of excising that part of the stomach which produces much acid, or sectioning a nerve which activates the stomach.

One important point: cigarette smoking will markedly delay the healing of any peptic ulcer.

Piles

see Haemorrhoids

Pleurisy *see* Pneumonia

Pneumonia

When discussing pneumonia a quick reminder of breathing anatomy is worth while. We take in air through mouth and nose, down the *trachea* (windpipe). In the chest this divides into two main *bronchi*, one for each lung. Then within the lung the bronchus branches out many times, out into air tubes which become smaller and smaller until they end up as terminal *bronchioles*. These lead into minute clusters of air sacs called *alveoli*, rather like a microscopic bunch of grapes. The walls of the sacs are surrounded by a network of very fine blood vessels. Oxygen passes across walls of the alveoli and those of the vessels into the blood, which will carry it round the body. At the same time the blood gives up, into the alveoli, carbon dioxide, the waste product of used up oxygen brought from all tissues. The carbon dioxide now is breathed out.

Pneumonia is inflammation of the lungs. Almost always it is due to infection by bacteria or viruses which have reached the alveoli when the lungs' natural defences have been lowered. Fungus also can infect, and occasionally irritant vapours will start the process. Sometimes solid particles, like bits of food or pus from the nose and throat, can be aspirated into the airways and carry microbes with them.

The alveoli react, as do all tissues when infected, by filling up with an exudate which seeps through from the blood vessels. Instead of only air they now contain fluid, which interferes considerably with the exchange of gases.

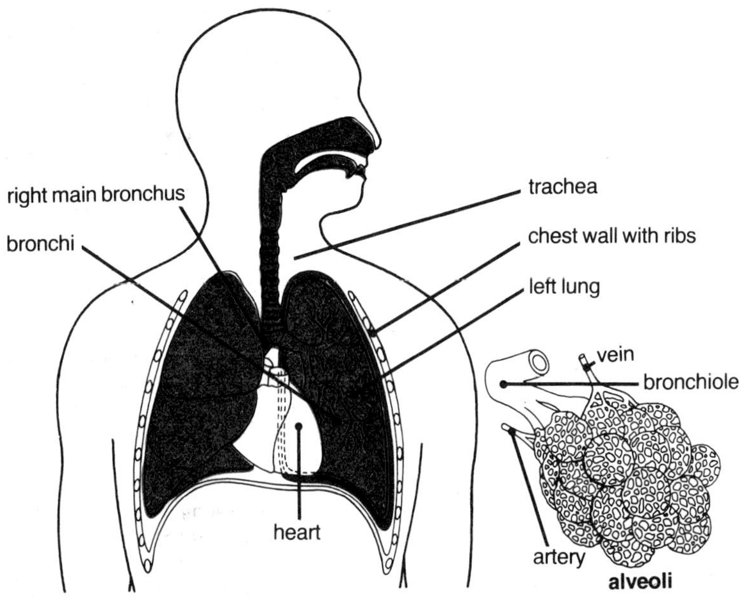

Pleurisy is the condition when infection and inflammation spreads from the lung surface into its covering membrane the pleura. This is a double membrane folded all round each lung, one sheet of it closely on the lung and the other against the inner surface of the chest wall.

Pneumonia proper generally gives its symptoms quite suddenly. But these may follow other symptoms of an illness in the nose and throat. A 'cold' or influenza can have been the bridgehead of microbes preparatory to lung invasion.

Fever, headache and shivering form the start. Cough follows rapidly, dry at first, then moist, with pus-laden sputum which may be yellow, green or even rust coloured. Now the patient becomes breathless as various parts of the 'spongy' pattern of the lungs become filled with fluid instead of air.

There are basically two ways in which this can happen. In *broncho-pneumonia* patches of infection are scattered round both lungs. On the other hand the infection may involve a whole zone, one or more of the lobes into which the lungs are divided (the right lung has three, and the left one two). This is *lobar pneumonia*. The difference is a matter for the doctor rather than the patient, each type having some different characteristics, and also tending to arise from different sorts of infection. One could generalise by saying that broncho-pneumonia is the less severe of the two, but as with all generalisations one finds many exceptions. The popular expression 'double pneumonia' merely means that both sides of the chest are affected.

The lung itself feels no pain. Rawness in the chest will be due to inflammation of the air tubes. But pleurisy is also a potent source of pain. The outer of the two pleural layers is very sensitive. Each breathing movement makes the layers slide against each other. In health this is a smooth easy affair, with a minute amount of moisture between them acting as lubricant. When they are inflamed and roughened their friction can be extemely painful so that the patient, though seeking more air, avoids taking a deep breath. If inflammation worsens, producing a fair amount of exudate, the patient paradoxically feels easier, for the fluid has separated the layers and they no longer rub against each other.

Modern treatment has almost erased the sinister symptoms and threat of pneumonia. Young children and those who are weak and undernourished may be very gravely ill. The elderly also are at much higher risk; their chest movements tend to be poorer, they cough up sputum less easily and their blood vessels are less elastic and effective in circulating blood defensively.

Antibiotics have revolutionised the outlook. Many patients have pneumonia so smoothly and speedily cleared that they do no realise that they have just had something which once carried immense danger.

Poisoning

The quicker you get a victim of dangerous poisoning to hospital the better. Call an ambulance. If possible let the hospital know in advance of the patient's coming and of the nature of the poison.

Swallowed Poisons

If the patient is unconscious: Follow the instructions for unconsciousness (p.210). Many poisons affect the body centre which controls respiration. If the patient is not breathing begin artificial respiration (p.26) without delay and before sending for the ambulance. Remember that you never give anything by mouth to the unconscious person.

If the patient is conscious: Ask him what happened (he may soon pass into unconsciousness). Protect his stomach and dilute the poison by giving bland drinks, tepid if possible, taken in slow sips (milk, barley water or plain water). While waiting for the ambulance put him in the recovery position as for unconsciousness (p.210) and keep him covered. Stay close to him lest he suddenly need artificial respiration.

Send containers of the poison and any liquid or tablets left over with the patient for the hospital doctors to see.

If there is a wait for the ambulance and if the patient is conscious try to make him vomit
BUT

a. Do *not* attempt this if in any way it delays getting him to hospital.

b. Do *not* attempt this if he has taken corrosives (strong acids or alkalis) or petroleum products. As it is drunk, petroleum sends vapours which could reach and damage the lungs. Corrosives burn the mouth and gullet. A return journey of these poisons in vomit would repeat the damage. A corroded, weakened, stomach wall might perforate during vomiting and let the contents pass into and burn the abdominal cavity.

Your only method for inducing vomiting is to keep the patient's head low and to irritate the back of his throat with your fingers or with the blunt handle of a spoon with folds of handkerchief wrapped round it. Never give salt or other chemicals.

Poisoning by Gases and Fumes
Though you should get the patient rapidly out of the contaminated atmosphere do not venture into this unless you are protected by a life line and a respirator.

For someone caught in a smoke filled room use a wet handkerchief round your nose and mouth as an emergency improvised respirator; take two deep breaths before you go in, then hold your breath as long as you can; crawl along the floor where smoke will be thinner. You may need a handlamp.

Preventing Accidental Poisoning
The rules are so simple, but so often disregarded. Keep all poisonous substances out of the reach of children, whose oral curiosity and love of experiment know no bounds. Have the medicine chest completely safe, inaccessible to and unopenable by children (p.155). Keep no pills or medicines on mantelpieces or in pockets, drawers, shopping baskets or handbags. Have none of the domestic cleaners, bleaches, turpentines and so forth in easily reached cupboards under the sink or dresser. Lock away all garden chemicals on a high shelf of the potting shed. Teach children to admire garden berries for their beauty but fear them if swallowed. Never keep any substance in an unlabelled container and never store a potential poison in a bottle whose shape suggests it could be wine or fruit squash.

Now that you have read this go round your premises to check. Now!

Pre-menstrual Tension

see Menstruation

Prolapse

Several parts of the body can get downwardly displaced from their proper position, but one uses the word 'prolapse' generally in relation to the uterus and the rectum (back passage). It also has been applied to the intervertebral disc (see Backache, p.32).

Prolapsed Uterus

The lower end of the abdominal cavity is encased within the bones of the pelvis. Its base is made of a shelf of muscles and ligaments which support or surround organs like the bladder, the uterus and the rectum.

A structure like this may weaken. Some people will suffer from a reduced muscle tone after middle age, and this is much more likely to happen to women who have had many children, especially if they have experienced difficult labours. The uterus then can sag down into the vagina. It may go even further, descending so that the neck of the uterus protrudes at the vulva. In the rare severe case the whole uterus can project out.

Generally this displacement happens gradually and in the early stages it gives no symptoms. Rarely a sudden sharp straining, as when lifting something heavy, may precipitate the prolapse. As the condition worsens the woman may feel an unpleasant dragging sensation and also a backache. The nearby organs are easily affected by the pull on the muscles. There may be constipation. With the bladder, however, the laxity can cause incontinence, especially stress incontinence, which is a leaking of urine on coughing, laughing, lifting or anything else which adds to pressure within the abdomen.

Operations to repair the defect are usually straight-forward and they form a significant part of a gynaecologist's work. There are times when this successful line of treatment must be deferred or avoided. A younger woman likely to have a pregnancy and childbirth which would undo the surgeon's success ought to wait. Some elderly or weak people are not fit to undergo operations. These women can wear an artificial support in the form of a plastic ring, called a pessary, which is inserted in the vagina. It is generally completely comfortable. However the ring is only a palliative and no substitute for the operation. It will not necessarily correct any accompanying trouble from the bladder or the rectum. The doctor or nurse has to find the correct size for

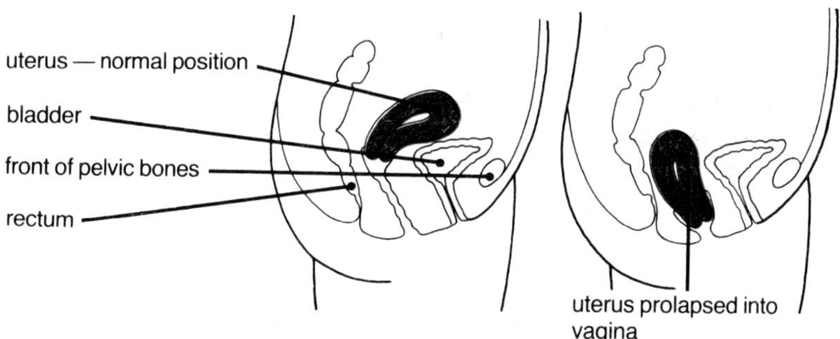

the patient. No ring should be left in indefinitely; it ought to be changed every few weeks or months.

Prolapsed Rectum

This does not happen very often. Its minor form may be found in children as well as in adults. A small amount of red projection comes from the anus, often after an excessive effort of strain with hard stools. It is only the inner membrane and not the full thickness of the rectum which is sagging, rather like the tucking out of a sleeve lining at the cuff. It is likely to correct itself spontaneously. (It is also quite liable to be mistaken for haemorrhoids by the uninitiated.) Taking steps to avoid further constipation and straining often forms the best treatment.

A difficult problem occurs when the bit prolapsing is the full thickness of the rectum. This is likely to happen with weakened muscles much in the same way as for uterine prolapse. Treatment is by operation.

Prostate Troubles

If elderly men consider the number of medical and surgical problems which can beset the reproductive organs of their female contemporaries they can be grateful that the only equivalent male trouble maker is the prostate.

To understand the prostate we must consider the rather complicated travel made by spermatozoa for ejaculation. Having been formed in each of the two testicles, they are passed to the *epididymis* on the testicle. From there they move up the long *vas deferens* tube which enters the abdominal cavity. It opens into the *urethra,* which is the tube leading from the bladder to the outside, within the penis. To be carried properly the spermatozoa need the fluid which forms semen. This comes from two sources. Most is from the *prostate* which is a gland lying just below the bladder. The urethra passes through and receives many little openings from the prostate. Just before the vas deferens reaches the urethra it is joined by a tube from another gland, the seminal vesicle, which also contributes a portion of the semen.

The point to note is that the urethra, leading urine from the bladder, begins by going through the centre of the

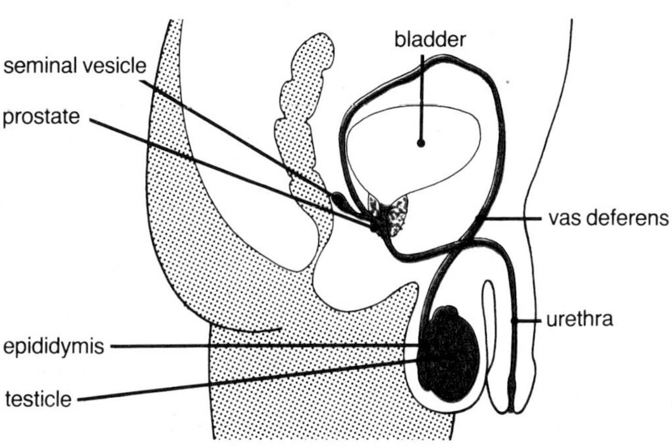

prostate. This is quite a large and firm structure, and it has a natural tendency to enlarge as men grow older. Occasionally the enlargement is not natural but is due to a tumour. Usually, however, there is no tumour, the gland merely gets bigger. There would be no harm in that if this increase in size did not press on the urethra, which in many cases it does. The emptying rate of the bladder then decreases, and the stream of urine becomes thinner. If things worsen the patient gradually has more and more difficulty passing urine or even beginning the stream. He may find as well that he feels a frequent need to go to the lavatory, or that he is troubled by a dribbling incontinence.

Unfortunately, because these symptoms progress gradually over a fairly long time, he gives them little attention and does not bother to consult his doctor. Urine which stagnates in the bladder may become infected, and this may involve the kidneys.

Then, perhaps, quite suddenly the blockage is complete. He cannot pass urine however much he tries. The bladder fills inordinately and he is in considerable pain. Cold weather, and a full meal with much to drink will predispose to the misfortune. Called at last, the doctor will pass a tube (a catheter) through the urethra and drain some of the urine away to relieve the pressure and the patient. He may not drain away all the urine at once, for a sudden complete release of such abnormal bladder pressure could be detrimental to the kidneys.

If there is difficulty or delay in getting the doctor, a patient could try to help himself by taking a hot bath. While there, relaxing completely, he might be able to pass some urine.

The real treatment of the enlarged prostate is surgical, cutting away the excess size. It is a straightforward affair which can be done in one of two ways according to circumstances and the judgment of the surgeon. The approach to the prostate gland can be by an incision in the lower part of the abdomen, or it could be through a fine operating instrument passed through the urethra.

Questions likely to be put by the patient are whether after the operation he will pass urine normally and remain sexually active. There are exceptions, but for the large majority sexual life should be unchanged and post-operative incontinence of the bladder will be slight and temporary. Fertility however could be impaired, but fortunately for most of these patients this would not be a serious matter.

The earlier the operation is performed the better, so no man should ignore the first suspicious symptoms. Another reason for this is that the less common condition of tumours of the prostate, a much more serious affair, can give similar features at its onset. It needs early diagnosis and treatment.

Psychosis

The word is often falsely used, giving rise to a lot of misunderstanding. Medically it covers the lay word 'insanity', and that again is sometimes incorrectly understood.

This severe mental illness in which the patient has lost touch with some aspect of reality should not be confused with neurosis (p. 163) where the sufferer recognises that he is mentally affected. The psychotic, whether in the belief that he is Napoleon or that powerful enemies are tracking him, or seized by the endogenous form of depression (p.84) is convinced that his state of mind is justified and corresponds with the world about him. It has been said that whereas the neurotic builds castles in the air, it is the psychotic who lives within such castles.

Sometimes psychosis may result from drug reactions, head injury or brain tumours, but very often no clear physical reasons are found.

Hallucinations, firmly believed in, can be a form of psychosis. The patient sees, hears or feels things which are not there and he reacts to them. Another abnormality may be shown as delusions, which can quite strongly disrupt the patient's life, and that of the people around him. Paranoia is the name for such mental disorder, with delusions of grandeur and power or with ideas of being persecuted. The victim may believe himself to be a personality of importance destined to change and rule his entourage (or the world). Or he may be distracted by the certainty that some group (or everyone) is systematically plotting against him. The study of history unfortunately shows how occasionally, with mixed delusions of grandeur and persecution, an otherwise well organised psychotic can reach power and create havoc.

Schizophrenia has often been defined as an illness of 'split mind'. Superficially this sounds clear and intelligible, but really it explains nothing. It is a form of psychosis, which may begin in adolescence and often has a large content of delusions. The patients tend to become introverted, withdrawn and inert. They have difficulty in communicating with others; their entourage cannot reach them by argument or emotion.

Sometimes one finds people using the term psychosis to describe an evil personality. This is grossly inaccurate and unfair. Another error is to label it as incurable. Treatment may have to be prolonged but it can succeed in many cases. Biological research is showing more and more how some mental abnormalities are related to subtle chemical conditions of the brain. This not only helps towards understanding psychosis but also in applying certain drugs for its alleviation.

The Pulse

Every time the heart beats, the blood it sends out hits the first large blood vessel, the aorta. This gives its walls an impulse which is transmitted down into all the arteries branching from it and into their divisions.

Some of these vessels can easily be felt pulsating when they lie just under the skin and just over a bone. At these points it is possible to assess the rate, regularity and nature of the heart beat.

The easiest place to measure the pulse is one or two finger breadths below the wrist, on the palm and thumb side.

Do not use you thumb which is not as sensitive as the fingers. Let three finger tips be in line together; if one of them misses the artery the other two will be there. Press only just firmly enough to feel what you want; do not squash the artery. It is a good idea to bend the patient's hand forward a little. This slackens ligaments and tendons crossing the wrist, making it easier for your to feel.

Another easy artery to reach is the small one which runs immediately in front of the notch of the ear.

Count the pulsations with a second hand watch for fifteen seconds; multiplying by four gives you the

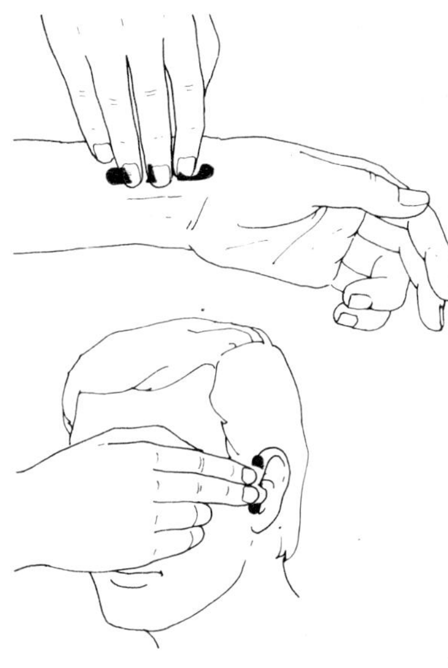

pulse rate. The normal pulse rate varies between 60 and 80 a minute. It tends to go up with exertion and emotion, to decrease with rest and relaxation. It should be regular. Only experience will teach you its normal force, therefore practise on all sorts of willing friends and relations.

Small children have faster heart beats than adults. The new born baby's pulse could be between 120 and 140. A healthy two-year-old child will average 100 and a seven year old about 90.

Pyloric Stenosis

see Vomiting

Quinsy

see Tonsils and Adenoids

Relaxation

Civilised man and woman are about the only animals who let nature down by not relaxing fully and frequently. Nearly fifty years ago Dr Grantly Dick Read advocated teaching mothers to relax so as to have easy and, often, painless labours. Since then a few changes have been made to these ideas, but his basic principles remain valid.

Interested people soon realised that one did not have to be a pregnant woman to benefit from relaxation. Some of its elements can be found in teachings like yoga or meditation but every man and woman can, and should, embrace relaxation. Even a very few minutes, once or twice a day, will give great refreshment. It costs absolutely nothing and needs no apparatus. It can be done at any time. It proves a restorative in demanding situations or at the end of the day's hard work. It may also be used to help those bothered with insomnia (p. 145).

The technique below is slightly modified from that described by Dr Dick Read in his book *Revelation of Childbirth* (Heinemann). It is simple and it is successful.

In true relaxing you are lying down and 'letting yourself go'. You are untensed, so limp on the bed that you might get a feeling of floating on air. Quite normal breathing is the only movement. It is not easy to manage this straight away. You can practice the following in rest periods.

Lie on the back on a wide couch or firm bed. A small bolster may be put under the head and shoulders and a smaller pillow under the knees. Arms are by the side, elbows half bent, hands half closed, knees slightly separated. The head lies loosely on a pillow.

Now relax the:

Shoulders by thinking of them opening outwards.

Arms by imagining them falling out of the shoulders, as though they did not belong to the body.

Back by imagining it sinking through the couch on to the floor.

Legs, knees and feet by feeling them falling outwards by their own weight.

Head by imagining it sinking into the pillow; the neck muscles are completely loose.

Eyelids by letting their own weight half close them.

Eyes by gazing into the far distance, rather than focusing on anything.

Face by imagining it 'hanging from the cheek bones', quite expressionless.

Jaw by letting it drop loose.

At first it may be necessary to relax these groups one by one. Then the different relaxed groups may be added to one another until the whole body is relaxed. Finally one becomes adept at relaxing all parts of the body simultaneously.

Breathing is allowed to follow its own natural rhythm without trying to guide it.

A pleasant, torpid, day-dreaming state often ensues. Any tendency to directed thinking should deliberately be diverted into a day-dream.

Resuscitation

see Artificial Respiration

Rheumatic Fever

There are no such things as 'growing pains'. The growth of a child is a normal event: pain announces an abnormality. The two do not go together.

If a child has limb aching and lassitude which the kind old lady next door dismisses as 'growing pains' ponder whether this might possibly be a case of rheumatic fever (also called 'acute rheumatism').

The sufferer is likely to be a child over the age of five or a teenager. Two or three weeks after a sore throat he begins to feel unwell, he loses his appetite, becomes pale and feverish. His temperature rises and he sweats. Now soon he feels pain in some of the larger joints (wrist, elbow, shoulder, ankle, knee, hip). They hurt with movement so that his sleep at night is not likely to be disturbed. The most characteristic feature is what doctors called 'migratory polyarthritis': different joints take it in turn to hurt, the pain moving day by day from one to another.

A rash, pink and with curved edges, may appear on limbs or trunks (but never on the face); it too is 'migratory', wandering and changing its outline and its sites daily. Sometimes small painless nodules develop just under the skin.

This average picture has variations. The basic sore throat may never have been present; it may have been replaced by a 'nasty cold' or by the most trivial of symptoms. The fever may not be high and the disturbance to joints may be so minimal as to be disregarded. On the other hand and very rarely, the child develops the chorea (St Vitus' Dance). Of insidious onset with restless fidgety movements, it can develop to uncontrolled muscle spasm and jerks.

The inflammation causing all these troubles is considered to be the body's sensitivity reaction to the poisons produced by the microbe known as Group A streptococcus, a common cause of sore throats. However any infection from this microbe anywhere else in the body could equally be the precursor of acute rheumatism.

Joint inflammations are bad enough, but the really serious risk in rheumatic fever is the concurrent inflammation of heart chambers and valve linings. It is this feature which the doctor watches and protects, watching the young patient with meticulous care. Inflammation within the heart instead of settling back to normality, may leave scars and deformities for life. Scarred valves are likely to interfere with the normal blood flow and thus to create heart strain and disease.

Treatment of rheumatic fever aims to reduce inflammation as much as possible and also to spare the heart. For the former aspirin in quite large doses, or sometimes corticosteroids, are effective. The heart is protected by keeping the patient completely at rest for a long time (sometimes many weeks) followed by a slowly controlled return to activity. This is a trying time both for the patient and for the parents, but justified by the results.

Even then the recovered patient is not always entirely free. He is at risk from another sensitivity reaction of his body to the poisons of any new attack by the Group A streptococcus. His doctor may advise the precautionary routine of taking penicillin for a very long time. And if about to undergo some medical adventure like a tooth extraction which is liable to liberate microbes in his system he ought to consult the doctor about the need for antibiotic cover.

Rheumatism

This word should be dismissed altogether as it is based on ancient and false medical concepts.

'Rheumatism' survives, as an etymological remnant in accepted terms like 'rheumatic fever' and 'rheumatoid arthritis', but when used all by itself the word 'rheumatism' is far too vague and unspecific. It is popular among many people who like to honour some of their pains with a fine sounding and sympathy producing name. Doctors do not care for it, but the word is so deeply installed in the language that it is difficult to do entirely without it.

A more positive postscript is that research is beginning to show more understanding of the causes of some 'rheumatic' illnesses. They appear to be related to an abnormal sensitivity of some parts of the body to chemicals produced by tissues elsewhere in the body. These sensitive parts react rather as in cases of allergy (p.14) except that the harmful substance has not come from outside but from within. It is like a nation beset by civil war. The medical term 'auto-immunity' has been given to such conditions.

Rheumatoid Arthritis

see Arthritis

Ringworm *see* Tinea

Roseola

Children under three years old are almost the only patients who have this peculiar and generally harmless fever. Suddenly they develop a temperature. They have a few other features such as red tonsils and throat, but nothing at all definite — and they seem relatively well. However, some small children are susceptible to convulsions when feverish, whatever the cause.

The fever lasts three or four days and then, very suddenly, a pink spotty rash shows on the trunk and the upper parts of the limbs. If they have not done so before the parents now call the doctor, only to find that with the appearance of the rash the temperature has fallen to normal and the child seems fit. The rash will clear within a couple of days; sometimes it fades almost as soon as it comes.

There is no treatment, apart from something like aspirin in suitable childrens' doses to ease the fever. (If the child does have a convulsion because of sensitivity to a very raised temperature, then this will be tended as described in the section on Fits, (p.113.)

Rupture *see* Hernia

Salpingitis

It might seem impossible to confuse body parts of such different sites and functions as the Eustachian tube, which helps to keep pressure stable inside the ear, and the Fallopian tube, which leads from each ovary to the uterus. Yet if either becomes inflamed, medical men call the resulting condition by the same name of 'salpingitis'. This is derived from the ancient Greek word for tube. Given the vast number of tubular structures in human anatomy one should perhaps be grateful that doctors have resisted the temptation to use the word for inflammation in many other organs all over the body.

What then is meant when someone has salpingitis? No problem if the patient is a man; it is his ear which troubles him. In the case of a woman this might refer either to her ear or to a Fallopian tube. However one can safely infer that the latter is meant. Inflammation of the Eustachian tube is generally quite mild, often accompanying the common cold and clearing spontaneously. That of the Fallopian tube is a serious matter (see diagram p.157).

Infection can attack the tube in one of several ways. It may reach it through the vagina and uterus, and some unfortunate examples can be the result of gonorrhoea or of lay attempts at procuring abortion. Or there may be spread of infection like peritonitis within the abdomen. Another but rare way is by the carriage of bacteria through the blood stream as could happen with tuberculosis.

The Fallopian tube is a narrow structure; when it becomes inflamed its tissues swell and block it. Pus is likely to be trapped inside and form an abscess. The end of the tube is so closely applied to the ovary that this organ often also becomes infected, when the whole condition is called 'salpingo-oophoritis'.

In the typical acute attack the woman has a high fever, discharge from the vagina and severe pain in the lower abdomen. Immediate treatment with the appropriate antibiotic is important. Sometimes the infection requires surgical removal of the infected part (in the same way as an infected appendix has to be excised). Even if operation can be avoided the scarring which results may leave the tube blocked and, since the ova cannot travel through it, impair the woman's fertility.

There is also a form of salpingitis which is not the sharp acute attack, but a slow, grumbling chronic form. It does not present the features of an emergency. The patient may even be able to carry on with her ordinary tasks but she feels unwell, bothered by aching in the back or lower part of her abdomen, by painful intercourse and sometimes by abnormal periods. A protracted course of antibiotics may help some of these cases, but others will need an operation.

Scabies

The impressive beast illustrated here lives under the skin. It is a mite and in reality only just visible to the keen eye, being about a quarter of a millimetre wide. It can be caught from contact of one skin with another. This has to be fairly close (e.g. sharing a bed); the friendly formal handshake will not do it. The mite also can survive about a fortnight in clothes or blankets, another reservoir of infestation.

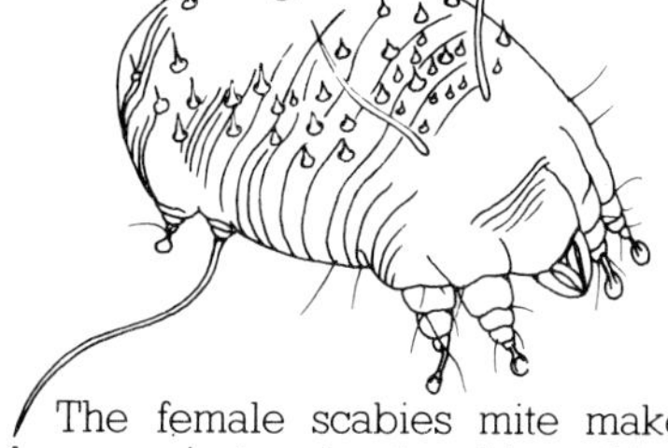

The female scabies mite makes burrows just under the skin and lays about fifty eggs in her lifetime. Symptoms of severe itching appear some six to eight weeks after her entry. She is more active when warm so that itching is felt at its worst when the patient is cosy in bed.

The little irregular burrows look rather like thread marks about an inch in length under the skin. The most common sites are at the wrists and between the fingers, but they can appear anywhere below neck level, including the buttocks and the genitals.

Very often there is a mild knobbly rash, and as well little blobs of pus where microbe infection has got in. Almost certainly there will be many scratch marks produced by the patient himself.

Scabies is not difficult to get rid of if the doctor's advice is carefully followed. This generally involves taking a hot bath at night, then briskly rubbing and drying all the skin below the neck. This opens up the burrows. Then the patient applies a medicated paint which kills the exposed mites. He puts on clean nightwear and goes to bed in clean bedclothes. He may have to repeat the process the next night, but should not be tempted to do it a third time, for the treatment is effective and a third application could be irritating. Some itching may continue for a few days due to the dead remnants of the mites.

Everyone in close contact with patient may need treatment at the same time. Also bed linen and clothing must be well washed; it is wise to apply a hot iron to parts like cuffs which lie against the skin. As for items like gloves which cannot be washed and ironed, it is sufficient to leave them unworn for three weeks; at the end of that time any mites stranded therein will have died.

Scarlet Fever

Medical name: Scarlatina

see also Fevers of Children

Scarlet fever is an illness more likely to alarm the patients' elderly grandparents than the younger generation of today. It is due to a special strain of the streptococcus bacteria, and over the last decades has become considerably less severe. This is not only through help from antibiotics but also because these bacteria themselves seem to have become less savage.

The incubation is brief: about three days (or a range of one to five days). It is a tonsillitis with a rash. What must be well understood is that this is an unpleasant infection, but whether or not it is accompanied by a rash does not relate to the severity of the infection. Where these special streptococci are concerned you should be just as concerned if no rash appears and just as calm if it does.

Symptoms are sudden with fever and sore throat. The rash appears within the next two days, first on the chest and sides of the neck, then spreading over the body. It is formed of very small ('pinhead'), bright red spots close together. However the area immediately around the mouth is often characteristically pale. The tongue shares in the rash. At first it bears a white fur over its intense redness, and then the furring clears to leave a raw looking tongue.

The skin loses its rash after about three days and then begins to peel. Peeling may continue several weeks, but the flakes which fall off are not infectious. The patient can pass the infection on for up to three weeks from the beginning of the illness. However if he receives antibiotic treatment like penicillin he becomes non-infectious within a day.

Antibiotics clear most attacks without trouble. A few can develop other troubles such as ear infections. The bacterial poisons may cause rheumatic fever (p.178) or kidney troubles, showing up a couple of weeks later. Sometime the urine is tested as a precautionary routine at that time.

Sciatica *see* Backache

Shingles

After a child has chicken pox the virus can settle in some parts of the body and lurk there quietly for many years without advertising itself. A favourite resting place is the beginning of the nerves of sensation which arise in pairs from the spinal cord at all the different levels formed by the vertebrae in the backbone. Each nerve serves one clearly demarcated area of skin.

Suddenly the virus may become reactivated, and spread along the nerve and its branches, causing a pain which at this stage has often fooled not only the sufferer but also many a doctor as to its true nature. Thence the virus enters the skin and produces the typical rash of redness and blisters, visibly mapping out the anatomical territory of the nerve.

The pain has been compared to the application of red hot gimlets. In an average case it and the rash last about a week. This is quite variable. Some patients get away with only three days of pain, and in some the rash leaves slight scarring and pigmentation of the skin. Others, especially the elderly, appear to be unfortunate, with symptoms lasting weeks. In some cases even when the rash has quite cleared the pain continues for months even and, rarely but tragically, for ever.

The neck and shoulder are common sites. By far the most likely parts to be attacked are in the upper back and chest. There is one area which gives special concern. Here it arises not near the spine but in a nerve direct from the brain, supplying the side of the face. If its distribution covers the level of the eye, then the rash could spread over the delicate conjunctiva which covers

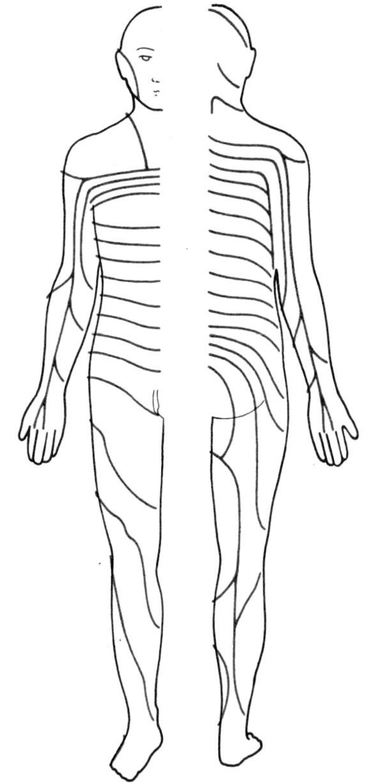

Front and back views of skin nerve 'territories' and therefore the zones along which the shingles rash and pain can develop.

the front of the eyeball. Blisters and scars here could do great damage to vision, and certain forms of eye drops or ointments are prescribed as protection.

The general treatment of shingles can be by one of various applications to the skin, and by tablets to relieve pain. Sometimes special drugs, if given early in the trouble, can mitigate the attack.

A very peculiar and quite inaccurate myth is that if the rash appears on both sides of the body, the patient will die when the two rashes meet in the middle. In fact it never does develop on both sides, and even if it did this would not be lethal but only twice as unpleasant.

Cases of shingles being caught from someone with chickenpox have been described, and vice versa, but these are very rare indeed.

Shock

The word 'shock' is unfortunate; in medicine and first aid it does not mean an emotional upset, rather it covers a collapse of heart and circulation which follows severe injuries. Heavy bleeding, large fractures, bruises and wounds and extensive burns can all lead to marked loss of body fluid; this decreases the circulated blood and the efficient working of the heart and lungs. Some purely medical conditions like heart attacks or overwhelming infections may also give the same results.

Here we are concerned with the first aid to prevent or, at least, to minimise the development of shock after injuries — for shock develops, it does not happen all at once. It may take minutes or hours according to the degree of injury. A fully shocked patient is pale, cold and sweating; his pulse and breathing are fast and feeble; he is torpid, dazed and may become unconscious. It is before he reaches this stage, preferably immediately after the accident and while you await the ambulance, that you should take steps to mitigate shock, even if he looks and acts relatively unaffected.

1. *Stop severe bleeding* (p.46).
2. *Treat the patient where he is.*

Many would-be helpers try immediately to lift the fallen man and to carry him, oblivious of the harm this could do. If the scene is the middle of a road detail bystanders to control approaching cars until the police take this job over. An exception could be the fast motorway where control is unlikely; here you may have to shift the patient fast and carefully to avoid worse mishaps. Also a house on fire, a room full of dangerous fumes, or a wall about to fall are no sites for treatment.

3. *Position him.* On the other hand let him adopt his most comfortable attitude provided this would not worsen a wound or suspected fracture. The optimal position is the head low and the feet raised (some 50 cm), and on his side. This would allow saliva, blood or vomit (by no means uncommon after injury) to flow from the mouth of a weak or drowsy person and not go into the windpipe. (*See also* Unconsciousness, p.210.)

However never move anyone who might have a broken backbone (See Fractures, p.117).

4. *Loosen tight clothing:* belts, braces, collar.

5. *Keep him warm* by loosely covering with a blanket or coat. If he is lying on a cold surface tuck material under him as well. You must *not* add an electric blanket or hot water bottles; this extra heat would draw to the skin vessels a large amount of blood which is needed deeper to keep heart, lungs and brain going.

6. *Dress any wounds* (p.220) with minimum of fuss and disturbance.

7. *Reassurance and comfort* play a great part. Talk calmly and firmly to him, sympathising with his predicament but showing confidence in his recovery. Never whisper to others in his hearing. Do remember that the apparently unconscious may hear what is being said and guard your tongue.

8. *Give nothing by mouth* to the severely injured. Any tablets or drink may be vomited, causing risk of choking especially if he gets drowsy or has to have an anaesthetic in hospital. If his thirst is great you can refresh him by letting him suck a moistened handkerchief.

Shoulder Troubles

It is interesting to compare the joints which unite upper and lower limbs to the trunk. At the hip the thigh bone has a 'ball' fitting into the 'socket' of the pelvis, and this gives a range of movement, which is relatively limited; strength and stability are the considerations. The arm however can swing right up over the head, and rotate considerably more than does the leg. Mobility is the primary feature.

For this the upper arm bone (humerus) is linked to two others, the collar bone (clavicle) and the shoulder blade (scapula) which to some extent move with it. These two bones can get involved in troubles which beset the shoulder (see diagram, p.91.)

The upper end of the arm bone fits into a very shallow socket made by the outer end of the shoulder blade, linked to the outer tip of the collar bone. The shoulder blade lies at the back, behind the rib cage. The collar bone is at the front, sitting over the upper end of the rib cage; its other tip linked to the top of the breast bone.

When the arm is raised sideways and upwards, the arm bone is rotating in this socket. But the socket moves as well, for collar bone and shoulder blade pivot upwards, thus contributing to the wide arc which takes the arm right over the head.

There are, for instance, some injuries which put out of action the major muscles pulling on and lifting up the arm bone, and yet the patient can move the arm a fair way from the side of his body by shoulder blade movement alone.

This coordination of bones carries its own disavantages. If shoulder blade or collar bone be damaged, then shoulder movement is greatly affected. The collar bone may break because someone falls on the outstretched arm. The force travels up the limb and jerks the collar bone which snaps. Immediately the shoulder joint is temporarily out of action as the weight of the arm painfully pulls down the collar bone's outer broken end.

Dislocation of the shoulder is relatively common, sometimes also likely to be due to a fall on the outstretched arm, sometimes caused by a blow near the joint itself. The socket is at its shallowest in the lower part, so the arm bone tends to slip down and a little forwards by the armpit space. If you suspect this has happened treat it as a fracture (p.117). There are some people who repeatedly have a shoulder dislocating itself because the ligaments supporting the bones have become lax. Some of them become quite adept at manipulating their arms to correct the dislocation themselves, but this is not a good idea, for with each dislocation there is a chance of damage to the bone or to the pack of nerves and blood vessels at the armpit; a medical examination should be made first.

Frozen shoulder is a common enough trouble for the expression to have become well known, without, however, being generally understood. It is a painful stiffness with all movements limited due to inflammation of the membranes enclosing the joint. Why this happens is not clear, nor why it gets better, which it will do but only gradually over months. The pain is extremely unpleasant, often spreading to the neck and elbow and preventing sleep.

Another trouble, called the *supraspinatus syndrome,* is due to some injury or inflammation near the point where a muscle (the supraspinatus) is attached to the top of the upper arm bone. As the arm moves upwards this point rubs against a bit of the shoulder blade at the roof of the joint. Characteristically the friction and therefore the pain happens not at the beginning, nor at the end of the full swing of the arm, but during the middle of its range.

In both these cases patients tend to struggle on a while before consulting a doctor. This is a pity for the sooner treatment is begun the easier is the cure. Sometimes injections of corticosteroids (p.79) are given, but often courses of physiotherapy, including special exercises, are prescribed.

Relatively remote troubles can create shoulder symptoms. Patients may be puzzled to find that the doctor examines chest, neck and abdomen to seek the diagnosis. By interconnection of nerves, trouble in the heart or near the diaphragm may give pain at the shoulder. Angina from the heart, pleurisy at the base of the lungs, or inflammation of the gall bladder are examples of these recondite causes, as is pressure on nerves of the upper part of the spine.

One more feature is worth stressing. A shoulder which is not fully used tends to stiffen up quite easily, especially in the elderly. This is a very important point in the treating of fractures around the joint or in cases of strokes which have weakened the arm. Old people with these conditions are well advised to take very seriously the doctor's advice about movements to maintain the freedom of their shoulder.

Sinusitis

There are several medical meanings to the word sinus. The one which concerns us here relates to the nose. The nose space opens into and above the back of the throat. It also has connections with other spaces to each side and above it. These are the sinuses.

They are hollows in the bone, with quite small openings into the outer and upper parts of the two nose cavities. They contain air and their fine lining membrane is continuous with that of the nose. Whether they have any useful function is debatable; it is certain however that when they get infected, and give us sinusitis, they can be a very great nuisance.

The largest sinus on each side is the *maxillary,* below the eye, between it and the upper teeth. A *frontal* sinus lies in the bone above each eyebrow. Then there are the *ethmoid* sinuses between the bridge of the nose and the inner end of each eye, and the *sphenoid* sinuses further back behind the upper part of the nose cavity. The names do not really matter; what does is the way they can behave if taken over by microbes.

Each sinus contains a slight amount of moisture. If infected the lining membrane swells, discharges more moisture which may change to thick pus. This drains away into the nose. At least it would drain away if it could, but all too often the swelling of the membrane completely blocks the

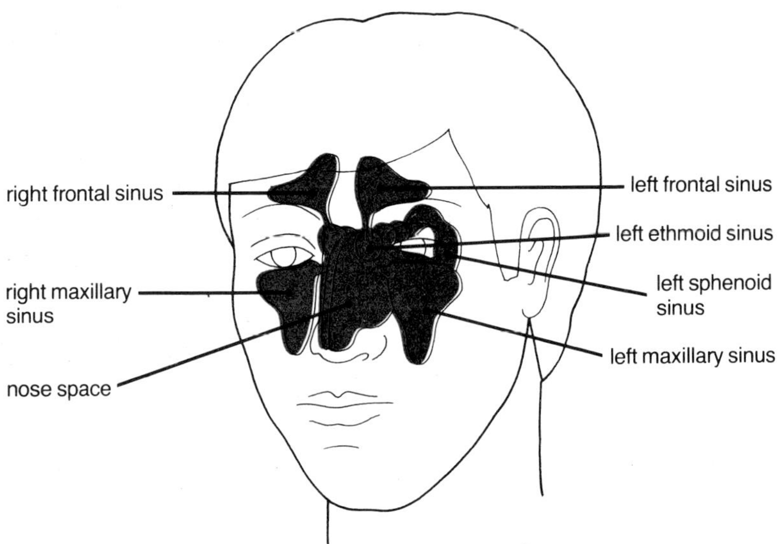

little openings which lead into the nose space. The pus is trapped, and builds up under pressure within the sinus. Headache, face ache and even a raised temperature may follow. Not infrequently the patient suffering from maxillary sinusitis believes he has toothache.

The maxillary sinus is a particularly troublesome one. Even if its membrane's swelling has not become bad enough to cause blockage, the situation of the drainage hole is unfortunate. It is so high up that a lot of infected fluid fills up the sinus before it reaches an escape.

One easy treatment of sinusitis is by nose drops which shrink the membrane and so ease drainage. This must not be done haphazardly; some drops may act very powerfully at first, but then rapidly irritate the membrane which reacts by swelling even more than before. Also, when satisfactory drops are used, a wise way (unless the doctor recommends otherwise) is for the patient to lie down on his back on a bed or couch with his head overhanging the edge directly downwards. Thus any drops instilled get the chance of spreading over those parts of the nose which bear the sinus openings.

Sometimes antibiotics are prescribed and very occasionally simple surgical help is needed to encourage drainage of pus.

The simplest reaction to sinusitis, that of trying to blow one's nose strongly, is not a good idea. It could force air into the sinuses, giving increased pressure and pain. A hot stuffy room also worsens the condition, for it tends to make the membranes swell further.

Slipped Disc *see* Backache

Smallpox

Smallpox is, or rather *was*, a virus infection which was found all over the world. The illness, medically called variola, was easily caught by contact with patients, their clothes, bedding or household articles or by moisture droplets in the air from the nose or throat. Major and minor forms occured, but the general pattern was an incubation of about twelve days, followed by three days of fever, aching and prostration and then the appearance of the typical rash. Small spots on the face and mouth spread to the neck, trunk and limbs. They were more profuse on the limbs, and relatively sparse on the chest and abdomen. The spots filled with a clear fluid which turned to pus, and then formed scabs which would leave permanent scars.

Complications included ulcers on the eyes, leading to blindness. Mortality in the severe form was very high. However those who recovered from any attack gained a life long immunity. There was no specific treatment against the virus.

In 1796 Dr Edward Jenner gave the first ever medical vaccination. It was against smallpox. He injected the fluid from the blisters of a milkmaid affected by cowpox, a disease of cows, into a healthy boy. Some weeks later he administered smallpox fluid to the boy who remained healthy. Vaccination (a name derived from the latin word 'Vacca' for cow) became established, though, of course, over the years Jenner's technique became considerably refined. It has saved countless lives.

However, vaccination itself was not without its occasional troubles, for it could have complications, including, in rare cases, encephalitis. It could produce unpleasant, and sometimes dangerous reactions if given during pregnancy or in cases of skin eruptions, or to patients generally debilitated or with some blood diseases or on such treatments as corticosteroids.

Over the last decades there was much medical concern lest, under our better hygiene and health control, vaccination itself might not actually be causing more risk than the disease itself. In the United Kingdom smallpox appeared as 'imported' cases, that is in patients who had come from countries where it was epidemic.

The answer to the problem seemed an idealistic, almost impossible, one — to eradicate the disease world wide. This gigantic task was initiated in 1967 by the World Health Organization. At that time smallpox was a severe problem in forty-four countries, some of immense populations. The work went ahead with a vigour and sophisticated planning which deserves far more publicity than it has received.

In 1971 the health authorities of the United Kingdom and of the United States announced that routine vaccination to children was no longer recommended. By that time the number of 'smallpox countries' was reduced to only one. The difficulties of control in some parts of Africa and India beset by communication difficulties and by fighting were very great but the planning won through.

In December 1979 the World Health Organisation announced that smallpox had been eradicated throughout the world and there was no evidence that it would return as a disease likely to be constantly present in any region or among any people.

The success of this operation had not been due to general mass vaccination but to teams of workers observing and controlling. Where smallpox was found patients were isolated, and a strong programme of vaccination of contacts was followed in the areas concerned

Where is the virus now? It is in research laboratories, whose numbers have been strictly restricted and where precautionary regulations are strong. It is felt that should, even now, a case of smallpox reappear the immediate vaccination of all contacts (from held stocks of vaccine) would give rapid control. Proper vaccination immediately after contact will prevent the disease. If given a few days later it will modify it to a minor form.

Smoking

It is not a matter of opinion but fact: smoking is very bad for you.

The cigarette devotee argues rather defensively. He feels that the warnings against smoking are similar to sermons against misbehaviour, and also will say 'statistics can be made to prove anything'.

In fact medical statements about smoking were never from a moral point of view, and their statistics never sought to prove a point. What doctors have found out about smoking is the result of painstaking enquiry, very fairly, very accurately, conducted. They wanted to know whether smoking had unusual effects, and if so what these were. The answers came back dramatic and unavoidable.

Burning tobacco slowly produces lots of chemicals, including tarry substances and also a gas called carbon monoxide. These do very nasty things to many parts of the body. In fact they are poisons. The tarry substances contain more than two hundred different compounds, of which many are scientifically recognised as producing cancer. Carbon monoxide strongly interferes with and reduces the amount of oxygen which the blood carries around the body.

Cigarette smokers have shorter lives than non-smokers. They are about twice as likely to die in middle age as are non-smokers. Studies comparing their life spans with those of non-smokers suggest that each cigarette shortens life by amounts varying from 5 to 25 minutes. But simple figures like this give no picture of the general loss of efficiency of the smoker, and the wretchedness to him (and to his family) of resulting illnesses.

Is this an overstatement? Let us consider what has been discovered about the action of cigarettes on various parts of the human frame.

Mouth and Stomach

Taste buds of the tongue are damaged. Food enjoyment is reduced.

Though cancer in the mouth and throat is not a common disease, its occurrence is up to ten times greater in smokers than in non-smokers.

Smoking interferes with the efficiency of the muscles which prevent back flow of stomach contents into the gullet (regurgitation).

Smoking does not appear to cause stomach ulcers, but it delays their healing so that they are more persistent (and more often fatal) than in non-smokers.

The Bladder

Cancer of the bladder occurs twice to three times as frequently in heavy smokers as in non-smokers.

The Heart and Circulation

Smoking does not appear to cause a raised blood pressure. However it greatly worsens the condition in someone who already has an abnormally high blood pressure.

It constricts blood vessels; it reduces the carriage of oxygen by the blood. This involves all the body but materially affects two of the most important organs: the brain and the heart.

Tests show decreased mental ability with heavy smoking.

Cigarettes reduce the efficiency of heart muscle and of the blood vessels which keep that muscle active and alive.

The risk of dying relatively young (aged 45-54) from heart attacks is at least trebled in the person who smokes fifteen or more cigarettes a day.

Pregnancy

A woman who smokes during her pregnancy is likely to have a baby with retarded growth at birth, weighing less than the baby of a non-smoker. Mothers who smoke are at greater risk of having a miscarriage or still-birth than are non-smokers. And the incidence of convulsions in their children is higher.

The effect moves on further. Children of mothers who smoked in pregnancy have proved a little retarded in learning ability compared to other children. Even at the age of seven their school performance was less good.

The Lungs

Cigarette smoke damages the protective anti-infection cells which line the air tubes of the lungs. It also reduces the power of the lungs to pass oxygen into the body.

Chronic bronchitis disables by cough and shortness of breath and is a frequent cause of death. Compared with a non-smoker the smoker of ten cigarettes a day has a five times greater risk of dying of chronic bronchitis. Twenty cigarettes a day increases this to ten times the risk.

The incidence of other forms of cancer seems to be decreasing in the last fifty years, but lung cancer is increasing and this appears to run parallel to the increase in smoking (sale of cigarettes). Compared with a non-smoker the person who smokes ten cigarettes a day increases the risk of lung cancer six times. The person who smokes twenty a day increases it eighteen times. The person who smokes thirty a day increases the risk about twenty six times.

How to Stop Smoking

Giving up (even after smoking for many years) will diminish the increased risks: after ten years of abstinence the ex-smoker will have lost almost all of the extra risk his past cigarette habit gave him.

Pipes and cigars carry less risk than cigarettes. One factor here seems to be that their smokers do not inhale as much as do cigarette smokers. However for the latter to switch to cigars or pipes may be relatively unhelpful if they have developed the inhaling habit.

The correct approach is to discontinue smoking entirely. Some advise planning to stop on a day fixed two or three weeks ahead. This seems illogical; the properly motivated person, he or she who at last understands what smoking really does to the body, decides to stop immediately. It is a big step to take. One can sympathise with what it means to the person who really enjoys each smoke, and even more with the addict who smokes to avoid the distress of not-smoking. To discontinue can be quite a hard task, but it is perfectly within the power of everyone. Once achieved the ex-smoker feels an improvement in health and a wonderful sense of freedom. (The financial advantage needs no stressing.)

1. Begin by assessing, quite honestly, how much you smoke a day. Calculate accurately what this costs a year. Imagine the sum spent on something desirable (holiday) or necessary (redecorations perhaps). The alternative is to go on smoking and share your money between the tobacco trade and the Chancellor of the Exchequer.

2. Stop fully. Do not try to tail off gradually.

3. Accept the fact that you may feel miserable, even bad-tempered, for the first weeks of your abstinence. This is the small and temporary price you, and maybe your family, will have to pay for the coming freedom. Suddenly the unease will clear, and you will pass tobacconists' displays with a pleasantly superior feeling of indifference.

4. Counter that desire to smoke which so often follows meals by brushing your teeth with a sharp-tasting toothpaste.

5. Tell *everybody* you have stopped smoking. Boast about it in fact, so that you would feel ashamed to be caught with a cigarette.

6. Others subconsciously might be jealous of your determination and try to coax you to have 'just one fag'. Ask them to help you by not making such offers.

7. When possible keep out of smoking areas. For instance travel in non-smoking train compartments.

8. Do not replace smoking by eating sweets; you would only put on weight. Do not rely on mouthwashes, chewing gum, special tablets or hypnotism. Their help is marginal. Rely on yourself.

All with consideration for their frames and their families will stop smoking. And feel fine.

Snakebite

The only poisonous snake in Britain is the adder. Its bite can be very painful indeed; though it may cause a transient collapse it is extremely rare for it to be fatal.

The adder is shy. It likes to hide in long grass or under shrubs, but in sunny weather ventures out. It bites only for food (attacking animals like mice) or if feeling threatened, as in an accidental encounter with human hand or foot. It strikes fast and may not even be seen as it does so. The bite shows as two small puncture marks where the fangs went in. These fangs are hollow, like syringe needles, and connected to a reservoir of venom at the back of the upper jaw.

Once inside the body the venom can damage blood cells and weaken heart beat. The bitten area becomes red and swollen and painful within a few minutes; the patient may become sick, dizzy, sweating and faint.

First Aid

1. Lie the patient down, and put the bitten part at rest.
2. Wipe away any venom still on the surface; if possible wash with soap and water.
3. Put on a clean dry dressing.
4. Reassure your patient who may believe an adder bite is fatal. But beware of increasing pain. If you have them give tablets of aspirin or paracetamol.
5. Now immobilise the limb *as if it were fractured*. Movement would increase blood flow within it and speed up the spread of venom through the body. It is this spread which can make the patient collapse.
6. Get the patient to hospital as quickly as possible.

Do *not* suck or cut the wound, apply chemicals or put on a tourniquet. These are out-of-date manoeuvres which do more harm than good.

Some suggest killing the adder by clubbing it, bringing the body to hospital for identification. This advice is weakened by the fact that the adder will have disappeared very quickly before you find a club, and that (outside a zoo) no snake other than the adder will bite. In any case you should be very cautious about handling the dead adder: its biting mechanism may yet function by a posthumous reflex action.

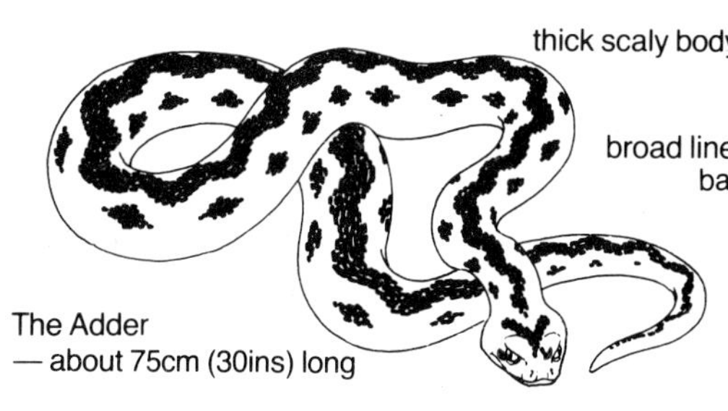

The Adder — about 75cm (30ins) long

Spastics

This is the unfortunate name given to children born with brain damage. The alternative medical term for the condition is *cerebral palsy* which is not much better.

Why should a baby have the misfortune to be born with harm to the brain? It is a grossly unhappy situation which happens about once in every four hundred births. The delicate, sensitive tissue of the brain reacts badly, and permanently, to certain forms of injury, especially oxygen deficiency. Some chance maldevelopment during the pregnancy, a difficulty during the birth or an illness soon after can create a lifetime of physical and mental handicap. It is important to note that the condition is not hereditary, nor is it due to any unusual food or drug taken by the mother.

The spastic's handicap depends very much on which part of the brain is involved, and how seriously. It can vary from a problem in walking to a complete inability to stand, combined with severe mental defect. In many cases attacks of epilepsy are another sign of brain damage.

The very small baby may not show features of the difficulties to come: only as he grows and develops his faculties will the deficits show up. Limbs may be weak with stiffened muscles. They may show tremors, purposeless, involuntary or poorly coordinated movements. Later, the child may prove unable to see, hear or speak well. Any mental retardation can seem far worse than it really is because these physical handicaps have isolated the child from the stimulus of contacts and experience. An early expert appraisal is very important.

Teaching, training and understanding form the only effective ways of help. There is no treatment which can reverse the damage. Certain forms of exercise may help and sometimes leg supports (calipers) help stability. In most cases the spastic child can be brought up sharing the family life with parents, brothers and sisters. Other children will be told of his difficulties and encouraged to play with him. Some schools specialise in handicapped pupils, which allows the child to mix with others who have similar problems. Far sighted parents will not let the attention needed by the spastic eclipse the equal, if different, needs of the other children.

Sprains and Strains

A sprain is a stretching and tearing of some fibres of ligaments which surround and support a joint. A strain concerns similar type of injury of fibres of a muscle anywhere.

The typical sprain is that at the ankle, when uneven ground or untoward movement while walking or running twists the foot sharply; generally it affects the outer side. A strain more characteristically happens to a limb which has been used in forced action, such as powerful throwing or kicking. In either case the area may become puffy and even bruised, from the rupture of small blood vessels. A blow on the muscle can also cause a strain, but then the word 'contusion' fits the case better.

How does one make sure there is no fracture (p. 117)? Sometimes this is difficult unless one is quite sure there has been no definite blow to a bone. If in doubt ask a doctor; sometimes he will be sure only after consulting an X-ray.

First aid to a strain or sprain consists in giving good support by firm use of a crêpe bandage. Each turn of bandage should overlap two thirds of the previous turn. But be careful to avoid tightness which would constrict the underlying blood vessels, especially around joints like elbows, knees, ankles and wrists. The bandaging should go over interleaving layers of cotton wool, which buffer the pressure. Warn your patient to remove the bandage if it becomes painful or causes a hand or foot beyond it to go numb or cold.

If you are dealing with the injury within a half-hour of it happening you may first try to reduce the swelling or bleeding under the skin by applying a cold compress. This is nothing more than a pad of folded cloth (a towel for instance) soaked in cold water, then wrung out, lightly bandaged with open weave material around the affected part and kept there some thirty minutes, while you keep the part elevated. If the compress warms up renew or dribble cold water on it.

Squinting

see Eye Troubles

Steroids

see Corticosteroids

Strains

see Sprains and Strains

Stomach Ulcer

see Peptic Ulcer

Strokes

The old word for a stroke is apoplexy, from a Greek verb meaning 'to strike down'. A present medical term for it is C.V.A. for cerebro-vascular accident.

A stroke is damage to part of the brain through a disturbance of its blood supply. A small vessel may rupture and bleed into the brain tissue, or a clot may obstruct it, cutting off the blood supply to the brain area it serves. Both events may happen with startling suddeness or more slowly over minutes or hours.

The effects of stroke will vary according to the area of brain involved. For instance, there may be impairment of eyesight, of speech, of word memory, of recognition of space and shape, of balance, of swallowing or of facial expression. In most cases, however, movement and feeling in limbs are the chief faculties to suffer. A leg or an arm, or both on the same side, may become numb and powerless. The victim may wake with this disability. He may be hit by it quite suddenly or he may find the handicap progressively developing. In some severe attacks he may lose consciousness, have convulsions or be incontinent. There is no absolute pattern.

Nor is there a predictable pattern about recovery. It can range from there being no improvement to a total return of function. Where there has been loss of power a great deal depends on assiduously following any advice given by the doctor on using an unaffected hand or arm regularly to exercise the affected limb gently and passively through its range of movements, and preventing the joints from stiffening. A great deal of careful nursing and encouragement is sometimes needed to help the patient in the recovery phases. It may take weeks or months to achieve optimal results.

First Aid
At the suspicion of a stroke get the patent lying down, if possible in bed, and put him in the recovery position as described in Unconsciousness (p.210). Loosen his clothing and cover him. Notify your doctor, describing clearly what has happened. Keep a careful watch on the patient lest he worsens; he may need help if he vomits or is incontinent.

Styes *see* Eye Troubles

Sunburn

If you get sunburnt it is your own fault. The lure of sun, especially on holiday, is all the greater in that it comes relatively infrequently. Few can resist the temptation of exposing as much of themselves to as much of available sunshine for as long as possible. This creates sunburn, which sometimes can be really severe, very painful and cause blisters.

People with red hair and fair skin are particularly sensitive, for their skin has relatively few of those cells which produce *melanin,* the dark pigment which forms under the effect of the sun's ultraviolet rays and which act as a barrier. The skin of coloured people already bears its complement of melanin. White skin has to develop its melanin gradually, during exposure, to get the desired sun-tan.

Preventing Sunburn
The skin is one whole organ; to some extent all of it will react to what is happening to one small area. If you gradually increase the zones exposed to sunlight then the total surface is tuned to accepting more sunlight.

Expose for about half an hour only on the first day. Then you can double the length of time each day, to one hour, two hours, four hours and so on. But still go carefully, for sunburn will show up only after, and not during, exposure.

You graduate the amount of skin you expose in the same way. Wearing sleeves and a hat with a wide brim is wise at the beginning. The effect of the midday sun is far more powerful than that in the early morning or late afternoon. Surroundings play their part for a good deal of sunlight can be reflected from snow, water and even sand. Wind increases the sunburn effect.

Sunbathing lotions and creams are designed not to increase the tan, but to protect by forming a barrier to ultra violet light. The thicker they are spread, the more effectively they work. With storage they lose their power, so last year's leftovers may let you down. Also marketed are preparations designed to give you a false, an imitation, tan. Make sure you realise which type you are buying.

A few medicaments like certain antibiotics or anti-depressants sensitise the skin to sunlight. If in doubt consult your doctor. Some people tend to develop blistery eruptions, especially on the lips, in strong sunlight. For these special sun-barrier creams can be prescribed.

Treating Sunburn
The first thing is covering under light clothes to prevent further exposure. Calamine lotion, especially in its oily form, is very soothing. Pain relieving tablets like aspirin or paracetamol

can help. If the burn is extensive and if it has produced blisters it must be taken seriously and medical treatment should be sought.

Sunstroke

see Heat Exhaustion

Swallowed Foreign Object

Any object capable of being swallowed and passing down the gullet will usually travel through the intestinal tract without giving trouble. It is rare for it to be held up, except perhaps in the first part of the intestines beyond the stomach (the duodenum) which has a loop like curve.

Craggy or pointed objects like small dentures, hair grips or open safety pins rarely penetrate the bowel wall, and sometimes larger ones could cause obstructions. Abdominal pains and tenderness are the warning signs. One must realise that children are prone to swallowing objects without telling their parents.

In the main no action need be taken after the swallowing. All that need be done is to wait with attention and watch the stools for the object's emergence, which may be some twelve to forty-eight hours after swallowing, according to the state of the bowels. Certainly purgatives should *not* be given and no attempt be made to induce vomiting. In certain cases doctors may decide to follow the object's course with X-rays, but this is rarely needed and would be possible only with something opaque to X-rays. Wood and most forms of glass, for instance, would not show up.

If something dangerously sharp has gone down one can try to 'buffer' it by giving stodgy foods (new bread, porridge) and reducing the amount of fluid drunk. The 'cotton wool sandwich' has a reputation for helping, if the patient can be persuaded to take it. Cotton wool is teased out into thin shreds between bread and butter slices.

The oddest foreign object in the stomach has the peculiar name of trichobezoar. This is swallowed hair from the habit some children have of chewing at their long locks. The strands stay in the stomach and gradually get matted together to form a large mass. Once the trouble is diagnosed (which is not easy) only surgery can clear it.

A fish bone stuck in the back of the throat is hardly a 'swallowed' object, but it can be considered here. A fine needle-like bone can easily embed itself deeply, with a bit sticking out, giving a lot of pain on swallowing. The sooner it is taken out the better, especially as it could cause inflammation and infection. Do not try to remove it yourself: the doctor has the correct lights, mirrors and forceps to deal with the situation.

Teeth

Because teeth are complex structures they can give trouble in many ways. Their two main problems are decay of tooth substance, and infection of the gums in which they sit.

The major factor is *plaque*, a gummy white coating on the surface, arising from chemicals in the saliva and food. Plaque holds bacteria which form acids. The acids erode the hard surface of teeth and then work deeper to create cavities.

Decay on the surface is painless.

After it has reached into the tooth sweetened foods or cold drinks may bring on toothache. Once the cavity leads into the central soft living pulp within the tooth things are much worse. Under pressure of infection and inflammation the pulp tissues may die and the tooth is denied its blood supply and nutrition. By settling at the base of teeth plaque will also lead to swollen, infected gums, and the teeth become loosened.

Toothache then is a feature of late and established damage and needs immediate attention from the dentist. The worst pain, accompanied by swelling of the face, comes from the dental abscess, a collection of pus at the infected point. Because of nerve ramifications one can easily be misled by the site of the pain; it can be felt in many areas around the mouth distant from that of the infection. Sometimes the pain of severe sinusitis (p. 186) imitates that of toothache.

The Dental Enemy

There is doubt that the most potent agents of decay are sweetened foods. Sugar can quickly incorporate itself in plaque, an offering to the bacteria which enjoy it, and create the destructive acids from it. Teeth and gums bathed in sugary solutions are at risk. Food residues from jam, honey, cakes, biscuits, chocolates, boiled sweets and sticky toffees are enemies of teeth.

If you have to eat sweets let it be with other foods, and not between meals. Far better is to replace them with raw vegetables, fruits and nuts. Dentists grieve sincerely over the constant damage being done to children by misguided gifts of 'sweeties'.

Tooth Brushing

The toothbrush is a much misused instrument. Some neglect it (the nation's yearly sale is said to average at one half toothbrush per head of population). Others choose and handle the brush with unnecessary mystique, seeking strange shapes and materials.

What sort of brush? Many specialists favour a quite straightforward tooth-brush: the bristle head to be flat and the handle straight and short for easier manipulation. Bristles of nylon are advised; for the average adult they should be of medium hardness.

When to brush. Ideally you should do this within a few minutes of every meal. If that cannot be managed, try at least to hold a mouthful of water and with cheek action jerk it to and fro around and between the teeth.

This several-times-a-day cleaning is valuable, but far more important is the at-least-once-a-day attack on plaque. It is wisest to do this at bedtime (and to eat nothing after!). Aim at removing the day's plaque accumulation as thoroughly as possible by brushing with care and thought. Take some three minutes to go over all tooth surfaces efficiently. An egg-timer would not be amiss in the bathroom.

How to brush. Try neither the up-and-down nor the back-and-forth strokes. Let the bristle head do rapid rotating movements. Think of all the surfaces of your teeth, back and front and biting areas, and make sure they all get their turns. Pay special attention to the rear teeth, which are likely to be skimped.

What goes on the brush? Paste dentifrice is considered to be less abrasive than powders. In fact the choice is one which varies from person to person. In this decision, as well as all others concerning the toothbrush and its use, your dentist is the right man to consult.

The Use of Floss

Dental floss, a fine silky thread which can be used to clean between the teeth, is a valuable adjunct to toothpastes. The dentist can advise about the different forms on the market.

Thin cleaning sticks, of wood, can do the same task. They must be used gently for this purpose and are not to be confused with toothpicks which most dentists do not recommend.

What about Fluorides?

It is quite definite that fluorides in one's system will harden tooth surfaces and reduce the cavity formation. They will not however heal an existing cavity. In some areas fluoride is a simple and natural constituent of water, which generations of inhabitants have been drinking with no other effect than better teeth than those of their fluoride-deficient neighbours.

Whether fluoride should be added to domestic water in other areas, is a matter for decision by the local health and water authorities. That fluoridation of water at the accepted concentration can do harm is a myth.

In the absence of fluoride in water one can take the drops or tablets of fluoride preparations available from chemists. It would be sensible first to get advice on this from doctor or dentist. Taking supplementary fluoride when the local water already contains enough might not be wise.

The effect of fluorides is on developing teeth, so it is especially important that children, from birth, receive an adequate amount. Once adult teeth have formed it is of less benefit. To some extent fluoride toothpaste is a help, but less so than that which is taken into the system. Fluoride will not pass across the placenta, so there is no point in the pregnant woman taking it for the sake of her developing baby.

Children's Teeth

Whereas the adult has thirty two teeth, children begin by developing their twenty 'milk teeth'. The first to appear at about the age of six months are the lower two front ones. Mothers tend to watch their coming with some concern. If the teeth erupt on time they are pleased at this normality. If they show early they will accept congratulations on the advanced state of the young child. However when teeth come out rather later than average they can be told the truth, that the date of appearance is of no real significance. The full set of twenty is likely to be present by the time the child is about two and a half years old.

Some years later they will be replaced and added to by the permanent teeth. The first of these will come at about the age of six. At twelve years old the child will have achieved all his adult teeth except the four 'wisdoms' at the very back of each jaw. These generally appear around the age of eighteen but very often they (and — by Old Wives' Lore — their owner's sagacity) are delayed until many years later.

Teething is also a matter full of myths. It is true that the first eruption of a tooth can give the poor child some trouble. His gum may be red and painful; he dribbles at the mouth and needs a bib and frequent face wiping; his appetite may decrease and his mood deteriorate; he may be exploring the mouth with fingers or with harder objects on which he wants to bite. He may even be a little feverish.

Generally he, and his parents, weather all this quite smoothly. Aspirin or paracetamol (in children's small doses) will help. Give something firm to bite on. Hard rusks come in here, as does the 'teething ring' which should be easily cleaned and sterilised by boiling and also must be far too big to be swallowed. Creams or jellies to ease pain by rubbing on the gum sometimes help.

What must be stressed is that the 'teething ages' are those where many children are exposed to new infections and illness. It is too easy to blame teething for all symptoms and so overlook a serious medical condition. Teething will not cause diarrhoea, vomiting, severe lack of appetite or fits. Another medical cause must be sought if these happen.

Early care. Milk teeth may be temporary but they are extremely important for on their healthy development depends the spacing and the position of the teeth to follow. From early on children should be taught the use of a toothbrush. Let it be of suitable size, with soft bristles, and use it gently. A small child cannot rinse his mouth out, so finish off with a wet brush to remove surplus toothpaste.

If children are taken to the dentist for regular checks they will get to know him as a pleasant friend and not a torturer, and will be conditioned to consult him more readily when they have grown up.

The Dentist

This overworked and skilled man has an unhappy reputation as one who inflicts pain. The truth often is that the chief culprit is the patient himself who has not followed the sensible advice of getting a six monthly check. Dental decay is far more easily stopped and corrected when found early. The dentist aims to teach tooth hygiene and to prevent trouble. He wants to preserve teeth whenever possible, and as painlessly as he can.

Many patients consult a dentist with the request: 'I have severe toothache; please extract the tooth.' To which the dentist might well reply: 'If your finger hurts, do you really want it amputated?'

First Aid to Teeth

Toothache needs a dentist. Meantime a useful first aid measure is applying a small pledget of wool soaked in oil of cloves. But try to keep it off the gum and do not use it more than two or three times a day.

Bleeding from a socket sometimes follows a few hours after a tooth has been extracted. Let the patient sit down, rest one elbow on the table, with the hand under the jaw. For at least ten minutes he bites hard on a really thick pad of gauze or linen which is placed across (not into) the socket. His elbow and hand help to maintain pressure. Do not let him rinse his mouth out, for this could wash away a clot which has formed.

Temperature and Thermometers

With the change to the metric system, Fahrenheit is giving way to Centigrade. Centigrade is far more sensible. Zero Centigrade, or 0°C, is the temperature of freezing water and 100°C that of boiling water (with some

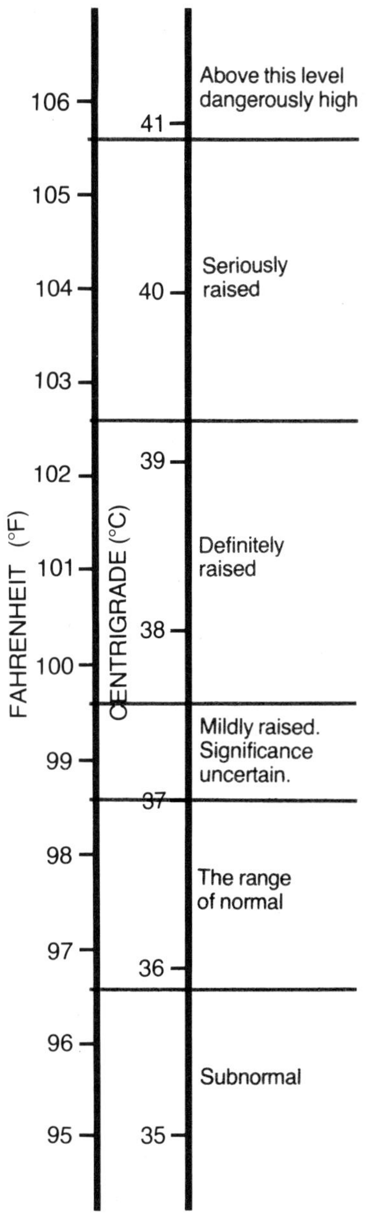

slight reservations about air pressure and specific gravity which need bother only a meticulous physicist). The scale on the left shows the comparative Fahrenheit readings. One degree Centigrade approximately equals two degrees Fahrenheit. The so called 'normal' for the body temperature of 37°C or 98.4°F is in fact only the average point of the normal range.

There is nothing absolute about temperatures. You could no more judge a patient's general condition by a single reading than you could dogmatise about a country's climate from one day trip to its capital. Regular interval readings and the general rise or fall of the temperature during an illness form the better guide, but there are so many other factors that some doctors and nurses depreciate laymen's use of the thermometer.

Here are some facts to guide (or to discourage). The 'normal' temperature range can be quite wide. Excitement, exertion or a recent hot drink can all raise the thermometer reading. Temperatures are relatively lower in the mornings and higher in the evenings. Certain medicines like aspirin can lower the temperature. During the fortnight before the onset of a period, a woman's temperature may be slightly higher than at other times. Quite young children tend to shoot fast into high fevers under circumstances which would only mildly raise the temperature of the older child or adult.

Follow a routine if you are going to use a thermometer. Hold it by its upper end. Wash it (*cold* water please!) and dry it. Shake down the column of mercury which may be raised from the last time it was used. It is here that so many thermometers

Take a firm grip of the top between finger and thumb. Hold it away from your body (and anything else). Bend the forearm up at the elbow

Rapidly straighten the arm right down.

Immediately, without stopping, give a hard jerking flick of the hand at the wrist.

If possible work well above a soft surface (e.g. bed-clothes) so that you hit nothing and risk little if you let go.

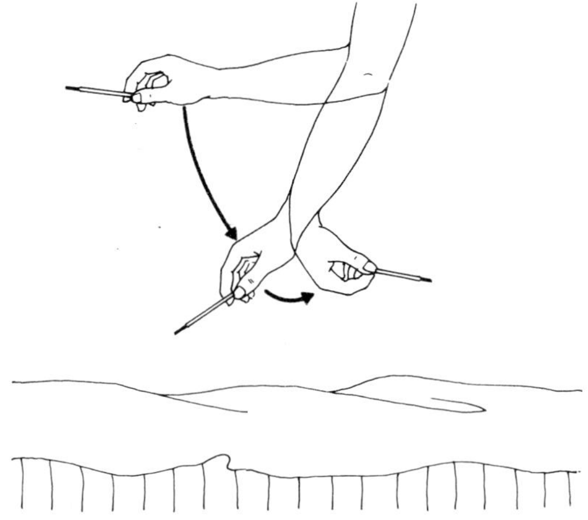

get broken by being knocked or dropped. But the method is easy (see illustration above).

Make sure this is done enough times to get the mercury line below 36°C or 95°F.

Put the bulb end (the bottom, with the mercury reservoir) under the patient's tongue and let him close his lips, but not bite with teeth. Let him or you hold the outer part and not move the thermometer for two minutes — even if it claims to be a 'half-minute' one. He must not speak during this time.

Now take it out and read it. The thin mercury line rising from the bulb is sometimes difficult to find. Holding its top rotate the thermometer very slowly and watch closely; at one point the mercury line suddenly becomes apparent. The temperature is the reading of its upper end against the engraved scale. Sometimes, for space reasons, not all the degrees are numbered; the bigger lines in between mark the full degrees and each smaller one indicates one fifth (or 0.2) of a degree. A small arrow is usually shown at the 'normal' body temperature. After use wash and dry the thermometer.

With a very small or an unruly child putting the thermometer in the mouth could be difficult. In this case use his armpit. Dry the area first; close the arm against it; hold it there gently for four minutes. An armpit reading is generally ½°C or 1°F below that taken in the mouth. Placing a thermometer in the rectum can be disturbing, and even dangerous, to the child so this use is not recommended.

Tennis Elbow

The accepted name for this condition has more style and receives more interest than its medical term of epicondylitis. It is a strain of muscles which straighten the forearm at the point where their tendons are attached to the bone. The attachment is by a bony knob at the lower end of the upper arm bone (humerus) on its outer side.

The grip of a tennis raquet, and the powerful swing of the stretched arm can certainly cause the small tears and inflammation of the tendon. In most cases however tennis elbow will come through a repetition of much finer actions, though always with some force, such as certain types of digging movements or a great use of the screwdriver.

Generally the onset of pain and stiffness is gradual and only slowly moves from being a mild nuisance to a crippling agony. The patient therefore delays consulting his doctor until the situation has become beyond him. Diagnosis is not difficult; there is tenderness accurately located over the tendons.

The doctor can reassure his patient that with rest, spontaneous recovery almost always happens . . . in due course. It may take two months; it may take two years. Faced with this uncertainty the patient sensibly asks if nothing can be done to speed up the cure.

Physiotherapy has been used in the form of massage or penetrating heat rays. Very helpful to some cases is injecting the tendon with corticosteroids (p.79) or a local anaesthetic or with a combination of both. Very rarely the case which refuses to improve needs an operation to free the stubbornly inflamed tendon fibres.

Testis Troubles

The testis is the male counterpart of the female ovary. It produces spermatozoa, which are the male reproductive cells. Like so many other organs it has a double function, for it also secretes a hormone, that is a chemical activator which works through the blood stream on other parts of the body. This secretion regulates the masculine characteristics of the body. The testis itself is under the governing control of other hormones produced by a gland in the brain, the pituitary. Its potential is not realised until it matures at puberty.

The two testes lie in the scrotum, the pouch which hangs behind the penis. Thus they are relatively external, and relatively cooler than if they were within the abdomen as are the ovaries. Spermatozoa will not develop at the higher intra-abdominal temperature. Some cases of poor fertility appear to be related to the wearing of tight and thick shorts which warm the scrotum, holding it firmly against the body. Frequent very hot baths have also been blamed for contributing towards infertility. (This is not a matter of potency at intercourse, which is unaffected, but of the number and quality of the spermatozoa.)

Descent of the Testes

The testis did not start its life in the scrotum. It had to travel there inside the foetus, having begun in the abdomen just below the kidney.

The testis begins its development in the foetus near the kidney at two months of pregnancy. During the remainder of pregnancy it migrates downwards within the abdomen:

at six months it is just below the level of the navel;

at eight months it is by the groin;

in the last month of pregnancy it descends into the scrotum.

Some testes do not make it. About one in every ten boys is born with the testicular journey incomplete. The scrotum may be empty on one side (or both). The doctor's examination may feel the testis at groin level, or may not be able to feel it at all, in which case it still lies within the abdomen. In a high proportion of these cases the testis will have satisfactorily finished its descent into the scrotum before the baby is a year old. Occasionally the uncertain testis appears to be in the right position but by muscle action slips temporarily up back towards the groin. This is disconcertingly likely to happen when the baby is tensing, especially if touched with cold hands.

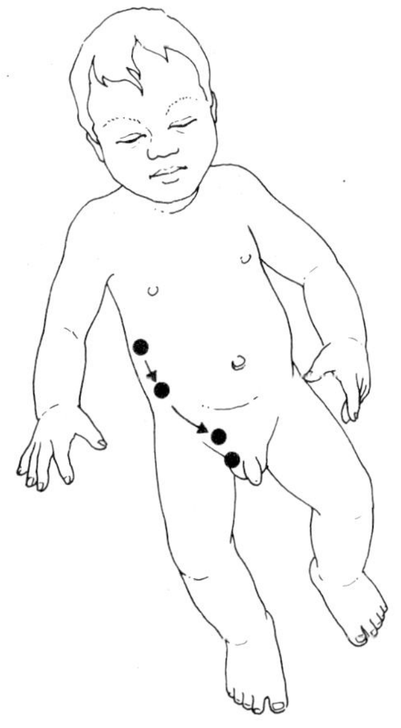

Sometimes a testis which has not ended up in the scrotum is not merely a laggard on the way (an *un*-descended testis), but has actually slipped off the normal anatomical route and lies fixed in some anomalous position around the groin (the *mal*descended testis).

A testis which is allowed to remain in the wrong position is going to have trouble. It will not develop spermatozoa properly. It is more vulnerable to damage from blows. It can twist on its upper attachments with torsion (which is described below) and it is more liable to develop tumours. If it has not reached the scrotum by the time the boy is a year old it is unlikely to correct itself and must be treated.

Injections of pituitary gland hormones have been used to stimulate the final move of the undescended testis, but they seem less certain than surgery which fastens the testis in its proper scrotal site. The operation is best done before the child is five or six if the testis is to function properly in later years.

Torsion of the Testis

As can be imagined from its history of migration, testes are not as firmly attached to their surrounding tissues as are most other organs. The testis more or less hangs from the tube which leads from it. Sudden movement, athletic stress or sheer misfortune can make this tube twist upon itself. The adjoining vessels, which serve the testis, twist with it and are occluded so that the testis becomes grossly engorged.

Generally the patient is a teenager; he will feel a very sudden and very severe pain, with sickness, and swelling of the scrotum. This is an emergency. Rarely, with luck, the doctor can reverse the twist, but in most cases an immediate operation is needed if the testis is to be saved.

Orchitis

Orchitis means inflammation of the testis. Such inflammation is likely to be from infection. The scrotum becomes red, swollen and tender —

but without the dramatic suddenness of torsion. Very often the infection is associated with and follows some other illness of the patient, like mumps.

The epididymis is an organ holding a long thin coiled tube attached to the testis, from which it receives and stores spermatozoa. Almost always it shares the inflammation. Therefore the whole condition is generally called by doctors not just orchitis, but epididymo-orchitis.

Rest, support to the testis, pain relievers and, where appropriate, antibiotics form the treatment.

Varicocoele

The trouble here is not so much in the testis as in the veins of the spermatic cord — a structure containing the duct leading from the testis. They dilate forming a soft swelling in the scrotum. Unless it gets big enough to be a nuisance it can be left alone. Some doctors believe that the increased warmth of the dilated vessels might be detrimental to spermatozoa formations by the testis. Treatment would be by injections to 'close up' the veins, or by operation.

Hydrocoele

This is another swelling in the scrotum, but it is tenser and firmer. It develops slowly as an accumulation of fluid within membranes which are wrapped round the testis. The scrotum gradually becomes evenly and smoothly larger. It is painless so the patient often lets it reach a surprisingly large size before consulting his doctor.

The fluid can easily be aspirated out, but it will form again. Repeated aspirations at intervals of a few weeks is a tedious business, so the alternative and definite treatment by surgery is generally to be preferred.

Lumps in the Scrotum and Testis

Tumours of the testis fortunately are rare, but when they happen they can be serious. Any lump should be shown to the doctor as soon as it is discovered.

Tetanus

'Suddenly a great hand seemed to take me across the chest, rendering respiration impossible. Another two such hands forced by head backwards towards my heels and my heels towards my neck, while my whole body poured perspiration. I felt some of the dorsal musculature give way with tearing agony, and this made the pain worse at the slightest movement'.

This dramatic account* came, many years ago, from a victim of tetanus whose recovery was something of a miracle. It describes the massive muscle spasms which the infection can force on the body. Back muscles being stronger than those at the front their contractions violently arched the patient backwards.

The infection begins with a bacterium which has the faculty of forming spores. These are dormant forms which can survive adverse conditions for many years until circumstances of temperature or moisture are favourable for their return to the ordinary active form.

Tetanus spores can be found almost everywhere, but particularly in soil and in dust. They exist within the intestines of animals and can be

*Reproduced from the *British Medical Journal,* by courtesy of the Editor.

found in those of men. Animal farming land forms tetanus areas, but the risk is not much lighter in cities.

A cut contaminated by soil can introduce the bacteria. The farmer's pitchfork, the housewife's potato-scraping knife, a bite from a pet, the dirt from a road accident and the rose thorn in a gardener's finger might all be sources of infection. There are notions that no nail will infect unless it is rusty; this is nonsense for the brightest nail can still carry tetanus. Another equally absurd idea is that a wound of the web of the hand always gives tetanus. The area of the body has nothing to do with it. However the depth and condition of the wound has some bearing. These bacteria live in the absence of air and do best in much damaged tissues. Deeply puncturing or severely lacerated injuries are particularly dangerous.

Once inside the body tetanus microbes produce a poison with a remarkable and powerful effect. Spreading along nerve paths, it reaches the muscles, increasing their tone. At first it stiffens them and eventually it subjects them to strong and painful spasms.

The incubation period from time of injury varies a lot from just one day to ten days, and not often more than a fortnight. Vague symptoms like headache, fever and sweating are the first to appear. Soon the stiffness shows up and it may begin near the wound. An early feature is tightness of the jaw muscles making it difficult for the patient to open his mouth, and giving the infection the alternative name of 'lockjaw'.

As the disease worsens so stiffness spreads. In severe cases a general rigidity of the body is punctuated by strong muscle spasms. They may come spontaneously or be triggered off by a stimulus like movement, touch, cold air or a noise. Apart from causing the distress of pain and exhaustion these spasms could make swallowing almost impossible, and threaten life by bringing on choking or by stopping breathing movements.

The urgent treatment is injecting a serum which neutralises any poisons circulating in the body. But it cannot affect those already settled in the nerve paths. Drugs must be used to relax the muscles. Antibiotics will be given and the wounded area may have to be cleaned up surgically to excise damaged or dead tissues.

The really sensible answer lies in immunisation (p. 138). Here is an example of a dangerous illness which is easy to catch and difficult to treat but very easy to prevent. Anyone who might get a dirt contaminated wound (and who can be excluded?) ought to seek the easy, harmless injections of 'Tetanus Toxoid'. They stimulate the body to prepare its own defences, ready to meet and overcome any attack by the bacteria. Up to ten years' protection comes from a series of three injections (spaced at six weeks between the first and second, with the third about six months after.) Tetanus immunisation is included in the routine recommended for babies. A single 'booster' dose tops it up after ten years, and also may be given as extra precaution after any injury which might create tetanus.

Do you garden? Keep an animal? Drive or walk on the roads? Do housework? Do repair jobs?

In fact do you move around at all?

If so are you immunised against tetanus? If not . . . why have you deferred? There can be no good reason.

See your doctor tomorrow.

Throat Infections

Do not confuse the simple straightforward sore throat with more definite infections like tonsillitis (p.207) or glandular fever (p.124).

Quite often it is related to a cold. Placed between the nose and the airway to the lung, the throat is liable to share infectious trouble of either. The steady sticky drip from the back of the nasal spaces can be a powerful irritant, leading to the scratchy burning feel of throatache with pain on swallowing. Heavy smoking or drinking sometimes play a part.

Usually the infection is due to a virus and then no antibiotic will be of any use. The only helpful treatment is that directed at the symptoms rather than the cause.

Applying antiseptics sounds a good idea, which is put in concrete form as one of the many sprays, mouthwashes and lozenges marketed for the throat sufferer. In fact they are not likely to do much good. The infection lies deep within the tissues, and these preparations just skim the surface of the throat very briefly. It is like hoping to depopulate a bee hive by going out three or four times a day to swat any bees moving by its entrance.

A little more sensible is the incorporation of a local anaesthetic in the lozenge or spray. That at least can deaden the throat and ease the pain for a little while. But then so could ordinary pain relieving tablets like aspirin or paracetamol taken in the ordinary way with water.

Gargling with aspirin has its advocates. This time the insoluble form is chosen: the tablet is allowed to break up finely in a small amount of water which is then used as a gargle. Each mouthful of the gargle is swallowed, and the slight sediment of aspirin particles left coating the throat has its soothing effect.

Thrombosis

Clotting of blood is a welcome protection when it closes up an injured blood vessel and stops it bleeding. *Thrombosis* is quite a different matter. It is the formation inside a blood vessel, or inside the heart's chambers, of something very similar to a clot, called a *thrombus*. At one point blood has changed from its fluid state to something like a lump of jelly, adhering to the vessel's of the heart's lining. Microscopically it consists of a meshwork of fine fibres with clumped up blood cells caught within it.

Why has it happened? Much has been found by research, but more remains to be discovered. A clot is not likely to form where the lining is quite smooth and healthy. But arteries are vulnerable to change; they become hardened and narrowed with age, and develop fatty deposits on their inside walls. It is here that a thrombus can form. Chemical changes within the blood can be a cause; certain drugs could predispose to thrombosis. An example is the oral contraceptive, but its newer formulations have greatly reduced this risk.

Another factor is slowing of the flow within the vessel, inactivity of a part of the body, like a limb, could be responsible. The action of leg muscles, for instance, keeps the blood circulating smartly, whereas inactive lying down leads to a sluggish flow. After operations or in long illnesses patients are encouraged by doctors and physiotherapists to move as much as they can.

There is many a thrombus existing and giving no symptoms. As long as it does not interfere markedly with the blood flow there is no trouble. But its presence is a threat. It may extend and ultimately block the vessel. Sometimes the body overcomes this by enlarging communicating neighbouring vessels, leading the blood to the same area originally served by the thrombosed vessel, just as traffic takes byways when a major road is obstructed. Occasionally however this cannot happen. If a major artery is involved very specialised treatment must be given, and this may include surgical measures to replace or bypass the stricken vessel.

Thrombosis in a vein is generally accompanied by inflammation and is then called *thrombophlebitis* (from the Greek terms 'phleb' meaning vein and '-itis' meaning inflammation). This occurs quite commonly in legs. If the trouble is superficial, just under the skin, as with varicose veins (p.212) it generally clears easily with simple treatment. But when the deeper leg veins are involved the matter could be graver and occasionally carry the risk of what is known as *embolism*.

A bit of any thrombus in a vessel or in the heart can break away and be swept off in the circulating blood. Such a piece is called an *embolus;* as its travels it may become wedged in an artery of smaller diameter. The blood supply to the tissues served by that artery is suddenly cut off. The consequences vary according to the organ affected. If at the back of the eye, vision is threatened. In the heart muscle it gives a sudden dangerous and painful heart attack. In some parts of the brain it could be a 'stroke'.

The outlook of many types of thrombosis and their complications has been considerably improved by the careful use of anticoagulants (p.18).

Thrush

There is a yeast like fungus called *candida* (alias *monilia)* which usually lives harmlessly in the intestines of human beings. There are occasions however when candida develops bigger ideas and gets out of hand. It can colonise on the skin, it frequently settles in the vagina and rarely it extends through the body.

Sometimes it get into the mouth and there causes a lot of trouble. This condition is known as thrush. It can happen to anyone, but the chief victims are bottle fed babies, adults of poor health and those with dentures.

It shows itself as slightly raised irregular patches of white, looking rather like milk curd. They come first on the tongue, then spread round the mouth to the gums, the palate and the throat. If they are wiped away they disclose a red, bleeding and ulcerated surface. The infection generally is mild but can be very irritating.

Fortunately treatment is easy, for there are special types of antibiotics which destroy candida. They can be swallowed as medicines or tablets, or be used in thick liquid suspensions which are rolled around in the mouth several times a day. It is important to continue their use for several days after the condition seems to have cleared to make sure that it does not recur.

Tinea

This is the name for a number of species of a microscopically small fungus which lives in the outer, dead layer of the skin and can be a considerable nuisance. Infection with tinea can affect different parts of the body.

In the scalp it is called ringworm, although it has no connection with worms of any sort. Scalp ringworm used to be common, but is now relatively infrequent. The fungus extends outwards from its point of attack, forming rings on the scalp. It leaves behind circular scaly patches, relatively (and temporarily) bald because of the way it causes hairs to break off. A similar formation of circular rings happens to infected skin beyond the scalp as on the arm or the trunk. Treatment includes taking tablets which make the skin develop a resistance to the fungus.

Tinea in the groins is called *dhobie itch* — a reference to Hindu laundrymen whose alleged poor hygiene was said to cause the fungus to get into underwear. The commonest site is between the toes. If you or your friends have this it is called *athlete's foot*, but your enemies have *foot rot*. The fungus is easily picked up from wet puddles on changing room floors. It loves moist, dark, warm places and areas between the toes are its ideal. The skin here becomes soggy, white, cracked and often painful. The trouble may eventually extend to other areas of the foot.

The treatment, applying prescribed ointments and sometimes dusting with powder between the toes, has to be done regularly and assiduously over a long period of time. Athlete's foot has the reputation of never completely getting better because patients tend to stop bothering about it as soon as it appears clear. However, some fungus is still lurking in the skin and treatment should be continued for some time after. Hygiene also plays a big part — in the avoidance of heavy shoes or socks which cause sweating and carefully drying between the toes, preferably with tissues or cotton swabs which are immediately burnt.

The most difficult cases of tinea to cure are those affecting the nails, which become thick, lustreless and discoloured. Treatment must be pursued with dogged optimism for many months.

Tinnitus *see* Ear Troubles

Tonsils and Adenoids

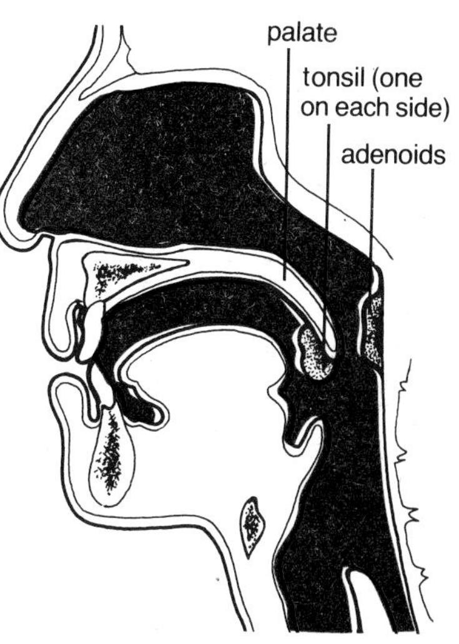

Tonsils are meant to get infected; that is what they are there for.

These two small masses at the back of the throat are composed of lymphoid tissue made up of cells closely associated with the white blood cells which defend against infection. This is the same type of tissue as in the glands which become large palpable and tender when the adjacent areas are infected. They act as traps to hold and destroy invading microbes. In addition they react to the chemistry of the microbes by producing substances which confer immunity.

With the mouth wide open each tonsil can just be seen where the mouth joins the throat; it is half hidden by a soft sideways fold coming from the back of the palate (the roof of the mouth). Just behind this region is the channel from the back of the nose. Were one able to look behind the palate one would see here also another mass of lymphoid tissue forming the adenoids.

Adenoids and tonsils are therefore perfectly situated to meet airborne microbes drawn in through mouth and nose. They are particularly busy coping with the many bacterial attacks which come to the small child, especially when he or she is moving from home into the outside world of school and young social life.

If tonsils are doing their job properly they should become 'infected'. Invaded by microbes they fight them, hold off their further spread and initiate the development of immunising products. The child then has an attack of tonsillitis.

Tonsils and adenoids are like fortresses set in a harbour to defend the land behind. When the enemy attacks they go into action. There is gunfiring and all the disturbances of battle. The enemy is repelled but later others may follow. Though the fortresses appear in stress they are fighting hard, and their defenders are gaining strength and experience. We must cherish them.

Adenoids may get so enlarged in these affrays that they interfere with nose breathing. But as the child grows they tend to decrease in size and even finally disappear. As for the tonsils repeated attacks of tonsillitis must be considered as almost normal in childhood. Their occurrence is highest between the ages of four and eight and they then tail off, to become infrequent after puberty. The huge majority of these fights between bacteria and body outposts are small, barely noticed, skirmishes with effective defence.

Unfortunately tonsillitis can at times get out of hand, cause pain and fever and sometimes complications like ear infection or kidney inflammation. The doctor will use his judgment when to restrict treatment to simple control of symptoms and when to prescribe antibiotics. He will also reassure the parents that the size of the tonsils (and they may become big enough almost to meet at the back of the throat) is no criterion of the severity of the condition. And he may have to counter their plea that the tonsils should be removed.

However, very frequent attacks and a constantly unhealthy throat suggest that the tonsils have become so damaged that they can no longer function properly and are the repository of disease-bearing microbes. The general practitioner and the throat specialist will consider whether tonsillectomy, the removal of tonsils, is necessary. Fortunately experience has shown that this situation is a relative rarity and that most children can be spared the operation.

A quinsy is a rather different matter from ordinary tonsillitis. Nowadays it is rarely seen for antibiotics prevent the development of this abscess, a collection of pus behind and around the tonsil. Tension and pain are great and the relief when the abscess is incised to let the pus out is correspondingly dramatic. Very often the tonsils are removed as well, for they are likely to be markedly infected and a possible source of later trouble.

Toothache *see* Teeth

Tuberculosis

Tuberculosis has decreased considerably but one cannot say that it has been eradicated.

The bacilli can live in dust; they thrive in shade but not in sunlight. Careless spitting and coughing, overcrowding, malnutrition, poor ventilation and lack of light spread the disease. Tuberculosis is caught and not inherited.

The tubercle bacilli can enter the body in one of two ways. They may come with food, such as unpasteurised milk, or they can be breathed in with the air holding fine invisible mists of droplets coughed out by someone who has an active tuberculous lung infection.

The Primary Attack

Many of us have caught tuberculosis without knowing it, and this generally happens in childhood. The bacilli could, for example, get into a spot of a lung and settle there to destroy the tissue. Symptoms may be absent or too indefinite to be regarded.

There is a great tendency to spontaneous cure. Unknown to patient and parents the child's protective white blood cells may contain and close off the infected site which may remain only as a small scar in the lung or enlargement of nearby lymph glands. The body's general defence system has effectively dealt with the situation.

This is the *primary attack* which many of us have undergone. We have caught and mastered tuberculosis without knowing it.

Rarely there. are less fortunate responses to this primary attack. If the child's health is poor and the defences low the bacilli might overcome the body's controls, spread through the blood attacking other organs like brain or bone. The infection becomes obvious. The term 'miliary tuberculosis' describes a severe and special form where there is wide scattering of the infection throughout the body.

Immunity and Sensitivity

Where, as in many cases, this primary attack settles naturally without treatment or recognition, some important effects remain. The body has now acquired a certain degree of *immunity* to any further tuberculosis attacks. It has also developed a *sensitivity*, allergic in nature, to the chemical substances of the bacilli.

The sensitivity is the basis of the *Mantoux Test* which injects a small amount of these chemicals into the skin. If temporary swelling develops at the injection site it demonstrates that either the patient has had a past, and healed, encounter with the tubercle bacilli or that he is in the throes of such an encounter.

B.C.G.

The letters stand for Bacille Calmette Guérin, the vaccine devised by two French bacteriologists. It is prepared from the bacillius but causes no disease; it stimulates the body to its reactive defences. B.C.G. will not always fully prevent tuberculosis but it will ensure that if the patient does catch the disease the attack will be considerably less severe.

In many areas school children between 11 and 13 years old are given the Mantoux Test. If the result shows that so far they have not acquired immunity they are offered B.C.G. Once vaccination has been successful a repeat of the Mantoux Test will produce the corresponding swelling in the skin.

B.C.G. should be given to babies born into a home where one of the residents has active tuberculosis. People in certain occupations may be more exposed to the catching of tuberculosis than others. Doctors, nurses or medical students, for instance, if they give no reaction to the Mantoux Test, can be vaccinated.

The Post-Primary Attack

Any further tuberculous infection which comes after the primary attack (perhaps when the patient has grown up) is the one which is far more likely to give trouble. Called the *post-primary attack* it could either be caught from a new exposure to the bacilli or develop from the re-awakening of lurking bacilli from the primary attack.

The body now reacts according to the balance of (1) its general health and immunity on the one hand and (2) the severity of the fresh infection and the degree of the allergic sensitivity to the bacilli on the other.

A post-primary attack does not have the same tendency to spontaneous cure. The body's acquired allergy to the bacilli has an unfortunately disruptive effect on the infected tissues, making them more vulnerable to the disease. This is the usual form of tuberculosis seen in adults.

Manifestations of Tuberculosis

The infection may be present a long time before giving definite symptoms. These, of course, will vary according to the organ which is affected. Cough, blood in the sputum, bone pain in a limb or in the back, enlarged or discharging neck glands could each be a feature, but the lungs are the most common site. Fever is generally slight; there may be night sweating. Loss of weight, poor appetite and lassitude are indefinite but real features.

Diagnosis is very much helped by X-rays which will show tissue damage and also the chalky calcification which so often forms around tuberculous lesions in the lungs. The laboratory will look for the bacilli in sputum or discharges.

Treatment

The classic triad of rest, good diet and fresh air remain important. Antibiotics specific against tuberculosis have created a wonderful advance. Since the bacilli can easily become resistant to one or other antibiotic several types are generally prescribed at the same time, and they may be varied during the course of treatment.

Cure is a slow affair of many months. It needs very good compliance from patients who must never give up or alter drugs and doses without medical consent. Patience and persistence are the watchwords.

Unconsciousness

When someone is unconscious his muscles lose their tone and become lax. If he is lying on his back or if his head is bent forward the tongue (which is muscular) tends to flop back against the throat and so block the airway to the lungs.

However, if one now fully bends the head back this movement carries the tongue with it, away from the throat, allowing a clear passage for air.

Another threat to the airway is choking from matter in the mouth, such as blood, displaced dentures or vomit — for the unconscious person can vomit.

Though the *cause* of his unconsciousness may be important it does not immediately concern you when giving first aid. Unconsciousness is an emergency in itself, whose *consequence*, whatever its cause, might be death from asphyxia. Your first and urgent measure is to prevent this.

Help to the unconscious follows a planned routine:

1. *Has the patient stopped breathing?* If so start artificial respiration (p.26) at once.

2. *Is he trying to breathe, but choking?* If breathing is harsh, difficult and obstructed bend the head right back (do this gently, with no side waggle) and carefully scoop your forefinger round the inside of the mouth to get out anything which might be lying there.

3. *Next immediately control any severe bleeding* (p.46).

4. *Check for possible fractures* before moving the patient. This is not easy, but you can feel all over from top of head to feet, firmly but gently pressing with the flat of both hands. Compare both sides of the body if you are uncertain of any bony irregularity you find. If you suspect a fracture leave out the next step, and keep watching his breathing to ensure that his airway remains clear.

Sometimes the circumstances in which you find the unconscious man suggests that he may have fractured the backbone. For instance he may have been thrown from a horse, fallen from a height or been hit in the rear. If so he must not be moved until the experts arrive.

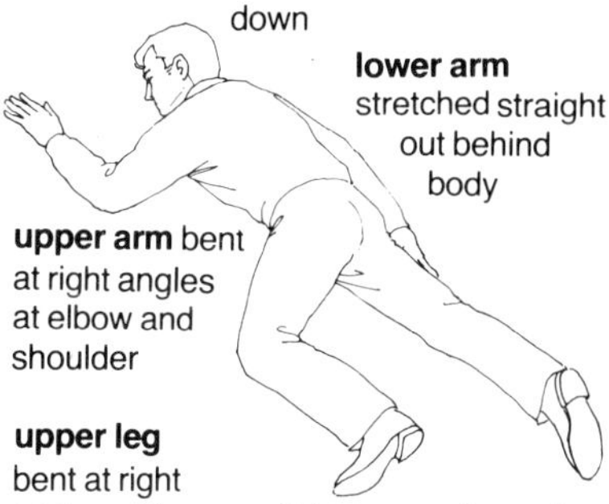

THE RECOVERY POSITION
patient lying on one side

head bent back with face down

lower arm stretched straight out behind body

upper arm bent at right angles at elbow and shoulder

upper leg bent at right angles at knee and hip

lower leg stretched straight out

5. *Put him in the Recovery Position* if you are reasonably satisfied he is unlikely to have a fracture. Move him gently and be careful you do not bump his head as you turn him.

This position keeps him safe with the airway clear. Any fluid in the mouth will flow out and not run into his windpipe.

Please note that you use this position also for weak, injured or comatose patients who may vomit or may be likely to lapse into unconsciousness.

6. *Dress any wound* (p.220) with the least possible disturbance to him.

7. *Cover him* with a coat or blanket.

Never try to give anything by mouth to the unconscious or drowsy person. This risks choking him for he cannot swallow.

Urticaria *see* Nettlerash

Vaginitis: Inflammation of the Vagina

A slight watery discharge from the vagina can be regarded as normal. Any heavy loss, especially when it is bloodstained or yellow, when it causes irritation or is malodorous is definitely abnormal and needs a medical check. Women should not defer seeing their doctor for quite unnecessary ideas of embarrassment or simply to avoid bother.

As occasionally the discharge accompanies another condition like diabetes or a bladder infection, the patient wisely brings a urine specimen to the consultation. (The doctor may ask for a specimen, passed in a special way, for laboratory testing.)

Trichomonas is the name of a microscopic single celled organism which can give a frothy white discharge. *Candida* is a fungus causing thrush (p.206), though correctly this word is reserved for the mouth infections from this fungus. Here the discharge will be creamy or yellow. Both these troubles are easily diagnosed and respond well to quite simple treatments by tablets or by the use of pessaries, which are medicated solid preparations to be inserted in the vagina.

Doctors' instructions need to be followed exactly. Men can carry the organisms without any symptoms, so sometimes husbands have to take tablets concurrently to avoid passing over to their wives a recurrence of the infection.

The name *senile vaginitis* suggests a trouble of rather ancient ladies, which is not at all fair. It refers to changes which can bother women over the age of forty five, that is after the change of life. Because of a reduction of their oestrogen hormone, their vaginal lining becomes dry, thin and irritating. Tablets or creams can correct this.

There are, of course, other causes. Every practitioner has seen the woman who is amazed, not to say abashed, when the doctor finds the cause of a discharge to be a forgotten tampon. Also some women believe they should use vaginal douches and deodorants and buy preparations which end up by causing inflammation.

To complete the list one has to include the less common causes like venereal infections and tumours. Also to repeat, emphatically, that an unexplained irregular blood loss must be reported at once to the doctor. The cause may be quite a simple one, but if it were a malignant growth the quicker it comes under care the better the outlook for cure.

Varicocoele

see Testis Troubles

Varicose Veins

Without muscle support around them and subject to the weight of blood between ground and heart level, no wonder superficial leg veins tend to distend. Women are unfortunate in that their hormone chemistry (especially during pregnancy) acts as a vein dilator.

Movement activates blood flow, preventing vein distension. Avoid long standing. Let women tap dance gently at the sink and ironing board.

Varicose veins look bad; they may worsen; they may cause ulcers (difficult to heal); they may even burst. The doctor will advise on treatment. Some elastic stocking supports are quite attractive. Injections can close up swellings, making the blood go round through deeper veins. Operations do the job more definitely.

Verucca *see* Warts

Vertigo

Vertigo, or true dizziness, is a loss of balance with the sensation that the body or its surroundings are moving. The victim may feel himself spinning, and wants to lie down for safety. He keeps his eyes shut to avoid seeing objects rotating about him.

Many things inform us of our position in space: movements of eyes; messages from joints and muscles, the semicircular canals (described in the section on Ear Troubles), the nerves leading from the inner part of the ear and the brain itself.

About nine tenths of the cases of vertigo are due to some trouble affecting that part of the ear (p.96) which deals with balance. This is the labyrinth, the name given to the complex of the cochlea and the semicircular canals. To begin with its position makes it vulnerable in cases of skull fracture. The nerve leading from the labyrinth, and those parts of the brain which record balance, are sensitive to *large* doses of some drugs like quinine and (for they must be included as drugs) tobacco or alcohol. Or they may be subject to abnormal pressures from organs alongside them.

Inflammation of the lining of the labyrinth structures and an over abundant secretion of the fluid it contains are common causes. The virus of many diseases like influenza or mumps occasionally affects the labyrinth, so that a community sometimes develops a small epidemic of vertigo. Happily with rest and suitable medicines such attacks clear in a few days.

Ménière's Disease is named after the French neurologist who, in 1861, was the first to describe it. The onset is generally in middle age and it has three classical components: vertigo, tinnitus (see Ear Troubles) and deafness. The last two may show up first some months before the vertigo. When it does come vertigo hits with great suddeness, sometimes even waking the patient up in the middle of the night. It lasts several hours and is accompanied by sweating and vomiting.

Intervals between attacks vary from weeks to months. Over the years they tend to space out and to become less severe, less long lasting. This comfort unfortunately is offset by the fact that there is a likelihood that the deafness worsens with each attack.

Attacks of vertigo are beyond home remedies, and medical help is needed. Treatment is uncertain for many drugs have been tried at different times. One simple line is sometimes advised to reduce the frequency of attacks and that is to avoid salt on foods.

Vitamins

Vitamins are present in food in minute amounts, but they are essential to health. Around them a lot of myth and magic has been built. Extremely happy in the thought that they are doing great things for their health people stock up with vitamin pills, vitamin drops and vitamin medicines. Commercial ingenuity is endless for one can find vitaminised aspirin, vitaminised shampoos and even vitamin enriched chocolates for pet dogs. Vitamin impregnated socks have not come on the market yet, but it won't be long now.

The truth is that although a deficiency can be harmful, it is extremely difficult in this country to lack vitamins. One might say it is almost impossible. The average commonplace, but good, mixed diet loads one up with more than enough. It is true that one may find examples of grossly poor nutrition, but then the circumstances are generally exceptional. The tea-and-bread-and butter feeder or the one who rigorously avoids fruit and vegetables can still be found, and will need an improved vitamin intake. The majority of us do not.

Nor are we likely to find much help in treating and preventing disease by extra vitamins. For instance vitamin C has not proved its case as a shield against colds. Vitamin E will not increase fertility in man. Nor does a blunderbuss mixture of the B group ease 'nerves'. There are however a few illnesses in which large amounts of certain vitamins are specially prescribed; these are very clearly defined and under medical suervision.

The haphazard vitamin swallower is not likely to do himself any harm, but perhaps his wallet will suffer. A dangerous overdose of vitamins is difficult to achieve except in the case of vitamins A and D. Here one must be careful. In gross amounts they can give unpleasant symptoms like headache, loss of appetite, vomiting, diarrhoea, muscle weakness and painful joints. What is worse is that a marked excess of vitamin D will move calcium out of bones, thus softening them and then will deposit it into organs like blood vessels, where calcium has no right to be. Such overdoses are likely to happen only to those who take large quantities of vitamin preparations with more optimism than knowledge.

Material bought over the chemist's counter just cannot replace or improve versatile shopping for a well mixed diet.

Vomiting

Being sick is a thoroughly disagreeable experience.

Muscles of the abdominal wall and of the diaphragm tense sharply; by increasing pressure in the abdominal cavity they compress the stomach. There is tightening up of the muscles which close the outlet from the stomach, and relaxation of those which should prevent food moving back into the gullet. The muscles of gullet and stomach walls churn violently so as to expel their contents. At the same time the sufferer sweats, goes pale and has a weakened pulse.

Vomiting has many starting points. As a symptom it is little help towards diagnosis of its cause. To begin with small children tend to vomit with many different sorts of illness. At all ages the cause can be in the stomach itself, in the abdomen or in the brain. There is, in fact, a centre in the brain which becomes involved in all vomiting forms.

A stomach can become irritated through poisons, infected food (or just too much food). Nerve messages from it reach the brain centre and from here pass further messages activating the muscles which initiate sickness. In a similar way inflammation or disorders of other abdominal organs like the kidneys, the liver, the gall bladder or the appendix will trigger off the vomiting centre.

Brain injury or meningitis will do the same. So can ear trouble or loss of balance as in vertigo (p.213), Ménière's disease (p.213) and migraine (p.160). And some of us know only too well how really disturbing sights or smells work through the emotions to bring about vomiting. The cause may also be more 'mechanical.' An obstructed bowel, unable to pass on its contents, will send it backwards to be vomited.

Rarely small babies, a few weeks old, suffer from what is known as *pyloric stenosis.* This means that the opening (pylorus) through which the stomach empties itself into the intestine becomes extremely narrowed (stenosis) and blocked. Why this happens is a puzzle. It affects boy babies more than girls, and generally the first born. Overdevelopment of the muscle ring at the pylorus is, it is believed, a genetic factor and therefore present at birth. Unable to pass his food on to.the intestines the baby is sick after each feed. This is no mere regurgitation but a very forceful ejection, described as 'projectile.' The food is shot out and does not just flow from the mouth. Understandably the baby appears constipated, passing no stools. This condition is an emergency. Treatment is generally a very simple operation on the stomach. But it must be done early before the infant has become severely deprived of essential fluids and minerals.

Another mystery form of sickness is that of some women in the early stages of pregnancy. By no means all women (or indeed all pregnancies of the same woman) have this trouble. Its name of 'morning sickness' indicates the way it can appear on rising and be a bother during the forenoon, to clear after midday. The easiest, and generally most effective, thing to do is to take a simple drink like tea or milk, with toast or biscuits, before getting up and to have small and frequent meals during the day. It is rarely necessary to prescribe medicines to control it, and certainly no woman should try any drugs without consulting her doctor.

Seasickness and travel sickness which affect a few people appear to be due to disturbances by movement of the fluid which fills the small balance and position sensing organs within the ear. On board ship visual impressions of a swinging horizon make things worse. A confusion of nerve messages about space and position activates the vomiting centre of the brain. The psychological expectancy of nausea may also play its part.

Lying back, relaxed, is the best position to take, and closing the eyes will help. However lighter attacks can be controlled by giving oneself a simple occupation. The victim should not fast but try to take small and frequent meals.

Very useful tablets are available against travel sickness. The dose should be taken about one hour before starting out. But the traveller should not also be the car driver, for these preparations can give a side effect of drowsiness.

First Aid

What domestic help can you give someone with severe vomiting? If you are calling a doctor (and you should if the sickness is continuing) keep a specimen of the vomit for him to see. Beware of any which looks very dark brown or black like coffee grounds, for this could indicate bleeding from the stomach.

Beware also of the vomiting of a drowsy or unconscious person. He may lack the control to prevent some of the vomit being breathed into his windpipe and choking him. Put him in the recovery position as for unconsciousness (p.210).

Repeated vomiting loses a great deal of fluid, and that fluid also carries away minerals important for the well-being of the body. This is specially harmful at the extremes of age, in the case of babies and young children and of the elderly. If possible try to replace the loss by drinks of water, or fresh orange juice with a half teaspoonful (no more) of salt to each glassful. Let the fluid be just tepid, and taken slowly in well spaced sips. This way it enters the stomach quietly, insidiously, and not as a cascade which could stimulate further vomiting.

Warts

The medical name is *verucca.* A wart is due to a localised virus infection of the outer layer of the skin. The virus encourages an exuberant multiplication of the skin cells, creating a hard raised patch, which sometimes becomes fissured. On the soles of the feet the wart is flatter because of pressure on it. It can be distinguished from a mole since it is the same colour as the surrounding skin.

Warts are a great nuisance and may be disfiguring and on the soles can be painful, but otherwise they are harmless. They can appear on any part of the skin; but the feet, the face and neck and the backs of fingers are the most usual sites.

Since warts are caused by a virus, they are contagious, that is they can be caught by contact. They may spread along adjacent fingers or be transmitted from one person to another.

Warts on feet very often arise from moist floors of swimming bath changing rooms. Plantar (i.e. on the soles) warts characteristically appear at areas receiving the highest pressure on the ground, the ball of the foot and the heel.

Treatment varies from the magical to the surgical. Many tend to disappear spontaneously and this has allowed the apparent success of many very odd cures.

Among the more orthodox lines the very simplest is the exclusion of air by keeping the wart constantly covered under waterproof adhesive strapping. Whether this works or not it is a sensible way of preventing spread to other people or other parts of the body. Most treatments consist of destroying the wart and here it is wise to avoid the D.I.Y. approach and let the doctor advise, since it is quite easy to damage not just the wart but also the surrounding skin. Various lotions and ointments, combined with a deal of patience are effective. More powerful is cauterising with electricity or freezing with liquid nitrogen or liquid carbon dioxide. Finally one can have the wart deliberately excised.

Around the face and neck one often finds warts of another shape. The 'filiform' wart projects like a thick pink thread. This may respond very nicely to the doctor tying a fine tight ligature at its base, and so 'strangling' it and its blood supply. A dressing is worn for a few days; when it is removed the wart comes away painlessly with it.

Wasp Sting *see* Insect Sting

Whitlows

This has become an old fashioned word. Originally defined as an abscess at or under the finger nail fold its meaning spread, first to cover infections at the sides of the nail and then to any abscess at the finger tip. The word is best forgotten and allowed to fade quiety away in its mist of vagueness.

Paronychia is the medical word for the infection which develops at the nail base. The acute attack begins with swelling and tenderness of the reddened skin. Soon after the yellow pus of a small abscess can be discerned underneath. Pressure builds up and pain increases.

In the early stage the formation of pus may often be aborted. Hot fomentations are advised by some but others believe they tend to make the skin soggy and prefer only prescribing antibiotics. Once pus has formed there is little doubt that it should be let out. The incision is simple and practically painless . . . when done by a doctor. No patient should try the short cuts of poking, piercing and squeezing for himself. These could almost guarantee spreading the pus further and deeper.

Waiting hopefully — and heroically — for the abscess to burst spontaneously is another way of asking for trouble. Fingers are precious and vulnerable; there is no justification in risking infection spreading to bone or tendon.

Chronic paronychia is a different matter. This slow smouldering infection is likely to affect those whose hands are constantly wet, like the conscientious housewife bereft of labour saving devices. The fold of skin over the nail base becomes puffy, dull red and sore. Pus does not usually form unless it is from a superadded acute infection.

It is no easy matter to treat and much depends on the nature of the infecting organisms. All too often they are not bacteria but a fungus called *candida,* the type which causes thrush (p.206).

Just because it has developed gradually and is not intensely tender it should not be disregarded. Antibiotics or ointments under medical guidance will help, but the cure is often lengthy. Throughout the patient must keep his — or, more likely, her — hands as dry as possible. Wearing rubber gloves may prove a false protection for they can retain moisture on a perspiring skin, or allow water to slip in from the wrist. If gloves are worn they should be long and cotton lined.

Any infection in the pulp of the finger tip can prove dangerous if not treated early. A puncture wound needs medical advice if there is any risk of tetanus (p.203).

Whooping Cough

medical name: Pertussis

see also Fevers of Children
and Immunisation

Caused by bacteria, this illness is dangerous to small children, who, if not protected by immunization, are particularly susceptible. It is also very contagious and isolation of suspected cases is important.

The problem lies in the word 'suspected' for the beginning of whooping cough resembles a simple, harmless cold. During the first week the child has a slight cough and, sometimes, a running nose but seems otherwise in good form. Now follows a week in which the cough gradually increases coming in short sharp paroxysms. In the third week the illness declares itself and the whole picture worsens.

The characteristics of the cough are that it appears at intervals in heavy spasms, is worse at night, and that at the end of each spasm the sufferer draws in a deep breath which may give rise to the harsh crowing sound called the whoop.

At their most severe the spasms bring up thick mucus and may be accompanied by vomiting. There is some risk here that the inspiration which follows aspirates into the windpipe some of the stuff from the mouth. In such cases the guarding parent is well advised to hold the child with head low to avoid choking.

Cough paroxysms may be triggered off by a child's excitement or even feeding. In such cases it is wise to try to give feeds just after a coughing bout is over in the hope that another one is unlikely to be building up. A soft diet, easily swallowed, is advisable.

Treatment with antibiotics may not help, especially if instituted after the illness has settled in. The relief of spasms is not easy, though the doctor may try sedatives or cough syrups in appropriate cases. Various unusual (if harmless) 'remedies' have been advocated with more optimism than science.

In the subsequent month the condition gradually eases, with coughing decreasing in frequency and severity, and the child is well again. However, for several weeks or months after, any trivial, unconnected cough, often surprises by producing a whoop much to the embarrassment of a parent who receives suspicious glances or comments from bystanders.

Fortunately many cases of whooping cough are not as severe as described above, with slighter coughing and little or no whoop. However, it is a threatening illness, especially to children under the age of two, with the risk of ugly complications like convulsions or pneumonia, and therefore protection of the small child by vaccine is really important. This is discussed in the section on immunisation (p. 138).

The immunised child sometimes can catch whooping cough, but then his illness is so mild that diagnosis is very often one of inference rather than of the ugly symptomatic certitude.

Worms

The world is full of worms trying to get inside man.

The live bodies of animals and man form warm havens in which many worms hope to pass all or some of their complicated life cycles. By good fortune (from their point of view) or by bad hygiene (from ours) they or their eggs can transfer from food, soil or water into living beings or from one living being into another. Some migrate about the body in a surprising pattern or settle down, cosy and nourished, in part of the intestinal tract.

Only a few types can be described here. The people of Europe and of North America are fortunate in that some of the nastiest of these parasites are to be found only in tropical and subtropical areas. Higher temperatures and humidity or lowered hygiene and education encourage their spread.

Those worms which bother man in European countries and in North America are far less frightening, though a considerable nuisance.

Threadworms

Thin, white and wriggly, threadworms are only about one centimetre long. Their eggs can lie around and be viable for weeks in ordinary housedust. Carelessness about what goes in the mouth is customary with children who are the chief sufferers. Swallowed eggs hatch in the bowels and take four to six weeks to become mature worms. The female, capable of laying a thousand eggs, moves to the lower bowel. At night it passes through the back passage to lay eggs on the skin just outside.

Apart from itchy, disturbed nights the patient does not suffer in health. Threadworms will not cause tooth grinding, nose picking, head banging or appendicitis — whatever the elderly folk next door may say.

It is not difficult to diagnose the condition by seeing worms on the area near the back passage or in the stools. With a microscope the doctor can identify eggs taken off the skin. Treatment by drugs is also easy. The hard part may be persuading the patient and the family to follow hygiene instructions meticulously. Sometimes all members of the household should be treated at the same time and the house be thoroughly cleaned over with a vacuum cleaner. Scratching in one's sleep will pick eggs up on the fingers; the nails should be cut short and at night pyjamas or knickers and perhaps cotton gloves will be worn. These clothes should be washed in boiling water daily. Bed sheets should be changed frequently.

The patient also washes his hands and nails with a soft brush after each lavatory visit and before every meal. He has his own towel or uses paper tissues.

Roundworms

The word 'roundworm' really applies to a whole lot of worms which are more or less cylindrical in shape. This includes the threadworms. It also covers *Trichinella,* a few millimetres long, whose larvae lurk in the flesh of contaminated pork. It could be caught by eating insufficiently cooked meat. At first the worms cause digestive upsets, but their main damage is the way they produce larvae which settle in cysts within muscles all over the body. The resulting disabilities vary greatly according to the muscles concerned. They are severest in the rarer cases affecting muscles governing breathing or those of the heart.

At the other end of the size scale is *Ascaris,* similar in length and appearance to the earthworms of our gardens. It is more common in the tropics but can infest in Britain. Unwashed raw vegetables or unwashed fingers contaminated after handling soil or animals can transfer the minute eggs to the mouth. Escaping from swallowed eggs, larvae begin a strange journey which may take two weeks to complete. They burrow into the walls of the intestines, get carried through blood vessels to the lungs where they emerge into the airways and thence up the windpipe. From its upper end they move into the gullet and so back to the intestine, now to mature as adult worms. Their presence may give no symptoms. However when infestation is severe the larval passage through the lungs could cause fever, coughing and breathlessness. A large number of worms in the bowels could produce colic or even obstruction. Some may be passed with the stools.

Though treatment for Trichinella is difficult, Ascaris is fairly easy to get rid of with the right medicine. It is clear how far more important than treatment is prevention by straightforward hygiene measures which prevent their entry into our bodies.

Tapeworms

These are very flat, but they make up for it by their enormous lengths. Contaminated beef, pork and fish each has its own type of tapeworm which can infest man if the flesh is eaten raw. It is the beef tapeworm which is likely to give bother in Britain. Larvae in the meat can survive slight heating so underdone steak has its risk. However meat inspection at slaughterhouses gives good protection against infested meat reaching the butchers' stores.

The larvae holds the head of the worm, a small but very predatory part. Pinhead in size it attaches itself to the lining of the gut of man by means of four sucker pads. In about three months a fully developed tapeworm will form from it. It is formed of separate segments rather like the components of a graded string of pearls, if far less pleasing. Tiny at the top, by the head of the worm, they grow in size and number gradually extending and curling in the intestinal space. Eventually up to a thousand segments form a ribbon-like structure of five or even ten metres long. The oldest and largest segments at the end will detach themselves while new ones are formed from the top. Some half dozen mature segments are passed daily with the stools; here they may be noticed, pale, flat and slightly mobile. Each is about 5 by 7 millimetres in size.

A tapeworm can live for many years in the bowels of man, surprisingly causing no symptoms other than occasional slight indigestion and, once the diagnosis is made, the patient's disgust at realising what he is sheltering inside him. The idea that the beef tapeworm causes weight loss or voracious appetite is quite false. The key to treatment is a medicine which destroys not only the segments but also the all important head of the worm.

Fortunately in Britain we are unlikely to be troubled by the fish tapeworm which causes anaemia by using up some its host's vitamins, or by the pork tapeworm whose embryonic forms can spread to create irritating and dangerous cysts in many parts of the body.

Wounds *see also* Abdominal Wounds, Bleeding, Chest Injuries, Dressings, Eye Troubles *and* Tetanus

A routine first aid approach to the wound which is not bleeding heavily is quite simple.

1. Sit or lie your patient down.

2. Wash your hands.

3. Collect together the material you need, and place it on a clean surface (opened out towel or handkerchief).

4. Clean around the wound, but not the wound itself. (If necessary you can keep this covered with a clean dressing or a swab.) Use soap and water on swabs of wool or gauze or, failing these, a clean handkerchief. Do this in separate strokes which overlap, always moving away from the wound edge. A fresh piece (or a fresh part of the handkerchief) is used for each stroke. Note that antiseptics are not used in first aid.

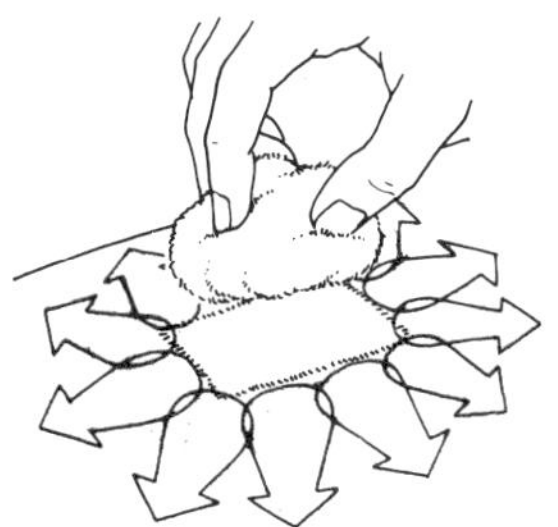

5. With the swab lightly remove any *loose* matter lying on the wound, but do not disturb any blood clots, for this might start bleeding.
6. Touching the material only by the edges cut gauze with clean scissors to a size large enough to extend beyond the wound onto the surrounding skin, and lay it on.

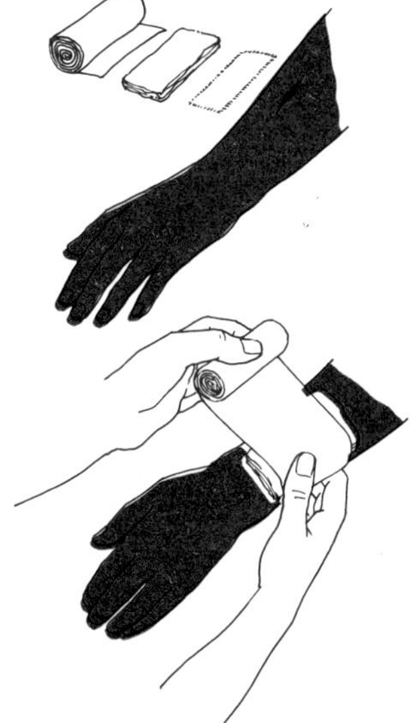

7. Cover with a thick pad of gauze or suitable material. Bandage gently but firmly enough to make sure that the dressing does not slip later.

Objects embedded in a wound. Do not try to pull them out for this movement may damage an adjoining structure like a nerve or a blood vessel. Put a dressing loosely over the wound. On this, and around the projecting object, build up a framework pad of gauze or wool. The object now lies within its centre and below its level so that the pad and bandage can be applied without it being pressed on.

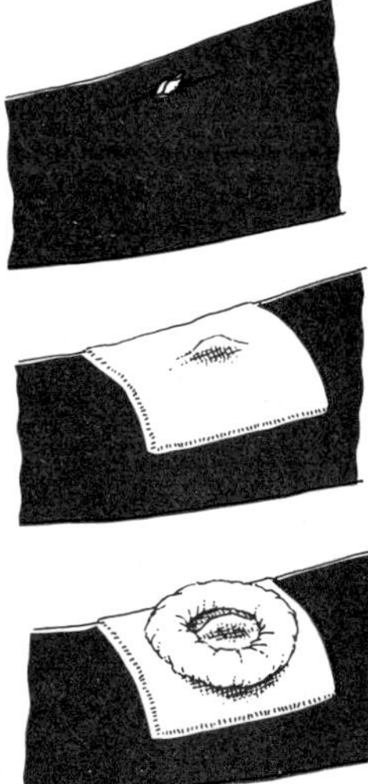

Tetanus (p.203) is a serious risk, especially if the wound is deep and punctured and if it has been contaminated with soil. Rusty pins and nails are often regarded as sinister objects if they have inflicted wounds. The fact is that the rust itself is not particularly dangerous, but that the object has become rusty suggests that it has been exposed to and contaminated with dirt.
An abrasion is superficial damage to the outer layer of skin which has been rubbed or scraped. Treat it like other wounds.

Useful Addresses

Al-Anon, c/o St Giles Centre, Camberwell Church Street, London SE5.

Alcoholics Anonymous, 11 Redcliffe Gardens, London SW10.

Anorexic Aid, Gravel House, Copthall Corner, Chalfont St Peter, Bucks.

British Red Cross Society, 9 Grosvenor Crescent, London SW1.

Disabled Living Foundation, 346 Kensington High Street, London W14 8NS.

Epilepsy Association, 3-6 Alfred Place, London WC1.

Royal Society for the Prevention of Accidents, Cannon House, The Priory, Queensway, Birmingham B4 6BS.

St Andrew's Ambulance Association, Milton Street, Glasgow C4.

St John's Ambulance Association, 1 Grosvenor Crescent, London SW1.

Useful Publications

Care in the Home (RoSPA).

Caring for Elderly Parents by Eleanor Deeping (Constable).

Incontinence by Dorothy Mandelstam (Heinemann Medical Books).

Incontinence and its Management edited by Dorothy Mandelstam (Croom Helm).

Notes on Incontinence (Disabled Living Foundation).

Nursing (Red Cross Association).

Revelation of Childbirth by Dr Grantly Dick Read (Heinemann Medical Books).